HEALTHIER CHILDREN

KEATS TITLES
OF RELATED INTEREST

HEALTHIER
CHILDREN

by
BARBARA KAHAN

Foreword by
Bernard S. Rimland, Ph.D.

KEATS PUBLISHING, INC. *New Canaan, Connecticut*

Healthier Children is not intended as medical advice. Its intent is solely informational and educational. Please consult a health professional should the need for one be indicated.

HEALTHIER CHILDREN

Copyright © 1990 by Barbara Kahan

All Rights Reserved

Library of Congress Cataloging-in-Publication Data

Kahan, Barbara.
  Healthier children.

  Includes index.
   1. Children—Health and hygiene—Popular works.
2. Children—Care—Popular works.   3. Diet therapy for
children—Popular works.   I. Title.
RJ61.K213   1989   649'.4   88-34756
ISBN 0-87983-475-7

Printed in the United States of America

Published by Keats Publishing, Inc.
27 Pine Street, New Canaan, Connecticut 06840

CONTENTS

DEDICATION

To the memory of my mother, Fannie Kahan,
one of the unsung heroines of the health and nutrition movement,
and to my father, another of the movement's
dedicated pioneers.

FOREWORD

I have a whole shelf—a long shelf at that—loaded with books on nutrition and related factors as they influence child health and behavior. Some of these books are quite good, and I refer to them and recommend them regularly. But this book is an unusually good one in a number of ways and it will render but a few of its predecessors obsolete. I admire the broad view Barbara Kahan has brought to her task. While a good many authors have placed heavy, sometimes complete, emphasis on the limited area they know best, such as food allergies, vitamin supplements, avoidance of junk foods and so forth, she has undertaken the very difficult job of addressing *all* these issues, and more. She has done a remarkable job. Further, her timing is right. After many decades of avoiding the issues the author addresses, society has begun—out of desperation—to pay attention.

School performance has been dropping precipitously for decades. So have college aptitude test scores. It is no longer news that high schools, and colleges produce graduates who cannot read or who can barely read. Hundreds of commissions have investigated the problem at the Federal, state, county, city, school district and individual school levels. The resulting reports cite the alarming statistics of widespread failure, then conclude with recommendations as familiar as they are futile: improve teacher quality, spend money, spend more money, spend even more money.

But it is crystal-clear that throwing money at the problem will not make it go away. As per-pupil expenditures in constant dollars have risen, student performance has continued to plummet. The nation-wide decline in student performance has been accompanied by an equally sharp decline in what was once called "comportment." Disciplinary problems are up, along with truancy, vandalism, drug use and delinquency. Hyperactivity has become so common that, in a number of cities, parents have instituted lawsuits against entire school districts for wholesale drugging of students with Ritalin.

While all this has been going on, a number of people have been standing on the sidelines, jumping up and down, shouting, trying unsuccessfully to be heard. Now at last, at long last, society is beginning to listen to these voices: "Nutrition," they are saying. "Junk food, depleted soils, pollution, herbicides, pesticides, heavy metals, cesarean deliveries, drugging of pregnant women, smoking!" the voices cry. Finally society is beginning to pay attention. Let's hope it's not too late!

Barbara Kahan's book is about these things. It is timely. It is comprehensive. It is easy to understand and to implement. I particularly like her strong emphasis on providing down-to-earth *practical* advice and information. I am delighted with this book. I think you will be too.

BERNARD RIMLAND, Ph.D
Institute for Child Behavior Research
San Diego, California

ACKNOWLEDGMENTS

I would like to acknowledge the help of the following in the preparation of this book:

My uncle Dr. Abram Hoffer, my nutritionist cousin Miriam Hoffer, and by brother Dr. Meldon Kahan, who each read the complete manuscript (and sometimes variations of it) for accuracy. Above and beyond the call of duty, they also made useful suggestions on style. The three of them have been extremely helpful and supportive, dealing with a torrent of words and questions without complaint and maintaining their much appreciated enthusiasm through thick and thin. I am deeply grateful to all of them.

The former staff of the Canadian Schizophrenia Foundation: my father Irwin Kahan, whose idea this all was in the first place and who in his kind and generous way has given me steady encouragement over the years; my dear friend Doris Rands, who is responsible for greatly improving the clarity, content and style of the book and has been a constant source of support; and Rene Foster and Pat Gilroy, who aided me on innumerable occasions by transcribing tapes, searching out addresses, photocopying, listening sympathetically and more.

The Canadian Schizophrenia Foundation, which gave me a grant from its Fannie Kahan Children's Fund to get started on this project and whose facilities and resources I used.

Debora Abood, Lisa Brownstone, Liz Kalmakoff, and my sister Sharon Kahan, who each gave me important feedback on different chapters and whose staunch support and friendship have meant so much to me over the years.

Many other friends who also took an interest in the book and helped me keep going.

The many people active in the nutritional/environmental field of health and behavior who have gone out of their way to be helpful and give me assistance, ranging from kind words to factual information.

Dr. Philip Zimmerman who kindly critiqued the chapter on nutritional supplements.

The staff of Connaught Library who continued smiling even when presented with long lists of requests for books and other material, and were always ready with an encouraging word.

Sandy Rogina and Jaki Russell, who have cared for my children with love and wisdom (and who also helped me by reading chapters of the book).

My children Tara and Brennan who often perked me up with their interest in the book and who have, for the most part cheerfully, helped me learn first-hand the ins and outs of healthy parenting.

All those parents and children who generously gave their time and energy to answer interview questions and questionnaires. (Some of these interviews were done by my brother Meldon.) Their pain and bravery have moved me deeply, and it is their thoughts and experiences which form the heart of the book. To all of them go my deepest thanks.

Evan Morris, the father of my children and my partner-for-life, who not only made the book possible with his support and encouragement but improved its quality a thousand-fold. A clear-headed and honest critic, a bright and positive force against discouragement, a willing listener, a great cook, an uncomplaining runner of errands, a research assistant, a wonderful parent and a loving friend . . . the list is endless. I am profoundly grateful.

AGES OF CHILDREN

To compile information for the book, a number of individuals were interviewed by my brother Meldon and myself and a questionnaire was distributed under the auspices of the Canadian Schizophrenia Foundation. Unless otherwise stated, the quotes in italics found throughout the book are excerpts from these interviews and responses to the questionnaire.

A list of ages of the children mentioned in the quotes at the time of the interview or questionnaire follows. Listed in parentheses are the time periods in which problems were first noticed. None of the names are the children's real names.

Ricardo: 11 years (2 years)
Pierre: 26 years (fifth grade)
Lyle: 27 years (high school)
Vanessa: 6 years (birth)
Marilyn: 22 years (6-7 years)
Shayna: 18 years (15 years)
Doug: 24 years (7 months)
Gordon: 4 years (2 years)
Bill: 10 years (1 year)
Nick: 11 years (1 year)
Dora: 12 years (1 year)
Tyler: 2 years (8 months)
Michael: 3 yrs. 7½ mths. (3½ years)
Richard: 6 years (infancy)
Albert: 15 years (5 years)
George: 7 years (6 years)

Raymond: 39 years
Nadya: 5 years (2 years)
Annette: 20 years (infancy)
Amy: 35 years (school age)
Ian: 16 years (pre-school)
Theo: 2 years (infancy)
Andrea: 63 years (childhood)
Michelle: 12 years (infancy)
Stuart: 10 years (infancy)
Jon: 30 years (20 years)
Erica: 20 years (13 years)
Suzanne Foster: 24 yrs. (12 yrs.)
Graham: 25 years (15 years)
Enid: 8 years (5 years)
Terry: 5 years (4 years)
Marla: 5 years (infancy)

INTRODUCTION

This guidebook has been written to help parents explore the benefits of a nutritional/environmental approach for children with learning and behavior problems. It is meant to be a starting point, providing information on how to pinpoint and correct negative nutritional/environmental influences, minimize common difficulties associated with this approach and track down useful resources. Many of the suggestions come directly from parents, including the author, based on first-hand experiences with our own children.

Parents whose children have learning and behavior problems are as diverse a group as any, a mixture of nationalities, racial backgrounds, income levels and occupations. Our children are also diverse. They may be speedy or lethargic, aggressive or timid, plagued by nightmares, unable to read at the age of nine or "loners." Some never seem to stop screaming; others at the age of five can't or won't utter a sound. They have been diagnosed variously as hyperactive, autistic, dyslexic, learning disabled, minimally brain damaged or schizophrenic. Multiple diagnoses are not unusual, depending on how many professionals they have been to see. Some of us have been told our children are going through a phase which they will outgrow, or that their problems are caused by poor parenting, emotional trauma, stress or social circumstance. Some children have been drugged, placed in special educational programs, psychologically tested and treated, and/or institutionalized. Even those children whose symptoms are less severe or are of recent origin have been the subjects of concerned discussions among family members, teachers and others who care about them.

Despite our differences—unemployed or working, single or part of a couple, parents of children with relatively minor problems such as irritability, or parents of children with more severe problems such as hallucinations—we have a strong common bond: we want our children to be as healthy and happy as possible. This is the reason many of us have decided to see if a nutritional/environmental approach will help our children.

Nutrition and the environment affect all of us profoundly—physically, mentally and emotionally—and their effects on children's behavior can be dramatic. A nutritional/environmental approach to children's problems, as described in this book, means taking account of what children eat, drink, breathe or are otherwise in contact with in order to make them healthy and well. For example, children might need to eliminate sugar from their diets, take vitamin and mineral supplements, reduce their contact with petroleum products such as natural gas and felt-tipped pens, or receive treatment for lead poisoning.

It is crucial to our children's well-being to recognize that they all have individual nutritional needs which must be fulfilled for them to be as healthy as possible. Diets composed mainly of processed foods (refined, sweetened, artificially colored, flavored and preserved, and exposed to various chemicals and contaminants ranging from relatively harmless to extremely toxic) do not fulfill these requirements and are at the root of many behavior problems.

It is not only the quality of the diet that is important, however, but the specific content as well; a basically good food that is bursting with nutrients and is well tolerated by most children may provoke a variety of physical and mental symptoms in others. In addition, it is important to remember that some children have much higher requirements for certain nutrients than other children, and in some cases may need to take nutritional supplements.

Environmental influences also play an important role in a child's health and well-being. Children are exposed to many different elements in the environment, ranging from relatively innocuous substances such as dust and pollens, which affect only some children, to substances which are toxic to some degree for everyone, as is the case with lead, cadmium and other heavy metals. In between these two extremes are a variety of other substances to which children are exposed. Some of these substances occur naturally, while some are the products of complicated chemical procedures performed in laboratories. There are substances which are difficult to avoid, such as gas in those parts of the world where gas heating is almost universal in the winter, while others, such as feather pillows, are more easily avoided.

All these categories include many items that are both useful and aesthetically pleasing. Unfortunately, how natural, useful, beautiful or common a substance is gives no indication of how it will affect any particular child. Every child is unique, and what each one reacts to and how severe that reaction is will vary from child to child. Substances as diverse as molds, aluminum, household cleaners, synthetic carpeting and fluorescent lighting have all been implicated in children's learning and behavior problems. Even color and sound can have an effect. In other words, anything that can be sensed by sight, sound, taste, smell or touch, and even some things that can't (for example, radiation and some gases) can affect children. Anything in the environment that can affect a child's body or mind has the possibility of affecting behavior.

It is strange to think that items so familiar and seemingly innocuous as apples or lemon-scented furniture polish might be at the root of a child's problems. But it does happen that some people weep for an hour after eating corn, just as breathing paint fumes puts some people into an irrational rage. Food additives turn many children into uncontrollable little demons, exposure to lead interferes with children's learning ability, and high sugar intake can cause erratic mood swings. It is a point worth stressing, because even though intellectually we may accept this, in practice we often forget. We are so used to attributing Jane's and Johnny's rowdiness to a hard time at school that we forget that Jane and Johnny may also be affected by their after-school snack of chocolate chip cookies or by fumes from the gas stove.

There is no "magic bullet" in this approach, no wonder drug, no instant cure. Rather than treating each health problem in isolation from the rest of the body, a nutritional/environmental approach concentrates on making the whole being well, improving health by improving each individual's nutrition and environment. Rather than regarding each person as identical to the next, a nutritional/ environmental approach recognizes that needs and reactions vary widely from person to person.

One of the guiding philosophies of this approach is that a healthy body will not only help ensure the optimum functioning of all its parts, including the brain, but will also be better able to cope with physical stresses such as viruses, bacteria, injuries and toxins, and psychological stresses ranging from the minor to the major. In other words, this approach is of use not only in dealing with immediate problems but in preventing future problems as well.

Although the focus of this book is on nutritional/environmental factors, it is not suggested that no other approaches should be used. There is no reason why this approach cannot be used in conjunction with other therapies.

A basic premise of the book is that we, as parents, have a right to understand fully all aspects of our children's problems and to play an active role in their recovery. However, it is important to note that many medical conditions should be treated with the cooperation or back-up of a doctor. In some cases a doctor's support can be crucial.

Attempting to improve a child's diet and environment, if done with common sense, is a remarkably safe approach and will not harm our children. At the very least, even if it turns out not to be the approach that solves all their problems, children will still benefit by becoming healthier. And at the best, given some time and some effort, our children may be counted among the many, many children who, after following this approach, have become pleasurable human beings, well able to cope with life's challenges.

1

FROM A
PARENT'S POINT OF VIEW

I took her in to her pediatrician. I had to ask. At nine months, kind of guardedly I said, "Is my baby okay?" He said, "Fine, fine."

I took her back to the pediatrician. I took her to another pediatrician and he said she was just fine, no problems whatsoever, that I was just being a concerned mother, overly concerned. "Apprehensive" is the big word. That's the way he felt—I was apprehensive. So he didn't suggest any treatment except to relax and enjoy her.

I had a little naked baby running around the yard in a very uptight Baptist neighborhood. And I was a Baptist, too, but I couldn't get across to these people that this child wouldn't keep clothes on. By the time she was 18 months old there was no keeping clothes on her at all. She was very hyperactive. She was terrified of grocery stores; she was terrified of the doctor's office. I couldn't just take her to the neighbors' and visit.

She had been rocking since birth. She would get on her knees and bump her head against the top of the crib and all night long you'd hear this bang, bang, bang . . . she'd keep me up all night with her rocking and banging.

I was just frantic over her head because this baby, by the time she was two and a half, had a four-inch-long bald spot on the top of her head, running from front to back, it was three inches wide, and had a bump to it that was at least an inch up, from beating her head—she put her head through all the wall boards, she knocked all the pictures off the wall.

[I was told] that I was neurotic. I should accept and enjoy this child and relax, she was all right. But she was like no baby I have ever seen. Her affect was flat. You didn't see great joy, you didn't see great sadness, just this flatness, and almost a distant look in her eye.

And then when she was four and a half I finally got some doctor who said, "There's something wrong with this kid." He did an EEG and declared her to be epileptic. He put her on phenobarbitol and she went straight downhill because that is the worst thing you can do, put a hyperactive child on phenobarb—it accentuates the problem. She was on phenobarb for a year and a half. This is where I blame myself—we had to fight her to give it to her so the little baby knew it was the wrong thing to take. Looking *back, she knew it was hurting her. It made her so groggy she fell down and busted her teeth.*

The phenobarb was hard to take her off of; we had to get a doctor in Chicago to do this because we couldn't get her off it she was so addicted. It took a number of weeks.

She was a problem. We couldn't take her to a shoe store; we got thrown out of Montgomery Ward's. No dentists would treat her, no doctors would treat her, and then when she was six we moved. I took her to a pediatrician and said, "I think there's something wrong with my baby." And the doctor said "I don't think there's something wrong with your baby, I know. It's terrible, and I would recommend an institution immediately." So then she sent me to a big neurologist downtown who declared her to be Down's syndrome. I doubted that so I asked for chromosome tests. It turned out she wasn't Down's syndrome. So everywhere we went we got a different story. We didn't get any help.

They put her on Mellaril [a tranquilizer] and she doubled her weight in sixty days. She went from a forty-pound five-year-old to an eighty-pound blimp.

I think everything we did made her worse. Every professional made her worse, made the family worse, especially me, because it's whoever goes in to see the doctor that gets the blame. So when I took her in they'd say, "Well it's your fault, obviously. Look how you messed up."

The biggest help we ever had was from a doctor close to us. He standardly prescribes Dexedrine and Dilantin for everybody who comes in that's hyperactive. He prescribed that for her and it made her worse and as an afterthought he says, "Why don't you try Ritalin?" We put her on Ritalin at the start of third grade. She went from a zero reader—kept all the same social behavior of a two- or three-year-old and didn't really progress in any way but reading—and became a grade-level reader within six months. Ritalin did help. She was on it for two years.

We took her to another doctor because she became a grade-level reader and that stopped. She still behaved like an animal, you could not take her to get her hair cut, you couldn't wash her hair, you had trouble giving her a bath, she wouldn't keep shoes on, she got kicked out of school several times, she never had a friend. This child never had a friend, she's almost twelve, she's never had a friend, because her social behavior is so bad. Now she's getting well.

It's been hard. In [the last town we lived in] it was the hardest because they were Baptists and I was a Baptist; you're supposed to raise a child as he should go and he'll go that way. It was very much a "spare the rod, spoil the child" atmosphere. You could beat Michelle to death and not change her a bit. Much of the time she's not functioning in a thinking manner. So you couldn't talk to her; you couldn't spank her—nothing would work. It was more a matter of trying to keep her from killing herself by putting her head through a window. Strange, weird, insane. How I explained her—I didn't try.

As for stores, many times if we wanted to buy shoes, I would call ahead and explain that I have a learning disabled child. L.D. covers a whole multitude of sins. It's a good catchall. I said, "She's different. She may cry a lot. There's nothing you can do. You're not causing her to cry. There's nothing you can do to stop her from crying. Just quietly go on your way fitting shoes. We'll pay for them as quickly as possible and get out of your store." I always called ahead. I never took her anywhere by surprise. I'd call ahead and I would tell them that she had problems. How many times I've thought of having it printed on a card and passing it out. I didn't always want to say in front of her. We took her out very rarely. We tried to teach her to eat in a restaurant. So we picked the same restaurant like McDonald's or maybe a quieter restaurant. We'd pick out something; we'd talk to her about it, we'd drive her by it, we'd look at it, this would go on. Finally we'd go in. Usually we would get the order placed. While it was being served, she would be so hysterical that we would leave, we would pay the ticket, we never saw the food. It was discouraging.

I don't have that many friends. I have friends at work—I'm a very outgoing person. But I don't bring them home—I can't bring them home. Michelle screams. This is all going to be changed, but this is how it's been up to now. You simply cannot have friends in. We used to try, we were big at cooking out in the yard. For Michelle's sake, we put in one of these big outdoor pools—the doctor told us that would help. It's thirty-one feet long, eighteen feet wide, it's decked and it's heated. So I thought, "Gosh, this is great, we'll throw some hamburgers on or whatever, cut a watermelon and have some friends over." But it didn't work. Because Michelle takes two people twenty-four hours a day just to keep tabs on her. So we don't have friends in the ordinary sense; I have many friends at work.

I have to credit Mayo Clinic because at least they came through and said childhood schizophrenia. They said, "No hope whatsoever." They said prognosis was just so poor. It was with tears in Dr. A.'s eyes he told me that. I have just loved Dr. A. because of the honesty and I felt he pegged the problem. After that I went to the library and read about schizophrenia; when you start reading things, then you start gaining some confidence, which you need, because, number one, you have to fight the school system. I'm a registered nurse, none of my nursing friends know about the orthomolecular approach—you have to argue with your neighbors—anybody sees you trying to do something and get out of the accepted pattern and get a kid well, they don't want to hear about your kid, they don't want to see your kid, they don't want to deal with your kid—they want you to hole up this kid somewhere. And particularly the school system; you have to fight it every inch of the way. I'm sure we will end up in one big lawsuit. I think I have grounds to win a lawsuit against my little city. I don't want any of the money—I will end up settling for a dollar, but I want the big satisfaction of them having to accept that there is a way to treat these children.

Things have gone from bad to worse now, and at eleven and a half she was the worst child I have ever seen. She was terrible. I say "was," because about seven or eight weeks ago, after having heard about the orthomolecular approach to mental illness and after just receiving the diagnosis at the Mayo Clinic of childhood schizophrenia, I started her on the vitamins. From reading. Some author, I don't know who, gave the "recipe," as I call it. How much niacin, how much vitamin C, B6, pantothenic acid, and B1, and some E, and how much I should give a child of her weight, which was 110 pounds. At this point I thought, "I'll try anything. If I kill her doing this, she has no life anyway. We've lost nothing."

Within three days of starting this, we had spontaneous speech for the first time. It was a miracle, it was beautiful.

This child was suddenly laughing appropriately. We never heard appropriate laughter, we never heard appropriate crying. We'd never seen any appropriate behavior in this child who was at this point almost twelve years old.

[After starting on a nutritional/environmental program] we have a different child. I keep using this term, we have a child "reborn," because that's what we have. She's not banging, she's sleeping through the night for the first time in her whole life; we're all so used to being woken up all night we can't sleep! We're laying there waiting for her to beat the walls, to cry, to scream, to fall out of bed, do whatever she does. But she's not doing it. We expect complete recovery.

We know she's very allergic to wheat, milk and eggs, we're not doing anything about that particularly—giving as little wheat as possible, we're not worrying about the eggs at all, we cut milk. I've had several of my friends say, "Oh, my word! It's not worth it, that's got to be the biggest hassle trying to keep off wheat, you're real crazy," and I said, "After living with a screaming little animal who couldn't possibly enjoy life and made me just heartbroken for all these years, that I should have to plan a four-day diet seems like nothing." The thousands and thousands and thousands of dollars—we've been to twenty-two neurologists and psychiatrists.

Parents get very tired. They need understanding. They don't need to be blamed, they need someone to say, "My gosh, it's been awful." In fact there are times right now even if someone looked at me real compassionate, who obviously cared, and said, "Gee, it's been really rough, hasn't it?" I'd probably cry buckets. Because I want someone to know it's bad.

That's with all parents—they need someone who is with them. And believe and try to understand that it's hard to live with and it's very heartbreaking. They don't need any criticism ever.   —Michelle's mother

---

From our own experiences as well as others, we all know that it is not easy being a parent these days. We are expected to ensure our children's health, happiness and good behavior, earn the money to feed and clothe them and us, maintain a clean and tidy house, lead an independent social life, and keep up with the rest of the world. We are to do this efficiently and uncomplainingly, despite the fact that many of us have to struggle along on an inadequate income, with family and friends too busy to be of help or in another city, and day care centers or babysitters too expensive, not suitable, or all filled. Even with two participating parents, it is hard to find the time and energy to do everything; yet many times, compounding the hardships, there is only one of us.

In addition to the money worries, housecleaning, child care and the odds and ends of living shared by all parents, those of us who have children with learning and behavior problems have to deal with an extra dimension of tensions, worries, disruptions, turmoil and heartbreak. Parenting a child with behavioral problems inevitably takes its toll.

My husband and I both took out our frustration and guilt on each other—now we are getting along well, with our son acting "normal."
—Gordon's mother

At one point it was very difficult for the family. Nick is the youngest of three and our middle child felt very rejected as Nick demanded so much attention. Also it caused problems between my husband and myself.
—Nick's mother

The presence of mentally disabled children has produced social difficulties, discouraging the normal children from inviting friends to the house and gradually making hermits of the parents.   —Annette's father

How dismayed I was when I learned that my illness had often forced my parents to disagree violently with each other, threatening their happiness. Here was my illness, sneaking in between them like ice under stone and slowly, insidiously breaking them apart.
—Suzanne Foster in her unpublished manuscript, *Stoney Lonesome Road: A Chronicle of One Woman's Battle with Schizophrenia*

Dr. Abram Hoffer, in the pamphlet *Research and Troubled Children*, published by the Canadian Schizophrenia Foundation, writes:

". . . parents who have to deal with a disturbed child become in a way abnormal. And they have to. It's impossible to remain a normal parent and to deal with a hyperkinetic child, because this would destroy the child. The parents have to yield in many ways and have to change their personalities and do things for their sick children that they would not do for their healthy children."

With impossible expectations laid on us, raising our children under difficult circumstances and being only human, we should not be surprised to find ourselves feeling, as many of us do, exhausted, angry, guilty, bewildered and overwhelmed. We should not berate ourselves for any feelings we may have, but rather recognize them, accept them and try to deal with them.

Following is a brief discussion of some of the most common feelings we all experience at one time or another.

GUILT

Ours is a world that likes to assign blame. If a child misbehaves or is strange or unhappy or unwell, conventional wisdom says it is the parents' fault (mothers in particular being the traditional scapegoats). This message is drummed into us by doctors and psychologists, the media, childless friends, relatives and strangers in the corner store.

Everyone hung that guilt trip on me. I thought I was responsible and I was supposed to undo it because I did it . . .   —Rick's mother

We were told that it was our fault, of course, that we weren't accepting him because he was adopted.   —Stuart's mother

He became so hard to handle—they said take him to a psychologist. I did, and the psychologist said all children's problems come from the parents. It shows that there's a real weakness in the home. They explained how it was my fault with Ed's behavior.   —Ed's mother

If only we were stricter/more relaxed, more consistent/more flexible, more caring/less giving. If only we weren't so obsessed with what they ate. If only we didn't yell so much, spent more time with them, stopped spoiling them rotten, had more patience. If only we made them follow their diet better. If only we'd sent them to nursery school/kept them home, if only they'd had siblings/been an only child, if only we'd had more time/more money/more energy. If only we'd taken vitamins during pregnancy, hadn't moved to such a high pollution area, had changed doctors sooner.

When you have a child like this and you're blamed constantly, you become

sort of hyperactive yourself. You're constantly searching for an answer, you're trying to sort things out and figure out why is this so, is there a design to this, is there some reason for this, why must we suffer like this? And we become pretty neurotic about it. I have observed this not only in myself but in many other people who have children like this or who seemed to be normal before they had these abnormal children. And they became abnormal themselves. You see it's a vicious circle. It's a self-feeding kind of thing. Then people say "Look at that. She's so overanxious she's causing this." But I knew this child would start screaming if the door was closed so I became very anxious about the door closing. And then it became obvious to other people that that was what was causing the child to be like that. —Stuart's mother

It is no wonder that with the finger of blame constantly pointing in our direction some of us begin to spend our days feeling anxious, defensive, and, ultimately, guilty. There may not be enough apples in the bag or hours in a day, but it seems there is always something stewing on the back burner to feel guilty about.

And, in most cases, we are feeling guilty about things that in fact we had nothing to do with. While we should of course accept responsibility for our true share of any problem, we should not take on responsibility that belongs elsewhere. And if we are doing our best to correct the situation, there is no need to feel guilty.

The guilt most of us feel, and the blame others most often attach to us, has to do with our parenting skills. However, it is important to recognize that here is a broad range in parenting styles and that one style is not necessarily better than another. We are all individuals with our own unique situations, and we should trust our own judgment about what is best for us and our children.

It is also important to recognize that in this imperfect world there is no such thing as a perfect parent, and there is no such thing as a perfect child. All of us make mistakes, and even if we didn't, there is no guarantee that our children would reflect our perfection.

Our children are subject to many influences besides us, genetic, dietary, social and environmental, and all we can expect of ourselves is to do our best. Healthy children are quite capable of adapting to a variety of less than satisfactory circumstances without being permanently damaged.

However, there are some children who are less resilient and more vulnerable than the majority of others, less able to cope in a positive way with the vagaries of everyday life. Many of these children have mental, emotional and behavioral problems, not because we didn't parent them properly but because they are subject to major physical and biochemical stresses, such as poor-quality diets, food and environmental sensitivities, heavy metal toxicities, hypoglycemia, unrecognized needs for greater than normal amounts of certain vitamins and minerals, and so on. And once some basic problems are corrected—their diet improved, nutritional supplementation instituted, contact with certain chemicals decreased—they will often delight us by displaying the fabled resilience of youth.

(Please note that children who are otherwise healthy can also exhibit severe mental, emotional and behavioral symptoms if they are abused physically, sexually or emotionally by their parents or others. Any parents who feel they may be treating their children abusively should of course seek help as quickly as possible, whether or not their children exhibit symptoms.)

Yes, it is important to parent as well as we can and to try to correct negative parenting habits. All of us will be responsible for some of our children's less-than-winsome ways, but in this we are no different from any other parent. Sometimes we are forced to do things we don't want to by necessity, mostly economic. If that's the way it is, that's the way it is; we don't have to like it, and some day we may be able to change it, but we should not feel guilty about it.

ANGER

Anger is a common reaction to a difficult situation and, directed appropriately and used as a goad to constructive action, can be a useful emotion. There are in fact many, many situations where anger is an extremely appropriate response. However, sometimes anger is directed unfairly at those who are closest to us, such as our children's other parent or the children themselves, who are probably not any more to blame than we are for the situation. Misdirected anger can be just as destructive as guilt, making it more difficult for all those concerned to work together to improve the situation.

It is important to express our anger, but we should be careful to make clear who or what is the object of our anger so misunderstandings do not occur, and to make sure that our anger does not get expressed in a harmful way. Kicking a punching bag or screaming at the wall or writing a stinging tirade in our nightly journal or trying to resolve a situation by stating clearly why we are upset and what we think should be done are all methods of dealing with anger that are not harmful and may be helpful. On the other hand, kicking the dog or mailing a hate letter or banging our heads on a concrete floor are not particularly constructive and will inevitably make a bad situation worse. Some of the information in Chapter 7 will be helpful in dealing with situations that make us angry.

Special mention should be made of anger directed at our children. There is no doubt about it, many children are capable of rousing intense feelings of fury and dislike in us, and to feel these emotions does not make us bad parents or abnormal in any way, as long as we do not let these emotions gain control of us.

I had trouble with Enid and it was more my trouble than it was hers. I was really hitting her hard. I was having a real hard time, I really didn't care if I ever saw her, I was really rejecting her and she was doing a lot of temper tantrums. I happened to choose a woman that I'm not particularly good friends with [to talk to] but was a good choice because she [told me] to go on out of the room and I said, just like a lot of people who abuse kids say, "They made me do it, they let me do it," and that's exactly what I said, too, "She made me do it." And she said, "Yes, she does make you do it, they do make you do it but you are the adult. Grow up, you are the adult and you have the ability to walk away. Once they reach the point where they are leading you into that they can't walk away, they are incapable of that, their emotions are raging right through them and they have no way, watch that danger sign and walk away, take the power out of it for the moment."   —Enid's mother

Enid's mother suggests that telling children what we are feeling, no matter what their age or level of understanding, will be a help:

Expressing yourself gives you a pressure valve that you've done it, you've expressed your feelings, plus the fact that, when you try and explain it to a kid that little, you're purifying what you are saying, you are making an effort to communicate with them so you're finding the words and you are putting it in [a] perspective that they will understand, and that helps you understand yourself. It's really important even with a one-year-old . . . even if they are just gooing and gawing . . . it really helps clarify all those issues . . .

DESPAIR

Some of us have been told that our children are hopeless, nothing can be done for them, and that either we should institutionalize them or accept that this is the way they will be for the rest of their lives. Others have gone from doctor to doctor, psychologist to psychologist, trying this approach and that approach with no improvement and sometimes a worsening of our children's conditions. Even those of us whose children exhibit only relatively mild symptoms may still have many fears that our children will never change and will grow up socially handicapped.

I think Cheryl had more temper tantrums than any of them, and she is really a nice gentle one now; and so sometimes when your kid has gone through a bout of temper tantrums, you figure you are raising this beast and you've done everything wrong and there is no way, you've blown it on this kid and they are never going to be socially adaptive and nobody is ever going to like them because they are so horrible, it's nice to know—once you have older kids you realize—that those things come and go . . .
—Cheryl's mother

I go into my slumps and come out of them and I find my son does too, no matter what I do, so I ride it out, accept symptoms and do not dwell on them. —Dagan's mother

The present is not necessarily a good predictor of the future. Children often do change for the better, either on their own as they get older or with treatment. Children who have prolonged severe symptoms when they are small can grow up to be happy, fully-functioning, well-liked adults.

Sometimes the change in children is so slow it is hard to believe it is happening. Sometimes we get so tired there seems to be no point continuing, because nothing will ever work anyway. However, it is important not to give up until we have explored all possibilities. The nutritional/environmental approach has helped many children, even those with extremely serious problems, and it is worth giving it a fair chance. And there are other approaches, both mainstream and alternative, which may be helpful as well.

When everything has been tried and there is still no sign of improvement, it is some comfort to be able to tell ourselves that it is not for want of trying, and that we have done our best. It may sound Pollyannaish but it is nevertheless important to say that if we keep our eyes and ears open and try to keep up with current developments, someday we may find an answer.

LACK OF SELF-CONFIDENCE

Many of us find that when things are not going well, for example when we have serious concerns about our children and our home life is in constant turmoil, our self-esteem suffers and we may feel that we are not smart enough/strong enough/capable enough to cope with our problems, that our only hope is to find outside help and that we have nothing to contribute to any solutions. There is certainly nothing wrong with reaching out to other people for help; in fact, it is important that we should. The more help we can get from others the better (see the section on support systems on page 27), but at the same time we must recognize the many valuable internal resources that we possess can often be the saving of a difficult situation.

The extremely important resources which all of us have to draw on in times of need are the knowledge and understanding we have gained from our own unique experiences and observations, our own feelings and intuitions, which are often more trustworthy than simple logic, a deep well of common sense, ingenuity and creativity, and a rock-solid core of strength. Often we do not recognize these qualities in ourselves and discover them only when we are faced with adversity; we can help them to surface by not denying their existence and by being positive about ourselves and our capabilities. Especially in hard times it is crucial to have faith in ourselves and to not put ourselves down. It is good and sometimes necessary to reach out to others for help, but we should never do it believing that everyone else is better or more knowledgeable than we are.

I [should] have had more confidence in my own ability. When Michelle was three, I was an Adelle Davis fan. I was on the right track—I had even bought the right vitamins. But I talked to her pediatrician about it and he said, "Martha, you're the biggest crazy person I have ever seen, you're full of baloney." He said, "You're going to kill that child." He said, "Nobody can take that much vitamin C and not get hurt." When we moved seven years ago I emptied my cupboards—I threw away exactly what has started getting her well. And she was three years old. If I had had confidence in my own ability—but I was a housewife and I thought, "Teachers know, and doctors know."

Then I graduated from college in '75—I started working and I thought, "Hey! I'm one of them and I still don't know everything." Shocked at how little I know, I looked around and they don't all know either.

—Michelle's mother

We have been fortunate in the selection of teachers, doctors and other professionals. They have been of great help. But underlying all of their advice has been the disturbing and ever-increasing awareness that so little is known about the problems of the developmentally disabled, or their solutions, and the unavailability of pat answers. Many opinions are offered, but no positive assurance is given. One is forced to enquire on one's own, study the literature, learn the experiences of others and explore all likely avenues to the solution for one's own child. It is necessary to rely on the old maxim that whatever works is right. More than one solution, even conflicting solutions, must be tried, and it has to be remembered that what works for one individual may not work for another. In appropriate cases one should not be afraid to go counter to professional advice or action when this is dictated by personal experience or the opinion of credible authorities.—Annette's father

[My suggestion to other parents is to] read everything you can lay your hands on. Don't give up. Be really stubborn and curious, observe your child very, very carefully. It's mainly through observation and fiddling with the diet that you can do it [unless] you've got a child who's reacting to an inhalant, or petrochemicals or something like that. Start when the child is as young as possible. Because it's a lot easier then, than after they go to school. Don't be put off by people telling you you're crazy. —Stuart's mother

LOOKING AFTER OUR OWN NEEDS

In addition to feeling guilty, angry and inadequate (just to mention a few common emotions) many of us are also simply exhausted, and this exhaustion in turn intensifies any negative feelings we may be having. And usually we are exhausted because all our energies are spent looking after our children's needs, and next to no energy is spent looking after *our* needs. However, it is crucial both for our sakes and our children's sakes that we not ignore our needs. An exhausted, stressed-out parent is not nearly as much help to a child as a rested, relaxed one.

Everyone, whether child or adult, has a variety of needs, including physical, mental and emotional. To look after ourselves properly we must make sure to get enough rest, eat properly (see Chapter 10), exercise (see page 263 in Chapter 18), deal with any ailments that come along no matter how minor, and, in some cases, depending on individual requirements, add vitamin and mineral supplements to our diets. We must learn how to minimize the effects of stress (see page 268 in Chapter 18), for example, by making time for relaxation and companionship; it is important to have at least part of the day where we can do things not because we have to or should but because we want to. We must make a point of finding someone sympathetic to discuss our troubles and joys with.

Unfortunately, many of us will find either that there are not enough hours in a day to accommodate all these needs satisfactorily or that there are major difficulties in the way, such as children who spend half the night screaming, effectively preventing us from fulfilling our sleep requirements. However, if we at least remain aware of our needs, we can slowly start integrating time for them into our schedules and spend a bit of energy doing some creative problem solving to figure out how to get around any obstacles in our way.

The biggest obstacle is often our own attitudes. Emotionally, it is difficult for many parents to accept that it is all right to take the time to do something that is important to us despite our children's objections. Children may prefer that we spend every minute of the day playing with them, rather than setting aside an hour to be on our own to recharge our batteries, but to a reasonable extent it is fair enough for us to ignore their wants for our needs.

On a very practical level, as outlined in various books such as *Confessions of an Organized Housewife*, by Deniece Schofield, we can increase the amount of time available to us, gain control over at least part of our lives and reduce frustration by following such principles as:

• PLANNING AHEAD. Use a calendar or other planning system to plan the most efficient use of time when scheduling errands, chores, cooking, visiting, entertaining and so on, and be prepared for these by making any required arrangements or getting in necessary supplies in advance.

• BEING ORGANIZED. Have a logical place for everything rather than frustrating piles of jumble; double recipes when cooking and freeze half for a future meal; follow a regular schedule so nothing important gets overlooked, thinking time gets reduced, and chores don't have a chance to pile up.

• SIMPLIFYING OUR LIVES. Decide which priorities are most important and concentrate on them. If it is hard keeping on top of everything, then reduce commitments, wash and clean only what is absolutely essential (mainly laundry, dishes, bathrooms and kitchens), get rid of clutter and objects that are never used.

• BEING REALISTIC. Do jobs in stages, don't try to do too much in too short a time.

• INVOLVING ALL FAMILY MEMBERS IN HOUSEHOLD WORK. Even very young children can do simple tasks, and of course older ones plus other adults should share the drudgery as well as the fun.

SUPPORT SYSTEMS

At one time or another all of us find ourselves in a situation where there is too much happening for us to deal with on our own, and we need the help of a support system. A support system is a resource that should be nurtured and well-cared for; especially when we are finding the going tough, a strong support system can be lifesaving. A support system is basically a fancy name for the network of people in our lives we rely on for help, advice and general encouragement. It can be as informal as occasional chats with the next-door neighbor, spur-of-the-moment phone calls or visits with friends, or Sunday supper get-togethers with our families; or it can be more formal, as with regular appointments with a counselor or monthly meetings of a parents' support group. We do not even need to meet people face-to-face to incorporate them into our network; a phone or mail relationship with a person involved in nutritional/environmental work can be extremely helpful and supportive. In other words, as well as family and friends, we can include many others in our network if we want or need to, such as health workers, people from helping organizations such as La Leche League (if we are having trouble breastfeeding), our children's teachers and other parents.

On a practical level, a support system may provide us with people to call on if we need help with such everyday things as cooking, cleaning, baby-sitting and transportation. On an emotional level, having people to talk to can help us feel better about ourselves and give us the energy to go on, as well as enabling us to gain a useful perspective on our situations. Sometimes just having someone who will listen and sympathize with us is all we need. Intellectually, people in our support system can help us clarify what our needs are, and give us information and suggestions.

An important skill to learn is how to ask for and accept help. Many of us know lots of people who could give us support and encouragement, but for various reasons we never get around to asking:

• WE MAY FEEL WE SHOULD BE STRONG ENOUGH TO DEAL WITH EVERYTHING OURSELVES. However, even the strongest of us needs help at one time or another and there is nothing wrong with admitting it; next time it may be our turn to help someone else.

• WE MAY FEEL THAT BY RECEIVING HELP WE WILL LOSE SOME CONTROL OF OUR LIVES. This may be true, but perhaps we should question whether this is such an important consideration when balanced against possible benefits, especially in a temporary situation.

• WE MAY FEEL THAT IF PEOPLE DON'T OFFER WE SHOULDN'T ASK. On the other hand, they may be assuming that if we don't ask for help we don't need help; what is obvious to us may not be obvious to others.

• WE MAY FEAR REJECTION. It is true that people have their own needs and problems and sometimes will say no to our requests for help. Although this may hurt, we should realize it is not a rejection of us but probably a matter of personal circumstance; we should not let this deter us from asking elsewhere.

Particularly valuable in our network is contact with others in the same situation as we are. These are the people who will understand best what we are going through, enabling us to share experiences and information and giving us mutual support and encouragement. We can do this casually with a once-in-a-while afternoon tea or on a more structured basis such as with a weekly parent support group.

We heard there's a Schizophrenics Anonymous in S. We started going in once a month to those. They were a tremendous help. It was the first time we had somebody to talk to, someone that could share our experiences. We listened to some speakers and my son was able to talk to other patients that were there. It was one of the most marvelous things that happened to us. I highly recommend that anybody should join . . .—Jon and Erica's mother

I usually listened to an interview program on our local station, and during one of my more trying mornings I heard a woman on the air describe a baby who sounded exactly like my own. Running to turn up the volume, I realized that she was from the Feingold Association. In search of both assistance and moral support, I attended the next meeting of the group and learned that many other parents had had a similar experience, and had at least helped, if not cured, their unmanageable children. —Theo's mother

And, of course, we should never overlook the support we can receive from and give to our children's other parent:

My husband and I are communicating as openly as we are able about the feelings we are having and we feel that we have been brought closer together as a result of our sharing and concern . . . —Michael's mother

Being a parent involves both pain and pleasure, not always balanced in equal amounts. It has its satisfactions but is rarely easy. Because we care deeply about our children and their happiness and well-being, it is particularly hard for us when they are obviously in distress and having difficulties. However, we must not get so submerged in the struggle of parenting a troubled child that we neglect our own physical and emotional needs.

Books referred to in this chapter and other suggested reading:
Confessions of a Happily Organized Family, Deniece Schofield. Writer's Digest Books, Cincinnati, 1984. Contains useful tips on getting organized, including how to get children to help out.
Confessions of an Organized Housewife, Deniece Schofield. Writer's Digest Books, Cincinnati, 1982. A commonsense book designed to help us gain control over our lives, at least in the area of housework.

The Hyperactive Child and the Family, John F. Taylor. Everest House, New York, 1980. In addition to brief discussions of nutrition management and medication, contains important sections on "Feelings and Relationships in Your Family" and "Your Child at School."

The New Our Bodies, Ourselves, The Boston Women's Health Book Collective. Simon & Schuster, Inc., New York, 1984. Contains a wealth of information and is a veritable treasure for women who want to improve the quality of all aspects of their lives. Sections include "Taking Care of Ourselves," "Childbearing," "Some Common and Uncommon Health and Medical Problems."

The Nutrition Detective: A Woman's Guide to Treating Your Health Problems Through the Food You Eat; Nan Kathryn Fuchs. Jeremy P. Tarcher, Inc., Los Angeles, 1985. While directed to women, this contains useful information for men also, covering nutrition and nutritional supplements, alcoholism, allergies, arthritis, blood sugar problems, fatigue, headaches, premenstrual syndrome, stressful living and so on.

2 FROM A
CHILD'S POINT OF VIEW

*A*t the age of five I began my schooling. Some of the things that stand out in my memory of those early years are quite strange, though of course I did not realize that at the time. I recall that the teacher's face would become distorted; I seemed to live in a world of my own, quite detached from those around me. Later, when we were learning to read I was very slow; the print would move, lines begin to run into one another. It was blurred sometimes too. I always seemed to be on the outside of things and had no friends, particularly at school or at the odd party. At home I had an uncontrollable temper and the least thing would set me off. Then after the short outburst I would be in floods of tears; laughter was a real luxury while I was growing up and something that rarely occurred.

From approximately the age of seven I remember having violent headaches; they would last for days sometimes. I also began falling down a great deal, and later on in my teens I realized that not everyone needed as much sleep as I did; I was always tired and lacking in energy. At school I was considered lazy and inattentive, I could not concentrate.

I must have been something of a complainer as I recall my father called me a "tragedy queen"; later a friend's mother called me a hypochondriac, a word I had to look up in the dictionary. I realize now that I used to irritate teachers, my peers, their parents and my relatives. Bit by bit I tried to withdraw into my own world. I would go off on my own and if upset I would go and sit with my dog or my pigeons and talk to them.

By the age of sixteen, when I went to college, the problems I remember were extreme fatigue, nervousness, inability to get along with my peers (for the most part). I still felt on the outside of things and was very easily hurt by people. I had violent headaches, dizzy spells, difficulty thinking, terrible depressions and anxiety. I prayed that I would die on many occasions.

I would often see little dots of light darting about me. It was rather like floating through the milky way except that the spots of light were only the size of pinpricks. I used to just watch them darting about in the room or if I was outside I'd lie on my back in the grass and watch them against the sky.

Sometimes I could not tell where my arms were, unless I looked to see. They would feel as if they were in a different place. By the time I was old enough to ponder on these things, something made me keep it to myself. I *never discussed or told anyone of my experiences. For the longest time, of course, I did not realize that everyone didn't see or feel as I did.*

On other occasions my tongue would feel as if it had swollen to enormous proportions in my mouth. Of course, when I looked in the mirror it was fine. Once in a while as I looked at my reflection in the mirror my face would seem to change and it would not look like me for a while, then it would change back again.

Very often the world would seem quite unreal to me. It was as if I were in a different dimension, as if I had somehow become not quite real. Occasionally I would feel sure that I could fly; this seemed to be a continuation of some very vivid dreams in which I flew over people's heads in an undulating fashion.

I would often hold lengthy and detailed discussions in my head complete with questions, answers and debate. This usually happened when I was in bed, though it could happen during the day as well.

A real daydreamer, people would say, as I gazed out of a window watching the world go from bright to dim and back again. I recall my English teacher saying that I had "a very active imagination" and that I could do well if only I would work harder. This really upset me as I tried very hard in school and spent hours and hours carefully doing my homework. My concentration was often spoiled by the ringing sound in my head, not a loud sound but like a million tiny bells in the far distance, a bit similar to the sound of leaves on a big tree rustling in the wind.

I don't really know what other people's sense of time is like but I somehow felt that my sense of time wasn't quite right, perhaps because my mind would go blank. Occasionally my ideas disappeared and I would have great difficulty in bringing them back and I would become very easily confused and forgetful. I was often afraid of things, especially new people and places. I seemed to have no natural sense of direction at all. I'd get lost very easily unless I knew the area very well indeed.

The fact that people always have expected so much more of me than I was able to cope with added to my anxieties; they'd say how fit and well I looked, that I had good common sense and intelligence and they didn't understand the headaches and the constant mental confusion. I wondered who I was at times.—Angela Eyre, reprinted from the *Huxley Institute-CSF Newsletter*, January 1981.

Most of us tend to assume that the way we experience the world is the way everyone experiences the world: that the sky is as blue, the lemons as sour, the cup of tea as hot and the late movie as sad to the person next door as they are to us. But to the person next door the sky may seem more grey than blue, the lemon tasteless, the cup of tea only moderately warm, and the movie boring rather than sad.

To us, the big blue pottery bowl with the red and yellow flower in the center is probably just that, a nice-looking big blue pottery bowl with a red and yellow flower. To one of our children, however, the flower may appear as a terrifying red and yellow monster.

To a certain extent, then, we all live in different worlds, with different physical perceptions and values. Because of this, living with children will be a great deal easier if we occasionally make the attempt to view life from their perspectives.

One major benefit of shrinking down to child size and entering our children's worlds is that we will have a better understanding of the reasons behind their odd or disruptive behavior. This understanding will make that behavior both easier to tolerate and easier to do something about. Because we respond to children's actions on the basis of our interpretation of those actions, figuring out the correct "why" behind what they do is crucial, so that we can react as constructively as possible. For example:

• DAWN IS CONSTANTLY TURNING THE BIG BLUE BOWL AROUND. We assume this is done just to annoy us; we react with anger and discipline her. When we finally realize she is turning it around because the flower is disturbing to her, we simply remove the bowl.

• LARRY ALWAYS LEAVES THE ROOM WHEN COMPANY ARRIVES. We decide he thinks he is better than the rest of us and feel resentful, until we discover that his apparent rudeness is caused by fear of people. Our irritation is replaced by sympathy.

• JASON REFUSES TO SEE THE DOCTOR. We attribute this to sheer perversity on his part. However, it eventually becomes clear that, from Jason's point of view, the real issue is not the doctor, but a scary ride in the elevator to the doctor's third-floor office. The breath we save from not yelling, threatening or pleading we can now expend on the acceptable alternative of climbing the stairs.

• DARCY IS INCREASINGLY WITHDRAWN FROM THE FAMILY. We interpret this as a desire to be left alone, but are horrified one morning to catch a glimpse of the turmoil beneath the quiet exterior. Now that we recognize the extent of her terror and depression, and keeping in mind that even very young children do commit suicide and acts of violence, we immediately take steps to prevent a tragedy.

In addition to changing how we react to our children, their awareness that we have at least an inkling of what they are experiencing will make life a little less lonely for them. And even more valuable than the comfort of a well-meaning ally will be the times when we are able to make sense of their experiences for them.

What Causes Different World Views?

There are many different factors involved in the fabric of our varied worlds. Age, gender, race, size, state of health, culture, religion, economic status, occupation and our own unique personal experiences are just some of the variables that shape each individual world.

Obviously if our children have been with us from babyhood on, many factors such as culture and economic status will be the same. If our children have been adopted at an older age, some of these other variables may have to be considered.

However, most of us following the approach to learning and behavior problems outlined in this book will want to concentrate on the differences caused by our children's own unique experiences and nutritional/environmental factors. At the same time, it is important to keep in mind the differences common to children by virtue of their age, and following is a brief discussion of this.

Children Are Not Small Adults

Because they are young and still developing mentally and physically, children live in a world different from the one adults live in. Some of these youth-related factors are fairly common to one degree or another to all children:

SIZE. Size affects how children relate to the world. Being much smaller than we are they may have to stretch to reach the water faucets, or find a stool when they want to get the crayons off the counter; in crowds they see knees instead of faces. What they notice in a room may be a few feet lower than what we notice, and their bedroom and the dog across the street seem bigger to them than to us. This explains why some things that are non-threatening to us are frightening to our children. For example, I can still remember bursting into tears when I was four years old at my first sight of Santa Claus, scared silly because he looked so incredibly tall and wide.

KNOWLEDGE. A child's world is affected by lack of knowledge both "factual" (What is electricity? How big is the sun?) and "social" (Is it all right to play hide-and-seek in a clothing store? Were those people joking or serious when they said to go out and play in the traffic? Why is it wrong to eat carrots from someone else's garden?). Children tend to act as the spirit moves them and take others at face value. Learning all the intricacies, nuances and unstated rules of acceptable behavior and personal interactions is, therefore, a long process. We are not born knowing the often arbitrary concepts of "right" and "wrong" or "appropriate" and "inappropriate;" it is not surprising that children sometimes act "bad." The world can seem a very puzzling place full of strange rules, random happenings, illogical reactions, misunderstandings and injustices. Some children may feel very insecure because of this.

POWER AND STATUS. Children have very little power or status in this society. Lack of size and knowledge are two reasons for this. Two more major reasons are their economic dependence on adults and their exclusion from all levels of decision making, whether at home, school or elsewhere. Children are rarely consulted or listened to, or even treated with respect, and generally depend totally on us to provide them with their needs and wants. Their reality is that we hold all the cards, and partly out of this frustration come the power struggles, the attempts to gain some control over their lives by fighting back with temper tantrums, hunger strikes, passive resistance, and whatever else seems to work.

PRIORITIES. Children have a different set of priorities than we do. Adults usually have many responsibilities such as a living to earn and homes to take care of, not to mention our children to look after. Children, as far as they can see, have only one major responsibility, themselves, which will often lead to a conflict of interest and friction. Playing snap, tag or goblins will seem much more important than getting the dishes done.

SENSE OF TIME. A child's time sense often differs from an adult's. Time is very subjective to children and it takes them a long while to develop any concept of time by a clock. This of course makes it very hard to fit them into schedules of any sort. Instead, children are present oriented, and their wants and needs are immediate. If they are hungry they want to eat right now, and find the wait for anything special like a birthday almost unbearable. They easily become totally absorbed in what they are doing at any given minute without any regard for what else they should be doing. Getting dressed in the morning can't possibly compete with the urgency of finishing the drawing of Supermouse.

THINKING PROCESSES. The way children think can also be different. Children's reasons for doing something may make perfect sense to them and be illogical to us (I asked my daughter why she'd done something and the only reply she could give was "because I didn't think you'd know"). And what makes sense to us (Go to bed now so you won't get sick) may seem illogical to them. (I can't go to bed now, I'm having too much fun!) Further, they seldom think of the consequences of their actions, which is sometimes disastrous to them and often inconvenient to us.

PHYSICAL. Children develop coordination as they grow older (using can openers, riding bikes, etc.), as well as strength, endurance, body awareness and sexual characteristics.

PERCEPTUAL. As they say, one child's music is some adults' noise. Things taste different and their sense of smell is more acute.

The above is a general summary of differences between adults and children. It is also helpful to find out about the differences more specific to each age group. Discovering that puzzling or annoying behavior is developmental and will pass can be very reassuring. Either talking to a parent who has older children or reading a book which gives details of common behavior month by month for younger children and year by year for older children will give us some guidelines.

At the same time as we take account of children's differences, it is important to remember that there are also similarities: children are beings with feelings, ideas and desires just as we are, and they have the same needs not only for physical security but for emotional security.

It is also important to remember that each child is an individual, and what applies to one may not apply to another even within the same family. Besides this, we must recognize that children are changing all the time; all of the differences listed above will be much more obvious the younger the child, and diminish as children get older. By constant trial and error they eventually learn to walk and to talk, they develop self-control and judgment, compassion and critical thinking.

Nutritional/Environmental Factors

Now that we have seen how different children's worlds are because they are children, we can consider the effect that nutritional/ environmental factors may have on them.

Although we may accept that nutritional or environmental factors are at the root of our children's learning and behavior problems, the specific role that these factors play is not always clear.

Sometimes she acts so good and is so cooperative and pleasant to be with, and other times I wish I could send her to the moon. I have tried asking her when things have calmed down what gets into her, and though she recognizes that her behavior was disruptive, her only answer is a sad and frustrated little "I don't know." I can only guess that at those times she is feeling so bad and so distressed from her food allergies or hypoglycemia that she just has no control.   —Jen's mother

Most obvious is how these nutritional/environmental factors affect a child's physical sense of well-being. Constant fatigue, aches and pains, runny or stuffed up nose, digestive problems, vague feelings of discomfort: any of these or other symptoms are enough to make some children cranky, irritable, restless, inattentive, lethargic, hyper, uncommunicative or even destructive.

In other children, nutritional/environmental factors not only affect their physical sense of well-being, but also interfere with their sensory perceptions, thoughts, emotions and motor activity.

Interference in any of the above areas can cause problems in both learning and behavior, which will, of course, also adversely affect children's social relationships (with friends, siblings, teachers, neighbors and others as well as with us). The following quote illustrates the difficulties that an auditory dysperception can cause:

He was an extremely fearful child. I could not be separated from him by a door. Every place I went, he had to be with me at all times. And it just drove me crazy—he would scream and scream and scream if there was anything between us at all. He couldn't play with any other children if the door was closed, if he were outside and I was inside.

Then we realized that he had no idea where sound was coming from. He was extremely disoriented. We were wondering if this was the reason for the severe separation anxiety. If we called him from, say, downstairs, he would run around upstairs trying to figure out where it was. If we were outside the window, and he was standing just inside the window, in the kitchen, and we called him, he'd run upstairs or downstairs. He could not identify the direction of sound.   —Stuart's mother

Perceptual problems can be caused either by too much, too little, or inaccurate information being sent to the brain by the sensory organs (eyes, ears, nose, taste buds, touch). Perceptual problems can also be caused by either misinterpretation or lack of interpretation of the information that has been received by the brain; in other words, the information has not been "screened" properly. For example, some children with ear infections may not hear as well as normally, sounds may be distorted, or there may be extra sounds such as a "whooshing" noise. Other children's ears may be in fine working order, with the audial message getting mixed up only after it arrives in the brain. A child's eyes may be functioning perfectly but still the child sees everything through a fog.

Common auditory dysperceptions in children include super-acute hearing, sounds muffled, sounds that aren't there, and hearing thoughts inside their heads or, more seriously, outside their heads.

Common visual changes are described by Dr. Abram Hoffer in his pamphlet *Research and Troubled Children,* mentioned in Chapter 1: "Primarily these children will have illusions. Things don't seem just right. People's faces oscillate or pulsate. Colors change. Sometimes they look at a face and see areas missing, blanks in what they are seeing. Rarely do they have hallucinations, but if they do, these can be quite disturbing to the child."

Sara's mother tells how Sara, who had both visual and auditory dysperceptions, told her doctor ". . . how words moved from left to right (never up and down); how words could disappear; how walls, pictures, floors, people, the ground etc. were all moving (very specific movement, walls, etc. back and forward, the sidewalk only up and down). She would hear someone calling her name with no one around; when lying in bed, the bedroom could turn upside down. . . ."

We discovered that his perceptions were off. The rugs would jump, he felt like there was a cloud between him and the wall, he was having trouble reading at school. The words were jumping. . . .   —Jon's mother

Problems with thinking involve two aspects. One is with the thinking process itself, involving lack of concentration and lack of logic, such as when a thought disappears before it is completed, repeats itself like a broken record, or is continually interrupted by random thoughts. A thought pattern that does not make sense is another example.

Second is thought content. What children are thinking about, whether it is devils, pirates, death, math problems, food or anything else from an infinite variety of possibilities, is not necessarily a problem. It is only a problem when children become obsessed with the thoughts and think of nothing else, so that matters of more immediate concern are ignored; if the thoughts are completely inappropriate, leading to inappropriate behavior; or if the thoughts are distressing to them (in some cases precipitating actions which may be harmful).

Nutritional/environmental factors can affect emotions, causing them to be inappropriate both in intensity and duration. For example it is one thing to be depressed for weeks because of a death in the family, and another to be depressed because of a missed movie, or for no apparent reason at all. Depression, euphoria, anxiety and flatness (lack of emotion) are common.

Motor activity (walking and jumping, talking and singing, cutting and drawing) may also be disordered. Some children never stop moving, jerking or twitching; many of these children are speeded up, acting like whirlwinds gone berserk, often walking sooner than others. Others move seldom and occasionally clumsily, sometimes due to poor coordination and muscle control.

It can easily be understood then, why children would have trouble both with their learning and behavior. It is not easy to read if the words on a page are moving or letters get mixed up, follow directions if only half the sentence registers, understand fractions if other ideas keep popping up to interfere, or explain a poem if thoughts keep being forgotten. We may think children are being disobedient when they quite honestly have not heard, or have misunderstood or forgotten our instructions. Or, more indirectly, sometimes children "misbehave" because of the sheer frustration of not being able to read, or write, when everyone, including themselves, wants and expects them to.

Personal Experiences

Even if our children were with us 24 hours a day, which they are less and less the older they get, they would still have their own unique personal experiences which, in addition to age and nutritional/ environmental factors, also color their world differently than ours. These experiences are sometimes partly responsible for learning and behavior problems, precipitating or exacerbating symptoms: Failing a year at school can contribute to, or cause, depression; a move to another city away from friends can cause resentment and rebelliousness; a divorce can cause insecurity. Many other things such as sexual abuse can also cause a wide range of severe symptoms. There are a million situations that can cause children to stop paying attention to schoolwork, lose their interest in learning, or to become "difficult" at home, silent, sulky or deliberately disruptive.

Even if we decide that personal experiences are only a small part of a child's problems, it is still important to be aware of them. In day-to-day living all factors affecting us, whether nutritional, personal experience or any other, are interconnected.

Walking a Mile in Our Children's Moccasins

In order to deal with children in the best way possible, we need to know how each one of them is experiencing the world physically, mentally, emotionally. A combination of methods such as the following can be used to gain an understanding of their lives, especially with respect to problem areas:

OBSERVATION. Observing children in difficult situations is one way of gathering information and getting an idea of where their difficulties lie. Observation can give us lot of clues to the "whys" of behavior that we might not otherwise be aware of.

Even adults don't focus in on a conflict and express it rationally. When you are in a crisis you are flipping out, you are not going to talk about it openly. Chances are [our children] are not going to come and say, "I had a fight with little Janie at the day-care, she wouldn't share her toys." They aren't going to do that, they are going to come home and they are not going to share their toys, or they are going to act out in some other way to be able to work it through. —Enid's mother

It is not always easy to interpret what we observe. For example, the same behavior problem at different times may have different causes.

We have seldom been able to find reasons for Annette's crying, screaming and other attacks of violent behavior. There are times, of course, when these attacks are clearly manipulative. On a few occasions they have been the result of the tantrums or angry speech of others, even though these were not directed at her. But we feel that most of them occur when she is suffering some extended period of undetected illness or indisposition, such as recurrent attacks of cold or flu virus, and premenstrual periods. —Annette's father

But it is important that we persevere with our observations, as the information we gain can be extremely useful.

Dr. R. Glen Green of Prince Albert, Saskatchewan has had a great deal of experience with children. In a personal communication he mentions some clues that can help us figure out what is happening with children:

"If the child does not like to look in the mirror, or if he spends a lot of time looking in the mirror, there is likely something wrong with his visual perception. Another sign is a child will watch his hands, or play with his hands, for several minutes at a time. Frequently, talking to himself or laughing is a sign and is due to perceptual changes."

There are other things to watch out for as well. Do they have a peculiar walk? Perhaps the floor seems uneven to them. Are they easily confused, can't concentrate, occasionally blank out? Thought disorders can be suspected. Are they clumsy and awkward? Visual and/or motor control problems may be at fault. Quiet and unresponsive? Depression is a possibility. Never seem to pay attention? Could be an auditory dysperception.

In addition to ourselves, other concerned people such as relatives, neighbors, baby-sitters and teachers will often have helpful observations and insights.

There are a few simple ways of checking out the possibility of perceptual problems:

1. Write down a few letters and numbers as Dr. Green does and ask the children to copy them. Suspect perceptual problems if children draw figures that are reversed, upside down or doubled.

2. Point out a picture and ask what they see. Suspect perceptual problems if children see things that aren't there or are distorted, if the picture seems to be moving or shaking, if the colors are different.

3. Say a word and have them repeat it. Suspect perceptual problems if they are not able to do this accurately.

4. Make sounds from different parts of the room while their eyes are closed and have them say where the sound is coming from. Suspect perceptual problems if they cannot locate the source of the sound.

5. Ask the following questions, as outlined by Dr. Green in the Canadian Schizophrenia Foundation pamphlet *Research and Troubled Children*:

   a. "Do words move when you read?"

   b. "Does your face move when you look in the mirror?"

   c. "Do pictures move when you look at them?"

   d. "Do you hear someone calling your name when there is no one there?"

   e. "Does the ground move when you walk?"

A positive response to any of the questions listed in number 5 indicates the presence of perceptual problems.

CONVERSATION. In addition to being good observers and testing out our suspicions, initiating conversations with children about their experiences will often be very helpful.

Asking why children are acting a certain way rather than assuming that it is because they are unreasonable/have no sense/are seeking attention may avoid a lot of high blood pressure. Terry's mother described how she and Terry's father took their four-year-old daughter skating one evening so she could show her father how much her skating had improved with her new skates. Once out on the ice, Terry started wildly jerking her feet and arms "like a puppet on strings." Terry's mother was getting increasingly frustrated at what appeared to be just acting silly and fooling around, but stopped herself from yelling and instead simply asked Terry what she was doing. The little girl replied, "Twirling, to show dad how well I can skate."

Another thing not to assume is that children will automatically tell us about anything out of the ordinary in their lives. Walls that move in and out may seem somewhat unusual to us, but be a normal fact of life to a child whose earliest memories may include walls that move in and out.

One example of how such a conversation might go is the following exchange which took place between George and his mother:

"After you've had that ice cream cone and I say to you, 'George, you are acting wild,' are you feeling good inside or are you feeling a little bit miserable?"

"Miserable."

"Oh, really. What is it like to be miserable?"

"Turning around in circles."

In general, when initiating a conversation, specific questions geared to each individual child, about school or daycare, friends and siblings, books and records, toys and TV, are best:

[Ask] "Did you see so and so, was so and so there, did you get a chance to play with them, what did you play, did you paint, what kind of artwork did you do," rather than ask, "Well, what did you do today." It just leaves them wordless; they don't know how to respond to that. Lots of times they just can't think of what they did in the day, it's just that it floated by them.
                                                                —Enid's mother

Other questions that might be asked are: What did you like best about today? What didn't you like? Did anything happen today to make you happy? To make you sad? Is there anything that scares you? If you could change anything you wanted to, what would you change?

In getting a good conversation going, there will be difficulties but perhaps fewer than we expect. Unlikely as it may seem, it could be that our children just naturally assumed that if we didn't ask, then we didn't want to know, and will be very responsive to active interest.

It is also important to recognize that even very young children are often able to give us at least a suggestion of what they are experiencing. Bill's mother wrote that when her son was an overactive four-year-old he told her, "Something inside makes me have to go fast—almost like a voice—I don't want to do things, but I do them anyway—the thing inside makes me."

However, in discussions with children, it won't be surprising if they don't immediately blurt out every thought, feeling and sensory dysperception they've had over the last three years. For those of us who have not regularly had discussions like this, it may take a bit of getting used to on both sides. Fortunately, children as well as adults get better with practice.

Following are some thoughts from Enid's mother that may help us improve communication with our children:

Bedtime is usually the time when kids will let things out, if you take the time to lay down with them for a half an hour just resting and chatting away. It may not happen for the first little while but after a while it does. I think that what they need is the time, you just can't sit down and say, "Well, what's bothering you." Generally a kid will either tell you what's bothering them or they will say, "No I don't want to talk to you about it," and if they say "no" you can say, "Well, when you are ready I'm here" or "You know you can always come to me."

I feel a real problem with my mother was that I would say something and she would just deny it immediately and as a young kid that is very frustrating because you know that what you said is the truth and if someone doesn't recognize it then what's the point of talking to them. When our kids tell us things we should believe them. It's really easy when they tell us things we don't want to know to negate it and to deny it and say, "No, that's not true that's not what is happening" or "You must be mistaken sweetheart," even things like "the day-care worker hates me" and you say, "Oh, she doesn't hate you" or "What are you doing in order to deserve that." We often don't come out with a simple, "Well, what makes you think that " or "Why do you say that?"

I really think that there's those three golden things that you do when you're communicating with someone, you look them in the eye, you give them focused attention (so it's no good talking to your kid while you are trying to cook supper) and physical touch (so that you are getting in contact with them on a real basic physical level). By doing that you let them know that you are responsive to them and what they are going to say or do.

One important point to remember when talking to children is not to minimize what they are feeling by saying it is due to their hypoglycemia/allergies/poor eating habits/whatever. Even though the hypyoglycemia (or allergy or junk food) may be exaggerating the problem, the problem may still be a valid one that needs to be dealt with. For example, being persecuted by the bully next door is still being persecuted by the bully next door whether one is suffering from a hypoglycemic attack or not. (See Chapter 12 for information on hypoglycemia.) The only difference may be that during the attack the problem seems hopeless and when the blood sugar level returns to normal the situation may not seem quite as bad. This is where parents can help by putting things into perspective.

At the same time it is also helpful to gently remind children when necessary that they always think the whole world is awful at 4:00 when their blood sugar level has dropped because they haven't had a snack yet, or that they can never sit still after eating hot dogs, or that their schoolwork always deteriorates when they have not taken their vitamins for a few days.

Something to keep in mind if children are resistant to our conversational overtures is that it may be best not to pressure them or demand answers; once they recognize we respect their privacy, they will probably be more willing to share their thoughts, feelings and experiences with us.

If despite our best efforts children are still not interested in talking about the things that are important to them, we will have to put on our guessing hats to figure out why. It may simply be that they are not able to express themselves very well. If the problem is that they lack either self-awareness or an adequate verbal ability, we can help them develop both of these qualities. In addition, it is important to remember that children can communicate through drawing, stories, music, drama and movement as well as conversation, and these methods of communication should also be developed.

One reason why children sometimes refuse to discuss things that bother them is the feeling that it will be too painful. For example, they may fear that saying their worries out loud will somehow make these worries all the more real. In this case it should be explained that talking will actually make them feel better and make the worries seem less serious.

Or the reason could be something completely different:

When Enid was in kindergarten she had a horrible year. She didn't talk to me about it and I think the reason why was that she didn't think I could do anything about it. She really didn't think I had any power in that situation; she identified that it was in school and out of my sphere.—Enid's mother

In some situations, strong and repeated doses of reassurance are all that is necessary. Some children may be afraid we will not believe some of their bizarre symptoms, while others may be afraid that we *will* believe them and go around telling everyone they are crazy. Still others may be too ashamed or too frightened of their symptoms to freely mention them.

Another possible difficulty is lack of a good rapport with our children. Perhaps they are having paranoid feelings, or perhaps the tensions produced by the illness have caused the relationship to deteriorate. In either case the development of two-way communication may be slow but—with time, patience and flexibility—not impossible. Encouraging a relationship with another adult that both we and our children feel good about may relieve some of the pressure and ease the situation, making eventual openness with us more likely. It is a good sign if children talk to someone, even if it is not us.

IMAGINATION. In those cases where children are unable or unwilling to tell us much, we will often be able to get a fairly clear picture of what is happening by using some imagination, which will increase our sensitivity to our children. There are certain exercises we can do to help:

• Think back to when we were children. Let all our memories come flooding in and remember the times we were misunderstood, the frustrations involved and so on. Shrink ourselves down a couple of feet, and go back 25 years in time . . . Remember not being able to reach anything? Or being in a crowd and seeing only legs? Or how huge dogs seemed? How rooms seem to have shrunk in retrospect? Being made to eat food that we absolutely hated? Forced to sit through boring classes?

• Imagine going into a room where everything is blurry, or seen through a fog.

• Imagine going into a room where everyone's face is changing.

• Imagine going into a room and being immediately aware of every single thing: the cracks in the walls, the flickering lights, the pattern on the linoleum, every sound from the dripping tap to the clinking knife to the people talking, the mixed smells of cooking and tobacco and perfume and sweat, not to mention the tensions and feelings hovering in the air.

• Imagine working and struggling at doing schoolwork and never getting it quite right.

• Imagine being taunted as a dummy or weirdo by other kids.

• Imagine an intense self-hatred and feeling of worthlessness.

• Think of three aspects of our children's behavior that we find bothersome, and, trying to see the problem from the children's point of view, list three possible reasons for each.

It should be noted that children's problems sometimes make them more vulnerable and put them at higher risk for being victimized, ranging in seriousness from being picked on by a teacher to being sexually abused by the next-door neighbor or family member. This is another reason why it is so important to develop good relationships (including observation, conversation and sensitivity) with our children from the time they are young, so that these problems can either be prevented or dealt with as soon as possible.

Again, it must be emphasized that not all our children's symptoms will be nutritionally or environmentally induced. It would be surprising indeed if certain extremely stressful situations such as a death in the family or divorce did not cause changes in children's learning and behavior patterns.

Children's Experiences

It is not easy getting inside someone else's skin, but once there, we may learn some extraordinary things. Following are more illustrations of the variety of experiences and feelings children with nutritional/environmental problems have had.

I remember when I was about nine or ten and I used to cry. I didn't want to, I just did.

There was one particular thing that I still remember, a short little fat man who had a bowler hat on. He was all in line. There was a short man and a very tall man, sort of the dimensions of Abraham Lincoln, long legs, stretched out body, top hat and his lines were all vertical, and the other one's were horizontal. I have never been able to understand that.

I had this feeling of being in a vacuum almost where I suddenly dropped into space. I was feeling like I was almost on a rock or near a rock and then it would get smaller and bigger. I think that the small was O.K. but with the big I was afraid . . .   —Albert

I can recall several experiences at age six or seven that could be described as being schizophrenic: feelings of jumping into bed, lest creatures crawl out of the wall, and feeling insistent and intense feelings of disgust for all new acquaintances for being very uppity, so to speak, and at that point became withdrawn for a long while, whereas before I had been very gregarious.
                                                                  —Marilyn

When I was about ten, I realized that I was not like other children. I lived in a fantasy world withdrawn from my peers, my younger sister and my younger brother. I liked to play by myself. I kept my doll house up in the attic so that I could be away from everyone else. I also knew that I couldn't concentrate on schoolwork and remember things as well as my classmates. About this time I would feel nauseated frequently in the morning. This nausea was often accompanied by fainting. The doctor said it was all nerves.

All I remember about the breakdown was a sensation of water cascading over my brain.   —Amy

As a child I was timid, withdrawn, felt rejected and unloved until my fifteenth year. I could never understand my mood swings as a child, just thought everyone was that way.   —Andrea

One day I asked her why she did not take my little dog for a walk. I said, "Mother's very tired, very busy and you've always done it before, why don't you?" She said, "I know this sounds dumb, but I just get terrified sometimes when I'm out like that."

There was the time I said, "Well, the thing is, you're really not standing up straight enough. Always look up, straight ahead, and that will straighten your body." And she said, "Oh, no, every once in a while I feel like I'm going to go head over heels and roll over. . . ."					—Erica's mother

He was so afraid that he was losing his mind. For a while he used to sit and watch TV just like a zombie, which was not like him. He wasn't talking to anybody, he was just sitting and watching TV.

He said, "Mom, that was all I could do, I couldn't read any more." I said, "What do you mean, you couldn't read any more?" "Well," he said, "I realized that by the time my eyes got to the end of a line I couldn't remember the words at the beginning of that line and then it got worse, like a primary grade child I was reading one word at a time and trying to hang on to the words that I read before." And of course at that point he was desperate because he thought, "My God, I am going crazy, my mind is gone."

He became more withdrawn, if visitors came to the house, even people he knew, he would just disappear quietly and be down in the basement. He was doing photography at the time and would disappear into this little darkroom for hours on end but didn't seem to be producing much out of it.

There again it wasn't until his recovery, when we could talk to him about it, that he told me what was happening in this darkroom. He said, "I just couldn't stand people. I was so afraid of everybody that that was the one place I could escape to and be safe." And he said, "I don't know which was worse, because I was so depressed and I suffered from claustrophobia. I was really scared in that little room with the windows all covered over in the dark." He didn't know which was worse—people or hiding from them.

Anyway, one time when he was down in this darkroom of his he took a razor . . . he just made these little crosshatches all the way up and down his arm, little tiny, tiny crosscuts and of course, when I saw that I was very frightened because I thought maybe next time he will dig a little deeper.

I was trying to find out why he would do a thing like that and he said, "I don't know, I just felt I had to . . . sometimes I would take a stone and bang on my arm or press something in." It was like he was incapable of feeling, like his feelings had all deadened inside and doing something like this, well at least he knew he was alive that way, forcing himself to feel something physically and a sort of a cry for help too.

I said, "You know I have been trying to understand. Could you look through these questions [in the Hoffer-Osmond Diagnostic Test] and mark with an X what was true three weeks ago?"

I was pretty shaken when I saw how many he marked "yes," some of these really weird and strange ones, like "Some of my organs feel dead . . . Sometimes my stomach feels dead . . . My body odor is much more noticeable than it once was . . . Always my thinking gets mixed up . . . At times I am aware of people talking about me . . . There are some people trying to do me harm . . . There is some plot against me."

During this time apparently he'd been scared of everybody, he'd been scared of the teachers and scared of the bus drivers. —Graham's mother

One day, while on the tennis court, I was beating my mother. I was playing well and felt good about it. Then Mother began to beat me and my spirits started to flag. We were in the middle of a rally when I looked up and saw the buildings at Yonge and St. Clair blowing up in slow motion. I was fascinated. I'd never seen anything like it before. First one building exploded, then another, dirt, bricks, mortar spewing off in all directions. Suddenly I was up in the air looking down on a single tennis court. There were two people playing. I recognized my mother and myself. The court was surrounded by charred debris. There wasn't a single building left standing. The only thing that was unaffected was the tennis court. I watched my mother and I playing tennis for a long time, then, in a split second I was back on the court again, no longer watching myself. I was aware of a large object coming towards me. It was a bomb. I threw my hands over my head and my racket spun across the court. There was silence. When I looked up the buildings were all intact and there was a tennis ball at my feet. My head was twirling.

It was an unhappy time. I refused to play tennis with any of my old friends. I didn't want to play with them. Their talking bothered me, sent me into a frenzy. I preferred to be alone. I frequented the park near our house regularly. I had nothing that I wanted to do, so I would just sit in the park for five to six hours at a time, thinking of nothing. The park was part of a dream that I had. It became my haven and I went there every time I felt upset. I was searching for something. I didn't know what it was but I thought I could find it there in the park.

This was the beginning of what I later called the fog, a heavy dead mood that plagued me for five long years. When I was in the fog, the world, when I noticed it, was like an out-of-focus picture, something unimportant and far away. People looking at me must have thought that I was an extremely lifeless child. All my senses would become greatly dulled and I would sit for hours in a kind of trance, thinking of nothing but feeling—feeling feelings, feeling emotion, sadness, eeriness, depression. It was a mood that seemed to open me up to every thought and idea straying through the world, open me up to the very universe itself as though my mind were just a big sieve with ideas going through so quickly as to create a blur of thought, a fog that poured in and out. There was so much of it and it moved so fast that I had no time *to think about what went through my mind, but only time to feel it going through. It was as though all my thoughts were separated by thick, heavy fog and when one thought groped around it could sense but not see another thought the way a person can sense but not see a person passing by on a foggy night. There were dim shadows of thoughts but nothing coherent, for the thoughts passed each other by without even meeting and forming a whole.*

The fog was a mood that made me feel very small and insignificant by showing me the immensity of everything that was not me. It literally hypnotized me, entranced me for hours on end. Its one good effect was that it drove all specific thoughts of depression and unhappiness away, glossed over my world and made everything merge into one kaleidoscope of emotion. Nothing stood out sharply or clearly. Everything was mellowed, sadness and happiness alike. When I was in the fog I could stand my unhappiness because it became the key that allowed the fog to have me. But I could never summon up the fog on my own. I always had to wait for it and at times of great depression I bitterly wished that it would come and get me.

My apathy grew. My indifference toward my environment, toward people, even my parents, grew steadily worse. Most of the time I was unaware of what was happening around me, so engrossed was I in my own lonely world. I simply did not care what people thought of me or of my appearance. They never had anything to offer me so why should I offer them anything. I preferred to be on my own.

I kept having horrifying nightmares, and in the morning when I awoke, I was unable to tell the difference between my nightmares and reality. Dreams became inextricably wound up with my real life and it terrified me, because I knew that some of them were dreams and some were not. The trouble was that I didn't know which were which.

The voices became so insistent that I had a real fear of killing my parents or myself. I had very little control over what I did. The voices would order me to kill my mother or anyone who interfered with me. At times when I felt I was more in command of myself I would warn my parents to stay away from me when I was in a hateful mood. I no longer trusted even myself. The voices were too powerful for me.—Suzanne Foster, from *Stoney Lonesome Road*

Suggested reading:
How to Talk So Kids Will Listen and Listen So Kids Will Talk, Adele Faber and Elaine Mazlish. Avon Books, New York, 1988. An excellent book on how to improve communication with our children. Includes chapters on children dealing with feelings, cooperation, punishment, autonomy, praise and roles; has exercises, checklists and lots of examples.

3

RESOURCES

There are many nutritional/environmental-related resources which can ease the task of improving children's health and behavior. These resources take many forms and include books and magazines, a variety of products and services, assorted groups and organizations and knowledgeable and supportive individuals. Unfortuantely, due to low visibility (that is, the resource exists but is not well known), cost or distance, it is not always easy to find the nutritional/environmental information, products or services we need. However, there are ways around many of these difficulties.

Low Visibility

Often more resources exist in our communities than we are aware of, and the main problem is finding out about them.

A good first step is to look under the appropriate headings in the phone book's Yellow Pages, and to check local newspapers, radio and television programs, newsletters (especially those of health or parent-oriented organizations) and community bulletin boards for announcements and descriptions of group events and activities, products and services. Many health magazines are packed with useful information, and often try to answer readers' questions. Some places have information centers which provide useful suggestions.

A good second step is to spend some time in the library, which in many cases will contain a wealth of reference material (including not only books and magazines but various lists of groups and organizations, clippings, consumer reports, government documents, and possibly films and computer services), as well as helpful librarians skilled in tracking down all sorts of information. If the material or information required is not in the library, the librarians will either be able to find it for us elsewhere or suggest where we might go to find it ourselves.

If still unable to find the specific nutritional/environmental resource we are looking for, the next step is to broaden the search.

Merely by mentioning our interest in nutritional/environmental matters to all our friends and acquaintances (including teachers, ministers or rabbis, doctors, and everyone else we can think of) we will often learn a great deal of important information and many useful tips. In addition, it never hurts to contact any groups we know of (such as health food and other stores, health and service organizations, parent associations, government departments, health clinics and hospitals, offices of elected representatives and university departments) and ask if they might have any knowledge of the particular resource we are looking for, or suggestions of where else we might look.

Another possibility is to put up notices on bulletin boards or in newsletters and newspapers outlining our needs, whether for organic goat's milk, homemade unscented soap or a nutritionally aware baby-sitter.

High Cost

Sometimes access to products and services is limited by lack of money. However, there are some ways to cut costs. In addition to taking advantage of sales, budgeting and refusing to impulse buy, other cost-cutting measures include the following:

• Comparison shopping. Prices sometimes vary significantly from one store to the next and from one area of a center to the next; for example, food in poor parts of a city is sometimes actually more expensive than in wealthier areas.

• Joining food cooperatives or buying clubs. Food co-ops are a tried-and-true method of saving money as well as obtaining higher quality food. A buying club can be as simple as a few households getting together and making joint orders to take advantage of bulk discounts; in some cases, by virtue of having a group name, buying clubs are eligible for the same discounts given to retail outlets.

• Buying directly from the source (for example, manufacturer or farmer) or from a wholesaler rather than at retail outlets.

• Growing our own food or making our own goods.

• Buying in bulk and avoiding convenience foods.

• Buying goods (such as clothing, furniture, kitchen appliances and special health equipment) second hand. Check retail secondhand outlets; classified ads in newspapers, newsletters and magazines; garage sales, rummage sales and flea markets; and notices on community bulletin boards.

• Bartering. Instead of paying money for products or services, it is sometimes possible to trade products or services. For example, we might be able to exchange fresh produce that we have grown ourselves for nutrition counseling, or spend time baby-sitting in exchange for a regular supply of additive-free bread.

• Taking off income tax all allowable health expenses.

• For those of us on some kind of special government assistance, taking advantage of any supplemental programs or allowances available for special health needs.

• Taking advantage of any discount policies that might be applicable to low income families, unemployed, seniors, members of certain organizations, etc.

• In some cases having a doctor's prescription will reduce costs. This will sometimes apply not only to some nutritional supplements but to items such as 100% natural-fiber untreated mattresses.

• Using health insurance to pay for medical services where possible. In Canada in some cases the provincial medical care commission will cover at least partial costs for treatment out of province.

• Arranging to pay in installments. If interest is charged, however, this may not be much help. A commercial group is more likely to charge interest than a nonprofit one.

• Buying high-quality products. Although cost is not always correlated with quality, this may initially be more expensive. But in the long run it is cheaper as the higher-quality product will probably last longer, need fewer repairs and work more effectively. Quality can be checked by looking up consumer reports (often carried by libraries), asking searching questions of the people selling the products, and asking those who have actually used the products how satisfied they are.

• Some local service clubs and charities will help raise funds to cover expenses due to special needs.

Distance

Although distance can be a problem, many places with both information and products can be reached by mail or telephone, regardless of how far away we live. (Some of these are listed in the section starting on page 50.)

When writing for information, double-check name and address for legibility. Especially when requesting information from a nonprofit volunteer group, it is a good idea to include a stamped, self-addressed envelope. (If writing out of the country, send International Reply Coupons rather than stamps.)

When telephoning, make a list of questions before placing the call to help keep thoughts together, and immediately write down the responses to ensure important details are not forgotten.

Some of the information to request either by letter or on the phone includes a description of the product or service, cost and discount policies, age restrictions that might apply, length of waiting list or delivery time, guarantees, servicing and replacement of parts, specific questions related to the service or product, names of related groups (especially ones located geographically closer to us) and any other nutritional/environmental information we are having trouble tracking down. (It never hurts to ask.)

As telephone charges can be expensive, it is worth checking to see if the place has a toll-free number or will accept collect calls. Many places are now using telephone answering machines, so have a message ready before phoning.

If the Resources Don't Exist

Sometimes, no matter how diligent the search, what we are looking for won't be found because it doesn't exist, or at least not in a form or location that is any use to us. In this case we should strongly consider initiating the resource ourselves. Sometimes this will not require much effort at all. For example, if there is nowhere in our area to buy organic whole-grain bread and we do not have the time or energy to make it ourselves, we might simply ask a local bakery if they would be interested in baking it for us. The chances of a positive response are increased if we lay some groundwork in advance, such as providing the bakery with the names of organic flour sources, a list of potential customers or an advance order for a specific number of loaves.

Or, if we would like to be part of a parent support group and there is none in our area, we can try starting one. To find other interested parents, some of the techniques used for tracking down resources will be helpful, such as placing notices on community bulletin boards or in newsletters and asking everyone we know to spread the word. We can also ask national organizations or other groups working in the nutritional/environmental field to pass our name and interest on to any parents in our area who contact them.

Not quite so simple but still possible to achieve are resources such as nutritional/environmental health clinics. Something of this scope requires dedication and hard work but has been done. Publicity, fundraising, a group of enthusiastic workers and intense information gathering and planning are some of the prerequisites for a project such as this.

Sometimes our role will be to pressure specific groups into providing the resources we need—for example, lobbying governments to fund an ecologic unit in a nearby hospital, urging school boards to provide at least one environmentally safe school in an area, or persuading a company to sponsor the costs of a child from a low-income family to travel to a nutritional/environmental clinic.

Whichever resource we decide to initiate, our best chance of success lies in joining with as many other interested people and groups as possible. Very often existing groups will be willing to support us in our efforts, at least to the extent of moral support and sometimes more. However, if no groups or individuals can be found to work with, we should not let this stop us, as there are many examples of individuals working wonders. And once we get started, the likelihood is that others will eventually join us.

Characteristics to Cultivate When Tracking Down or Initiating Resources

When having trouble finding the resources we need, there are two main characteristics worth encouraging in ourselves.

The first is *persistence*. Chances are we will not find what we want with the first or even second or third or fourth query made. Tracking down resources or initiating them is often a lengthy process, and if the search is abandoned prematurely we may miss something that might have helped us and our children.

In our search, particularly when dealing with large impersonal bureaucracies such as government agencies and departments, it is important to be prepared to deal with obstacles including:

• Letters that are not answered and phone calls that are not returned. Don't hesitate to phone or write again.

• People who are grouchy, impatient or generally unhelpful. Assume they simply got out on the wrong side of the bed and carry on regardless, politely but firmly; however, in extreme cases being rude in return will sometimes be the most effective method of ensuring a more cooperative attitude.

• Bureaucratic run-arounds and red tape. If despite the best of efforts no progress is made, ask someone with more clout, such as a politician, doctor or head of an organization to help.

• Misinformation. It never hurts to double check information, especially when dealing with vague and confused bureaucracies.

In the face of obstacles like these, it is easier to be persistent if we can manage to maintain our patience and sense of humor and develop a thick skin. Being persistent means being assertive and stating our needs as often and as loudly as necessary until we get a satisfactory response.

The second characteristic to encourage is *being organized*. One simple method of keeping track of contacts, ideas and information is to use index cards kept together in a file box. Writing everything down in a loose-leaf binder with sections can also work well.

Resources List

Most of the places listed on the following pages have brochures or catalogues describing their products or services which they will send on request, and all (with the exception of some of the treatment facilities) offer mail-order services.

FOOD

Most of the places listed in this category supply organic food (check with each place individually if this is a concern), and many of them also have food for those with special dietary needs such as gluten-free flours. Some sell products other than food, such as books and nutritional supplements.

In addition to the places listed below, other possible sources of high-quality food or food for special needs are:

• Local grocery stores (some of them have special health food and specialty sections)

• Growing our own (in our backyards, balconies, community plots, in the basement or kitchen or rented greenhouse)

• Food co-ops and buying clubs, health food stores, farmers' markets, and directly from the farmer or food manufacturer

Sometimes, if we are willing to buy on a regular basis or in quantity, it is possible to make special arrangements with stores to make food goods to our specifications, for example, arranging with a baker to make a supply of bread containing no milk products. We do not of course have to limit ourselves to stores, as there are also individuals willing to make us up batches of, for example, additive-free canned goods, or, if time is more of a problem than money, premade frozen dinners containing the ingredients of our choice.

Canada

CRS Workers' Co-op
1239 Odlum Drive
Vancouver, B.C. V5L 3L8
(604) 251–1585
Contact: Anita Pollard/Anne
Romanow

Mary Jane's Limited
377 Duckworth St.
P.O. Box 5386
St. Johns, Nfld. A1C 5W2
(709) 753–8466
Contact: Sharon Dean, General
Manager

The Root Cellar
34 Queen Street
Charlottetown, P.E.I. C1A 4A3
(902) 892–6227
Contacts: Gail and Joseph Kern

Wild West Organic Harvest
Cooperative
2471 Simpson Rd.
Richmond, B.C. V6X 2R2
(604) 276–2411

United States

Allergy Resources
62 Firwood Rd.
Port Washington, NY 11050
(516) 767–2000
Contact: Christine Beaman

Erner-G Foods, Inc.
P.O. Box 84487
Seattle, WA 98124–5787
(206) 767–6660

Jaffe Bros.
P. O. Box 636
Valley Center, CA 92082
(619) 749–1133

Walnut Acres, Inc.
Penns Creek, PA 17862
(717) 837–0601
Contacts: Robert Anderson/Paul
Keene

NUTRITIONAL SUPPLEMENTS

Most of the places listed in this category offer a range of supplements
(vitamins, minerals, etc.) free of many common sensitivity–causing
substances such as sugar, starch, wheat, soy, yeast, corn, artificial
colors, flavors, preservatives. (Check individually for specific details.)

United States

Bronson Pharmaceuticals
4526 Rinetti Lane
La Canada, CA 91011
(818) 790–2646

Freeda Vitamins
36 East 41st St.
New York, NY 10017
(212) 685–4980
Contacts: Dr. Philip Zimmerman/
Mrs. Sylvia Zimmerman

Nutri-Cology, Inc.
400 Preda St.
San Leandro, CA 94577
(415) 639–4572
Contact: Customer Service
Department

Britain

G & G Food Supplies
51 Railway Approach
East Grinstead, West Sussex RH19
 1BT
(0342) 23016
Contact: Jeremy Stephens

Larkhall Laboratories
225 Putney Bridge Road
London SW15 2PY

Vitamin Service
Dellrose Cottage
Littlewick Rd., Lower Knaphill
 Woking, Surrey GU21 2JU
Brookwood (STD 04867) 88845
Contact: Mrs. Peggy Aschwanden

TREATMENT CENTERS

The following centers all have a nutritional/environmental approach
to health.

Alan Mandell Center for Bio-
 Ecologic Diseases
3 Brush Street
Norwalk, CT 06850
(203) 838–4706
Contact: Joan Jewell

Olive W. Garvey Center
3100 North Hillside
Wichita, KS 67219
(316) 682–3100
Contact: Hugh D. Riordan, M.D.

Gesell Institute of Human
 Development
310 Prospect Street
New Haven, CT
(203) 777–3481
Contact: Harvey Lederman, M.D.,
Medical Director

North Nassau Mental Health Center
North Nassau Division of Nutritional Medicine
1691 Northern Boulevard
Manhasset, NY 11030
(516) 627–7535
Contact: Yvonne Meyer

Philpott Medical Center
17171 S.E. 29th Street
Choctaw, OK 73020
(405) 390–3009
Contact: William H. Philpott, M.D.

Princeton Brain Bio Center
862 Route 518
Skillman, NJ 08558
(609) 924–8607
Contact: Marie Arcaro/
 Judith Drumm

INFORMATION

The organizations listed in this category are for the most part
information-oriented. Many of them publish regular newsletters,
sponsor meetings, and distribute books, pamphlets and other literature dealing with a variety of nutritional/environmental topics. Most
will try to answer specific questions and do their best to help in

whatever way they can. Some of them also function as support groups, some as pressure groups, and some provide services such as counseling and doctor referral. Many have branches or affiliates around the world—check individually for names and addresses.

As the majority of these groups are volunteer-staffed with limited budgets, include self-addressed envelopes with stamps or International Reply Coupons when making requests for information.

United States

The Allergy and Asthma Foundation of Lancaster County
2445 Marietta Ave.
Lancaster, PA 17601
(717) 293–1527
Contact: Dr. Stephen D. Lockey, III

American Academy of Environmental Medicine
P.O. Box 16106
Denver, CO 80216
(303) 622–9755
Contact: Judith A. Howard/Robin R. Savely

American Academy of Otolaryngic Allergy
1101 Vermont Ave. N.W., Suite 302
Washington, DC 20005
(202) 289–4607
Contact: Sandra L. May

Candida Research & Information Foundation
P.O. Box 2719
Castro Valley, CA 94546
(415) 582–2179
Contact: Gail Nielsen

Feingold Association of the United States
P.O. Box 6550
Alexandria, VA 22306
(703) 768–FAUS

Human Ecology Action League
2421 Pratt Ave.
Suite 1112
Chicago, IL 60645
(312) 665–6575
Contact: Marj Beck Gibson

Human Ecology Research Foundation of the Southwest
8345 Walnut Hill Lane
Suite 205
Dallas, TX 75231
(214) 361–9515
Contact: Katheryne George

Huxley Institute for Biosocial Research
900 North Federal Highway
Boca Raton, FL 33432
(407) 393–6167

Institute for Child Behavior Research
4182 Adams Ave.
San Diego, CA 92116
(619) 281–7165
Contact: Bernard Rimland, Ph.D.

La Leche League International
P.O. Box 1209
Franklin Park, IL 60131–8209
(312) 455–7730
Contact: Mary Gisch

Nutrition Survival Services
P.O. Box 31065
4703 Stone Way N.
Seattle, WA 98103
(206) 547–1814
Contact: Sally Rockwell

Well Mind Association
4649 Sunnyside Ave. N.
Seattle, WA 98103
(206) 633–2167
Contact: Elaine Stannard, President

Canada

Allergy Information Association
65 Tromley Drive, Suite 10
Islington, Ontario M9B 5Y7
(416) 244–9312
Contacts: Mary Tutty/
  Susan Daglish

Canadian Schizophrenia Foundation
7375 Kingsway
Burnaby, British Columbia
  V3N 3B5
(604) 521–1728
Contact: Steven Carter

Candida Research and Information
  (Canada)
#2102, 155 Marlee Avenue
Toronto, Ontario M6B 4B5
(416) 789–1562
Contact: Maggie Burston

Consumer Health Organization of
  Canada
P.O. Box 248
108 Willowdale Ave.
Willowdale, Ontario M2N 5S9
(416) 222–6517
Contact: Libby Gardon, President

La Leche League, Canadian National
  Office
493 Main St.
Winchester, Ontario K0C 2K0
(613) 774–2850
Contact: Jannie Van Noppen,
  Director

The Morris Centre
676 Stella Ave.
Winnipeg, Manitoba R2W 2V9
(204) 589–6101
Contact: Sister Theresa Feist

Britain

Foresight
The Old Vicarage, Church Lane,
  Witley
Godalming, Surrey GU8 5PN
042 879 4500
Contact: Belinda Barnes

Hyperactive Children's Support
  Group
71 Whyke Lane
Chichester, Sussex
Contact: Mrs. Sally Bunday

La Leche League of Great Britain
BM3424, London WC1 6XX

Schizophrenia Association of Great
  Britain
The International Schizophrenia
  Centre
Bryn Hyfryd, The Crescent
Bangor, Gwynedd LL57 2A6
(0248) 354048
Contact: Mrs. Gwynneth
  Hemmings

Australia

Orthomolecular Medical Assoc. of
  Australia
14 Banksia Ave.
Beaumaris, Victoria
(03) 589–5733
Contacts: Dr. Ian Brighthope/Mr.
  John Stroh

SOMA Health Association of Australia Ltd.
G.P.O. Box 3745
Sydney, NSW 2001

MEDICAL-RELATED SERVICES

United States

Doctor's Data
P.O. Box 111
West Chicago, IL 60185
1–800–323–2784 or (312) 231–3649
service: elemental analysis of hair,
urine and blood; amino acid analysis

Dr. Hal A. Huggins
P.O. Box 2589
Colorado Springs, CO 80901
(303) 473–4703 or 1–800–331–2303
service: education and treatment of
those with mercury toxicity from
dental amalgam fillings
Contact: Ginny Haynes

Canada

J. D. Campbell Enterprises
Box 1628
Victoria, B.C. V8W 2X7
(604) 383–3498
Contact: Joseph D. Campbell,
Ph.D.
service: life style, diet and hair mineral analysis service with
recommendations and guidance

PRODUCTS FOR THE ENVIRONMENTALLY SENSITIVE

The places listed here carry such products as additive-free, 100% natural fiber bedding, fabric, clothing and mattresses. In some cases they also carry products for personal care and home cleaning that are less likely to cause reactions than the usual ones.

Allergy Resources
62 Firwood Rd.
Port Washington, NY 11050
(516) 767–2000
Contact: Christine Beaman

The Cotton Place
P.O. Box 59721
Dallas, TX 75229
(214) 243–4149
Contact: Barbara Sherry

The Janice Corporation
198 Route 46
Budd Lake, NJ 07828
(201) 691–2979, 1–800–JANICES
Contact: Pam Ledoux

BOOKS

Books are one of the most useful resources around, containing vast amounts of helpful information. If we are looking for a particular book and it is not in the library, the library can request it for us on interlibrary loan. If we prefer to buy it, many bookstores will special-order it for us if they do not already stock it. Complete information, including publisher, will speed up this process; check *Books in Print* (in most public libraries) for this information. When money is a problem, request a paperback edition rather than hardcover. (Sometimes the same publisher will do both and sometimes hardcover will be published by one publisher and paper by another.) For those of us who do not live near any bookstores, some shops will send books by mail. Many health books, such as the ones listed in this volume, are also distributed by health food stores and by many of the organizations listed on the previous pages. If all else fails, we can write to the publisher and find out who does distribute their book, or arrange to buy the book directly.

Suggestions for further reading:

How To Survive Without a Salary, Charles Long. Horizon Publishing, Toronto, 1981. Anyone interested in cutting costs will find this book extremely useful.

Back to Barter, Annie Proulx. Pocket Books, New York, 1981. A comprehensive book on bartering, from individual barters to barter clubs.

4
WORKING WITH DOCTORS

Good doctors with a nutritional/environmental orientation are an invaluable resource to be cherished and consulted whenever possible. Many children, especially those whose problems are particularly serious or complex, will benefit greatly if we are able to find a knowledgeable and sympathetic doctor to work with.

Working with a good doctor enables us to find out what is wrong with less difficulty and more speed than working alone. Doctors have access to lab tests that we do not, an awareness of a broad range of possibilities to consider or rule out that we may not have heard of, plus experience gained from dealing with many cases similar to our children's. Good doctors can save us a lot of time and grief by eliminating at least some of the guesswork involved in tracking down the specific nutritional/environmental factors causing a child's problems.

I don't advise you to treat your child yourself. It's better than nothing. I'd do it any time rather than take an ordinary doctor's treatment, which is the tranquilizers. But I think we do need physicians; there's no substitute for a physician. You need the lab work. —Michelle's mother

On the other hand, no doctor can know our children and their backgrounds, eating habits and attitudes or our families better than we do. No doctor can care more about our children than we do. It is important to always remember that we are just as smart as our doctors, and by reading, talking to people, observing and thinking we can gain a great deal of knowledge in this area ourselves. One doesn't need a medical degree to understand medical subjects.

The ideal to aim for is a partnership with our doctors, in which each of us has an interest in and a responsibility for the health and well-being of our children.

Finding a Doctor

I think the first thing [parents] should expect is a physician who will take the time to listen to the complete history of the child's problem areas and then who will be willing to explore to find the causes rather than simply to prescribe medication which might cover up symptoms.   —Dr. Hugh D. Riordan

The best choice for a doctor is one who accepts that nutritional and environmental factors can cause learning and behavior problems, has seriously studied all aspects of a nutritional/environmental approach, and has had some experience using it. In addition, such a doctor will not have an analysis that lays the blame for our children's problems on us.

Number one rule I've had for about five years—when you walk into a doctor's office and he says, "Oh, my God, you've made a mess of things," or in any way insinuates that it was your fault, you know that he has no idea what he's talking about, and you pack up your bags before you run up a big bill and get out, and maybe refuse to pay because he obviously does not know what he's talking about, he's not up-to-date at all in anything.
                                                        —Michelle's mother

Preferably, a doctor will consider all aspects of nutrition and the environment, and not feel that most problems have a single basic cause, whether this be hypoglycemia, allergies or lack of a vitamin or mineral.

It is also important to try to find doctors with whom we and our children can establish a good rapport. The existence of a good rapport makes it easier to ask questions without feeling foolish or pressured by time, to be candid about feelings, worries and symptoms, and to feel confident in the doctor's judgment and abilities. These factors do not in any way indicate how knowledgeable a doctor is or how good at diagnosing or treating health problems; however, how comfortable we feel with our doctors and how good we feel about them will help determine to what degree we and our children follow the treatment program.

Locating a nutritionally and environmentally aware doctor may not be easy, particularly for those of us living in a small city or rural area. However, we might be lucky and find there is one not too far away from us. Every time we contact a group concerned with the effects of nutritional and/or environmental factors on health (see pages 53–54 in Chapter 3) we should ask for names of sympathetic doctors. Some groups keep lists of nutritional/environmental doctors. Mentioning our search to as many people as we can is also helpful in finding a doctor.

It is very difficult to find a doctor who will listen to a mother's complaints with any degree of compassion and understanding. If you can find a doctor who has a child with problems, see him. Contact with other parents whose children have problems is another way to find a doctor. People who run health food stores are often able to come up with a name for referral.
—Dr. R. Glen Green

Before deciding on a doctor, it is a good idea to find out what the experience of others has been with her or him. (We should of course keep in mind that at least part of people's reactions will be determined by how a doctor's personal style suits their own personalities, and that our requirements in that area might be quite different.) We can also check a doctor out by phoning in advance or having a preliminary visit and asking about attitudes on nutrition, the environment, and any other issues we feel are important. If we or our children are not happy with a doctor after a few visits, we should not hesitate to look for a different one.

In our search for a doctor, it is a good idea to remember that there are many types of doctors. We don't have to restrict our search to general practitioners. There are also pediatricians, allergists and internists who might be sympathetic, and even some psychiatrists, as well as doctors, such as homeopaths, chiropractors and naturopaths, who have been trained in other systems.

We should also keep in mind that it is not necessary to rely solely on doctors. There are other professionals who can give us valuable assistance, such as nutritionists, reflexologists, social workers, psychologists and acupuncturists. In addition, knowledgeable laypeople, especially other parents, will often be able to help us.

We can choose what role we want doctors to play in getting our children better according to the variables involved, such as the particular doctor, the individual child and the nature of the problem. Some doctors we will want to have as primary supports, others as secondary supports.

A doctor who is a "primary" support will be fully involved in all aspects of diagnosis and treatment in accordance with our aims of trying out a nutritional/environmental approach. The role of other doctors may be limited to doing specific lab tests for us, giving us referrals to other doctors, handling the regular medical problems that crop up, such as mumps and flu, giving advice, or acting as backup in case we run into situations where we feel out of our depth.

If we can't find a doctor close to where we live, we may have to consider traveling to another center.

I would still try to go to the very finest. I would say to myself that it's still a new enough thing that I would not try to save any money on transportation. I would get back to either Manhasset or the Brain Bio Center or Dr. C. or these top men in the field. Because I think the ones that are just learning have quite a bit to learn, at least from our experience.

—Jon and Erica's mother

If we cannot find a knowledgeable and experienced nutritionally/ environmentally oriented doctor near us and cannot afford to travel, there are some other possibilities to consider, which, though not a first choice, might still provide some help. For example, some doctors may be willing to give us advice and information through the mail or on the phone. It certainly never hurts to approach doctors in this way, and the worst that can happen is that they will not respond.

Another possibility is finding traditionally oriented doctors who are open to new approaches, and will work with us in learning about the nutritional/environmental factors affecting our children's health. If they are interested, there is much information available to them, including training courses given by some organizations.

We should not overlook the possibility that our own family doctors might be interested in working with us. Approaching them will in some cases produce worthwhile results.

My family doctor is extremely interested in the case and when he first realized I was going elsewhere with Stuart, he asked if he could still be our family doctor. So I said, "fine," and he's been quite interested. He knew nothing about vitamins. He was very suspicious and still is, of course, about any doctor who "peddles" vitamins, but at the same time, the first time I went to talk to him I don't think he even knew what the word pyridoxine [vitamin B6] meant, and the second time I went to talk to him six months later he was telling me all sorts of things about pyridoxine-dependent children.

—Stuart's mother

Building a Relationship with Our Doctors

The type of relationship to aim for with our doctors is a working relationship with mutual respect and tolerance, or in other words, a partnership. To achieve this requires that we share responsibility for our children's health by actively questioning, learning, thinking critically and taking part in decision making. At the very least, we should ask our doctors to explain anything we don't understand or are unclear about. (It is often useful to prepare for a visit to the doctor's by making up a list of questions or comments.) We must also recognize that each member of the trio that includes us, our children and our doctors has a valuable contribution to make to our children's well-being. Doctors have general medical knowledge and expertise, and we (and our children) have specific knowledge of our children, including each one's unique characteristics, nutritional and environmental histories and individual circumstances.

Doctors who keep us fully informed, answer our questions, value our input and give us moral support will be fulfilling their role in the partnership.

Following are two quotes concerning doctor-parent relationships, one from a parent and one from a doctor:

My attitude about doctors is that I use them for what I need them. I think you have to know what you need in advance and you can't let them sway you too much. I think you have to go to a doctor with the viewpoint of getting their information and then you have to come home and assess it. You have to be quite clear about what you want and what information you want and if you're a little bit fuddled then you should say, "Well, I have to think about it," and come home and think about it because you get really easily swayed. —Tyler's mother

In general, my main suggestion for parents and children concerning problems of this nature is to fully educate themselves in both prevention, nutrition and other areas of health. I must stress that, as a doctor, I am not here to wave a magic wand over patients to make them better. The doctor is there to analyze, to diagnose and to recommend the treatment which is carried out by the parents or by the patient. I am of the belief that people who do take responsibility for themselves, in general will do very well. The patients who I have difficulties with are the ones who expect the doctor to take full responsibility for their condition. In order for any kind of treatment whatsoever to be given to patients, it is absolutely essential that the patient understands exactly what is going on within themselves so that they can contribute to their own health. So, it is vital that they educate themselves in not only their own condition, but also in prevention as well. —Dr. Zoltan Rona

Suggestions for further reading:

Clinical Ecology, Lawrence D. Dickey, editor. Charles C. Thomas, Publisher, Springfield, Illinois, 1976. Very informative and, at 800 pages, thorough; a particularly good book to recommend to interested doctors.

Orthomolecular Psychiatry, David Hawkins and Linus Pauling, editors. W.H. Freeman and Company, San Francisco, 1973. Linus Pauling, two-time Nobel Prize winner, writes in this volume (in an article reprinted from *Science*) that "Orthomolecular psychiatric therapy is the treatment of mental disease by the provision of the optimum molecular environment for the mind, especially the optimum concentrations of substances normally present in the human body." Sections include "Theoretical and Experimental Background," "Clinical Diagnosis," "Treatment," and "A Practical Clinical Model." Given the vast amounts of material covered, it would be worthwhile reading for interested doctors.

Patient Beware, Cynthia Carver. Prentice-Hall Canada Inc., Scarborough, Ontario, 1984. A very helpful book for anyone dealing with doctors; gives much practical advice and general information. Covers everything from "The Doctor's-Eye View of Patients" (Chapter 1) through "Finding a Good GP" (Chapter 6) to "Changing the Medical System Itself" (Chapter 15).

A Physician's Handbook on Orthomolecular Medicine, Roger J. Williams and Dwight K. Kalita, editors. Keats Publishing, Inc., New Canaan, Connecticut, 1977. Contains a collection of articles covering a broad spectrum of the nutritional/environmental field, of interest to laypeople as well as doctors and other professionals.

5
INTRODUCING THE PROGRAM

Very often the hardest part of following a nutritional/environmental program is getting started. Changing children's diets (such as reducing sugar and refined foods or eliminating sensitivity-causing foods) or changing children's environments (such as removing synthetic carpeting from the house and reducing exposure to petrochemicals) cannot be done instantly. Time and energy, both of which are in short supply for many of us, are required. However, keeping firmly in mind the goal of a healthier and happier child will give us extra energy, and a bit of organization and planning will save us time. By maintaining a sense of humor and a perspective, introducing the program might even turn out to be an interesting challenge rather than simply more work and drudgery.

Following are a few suggestions for reducing some of the difficulties involved in introducing a nutritional/environmental program to our families. (Some of the suggestions mentioned here are also discussed in Chapter 1.)

Make the Program a Priority

Although following the program will eventually become part of the routine, in the beginning it can be something of a disruption. For this reason, consider temporarily reducing other commitments and concentrating energies on implementing the program.

Introduce the Program During a Low-Stress Time Period

Any change, no matter how positive or necessary, is stressful. Because of this, it is best to start the program during a relatively calm period of time when there is not too much else happening. For example, starting the program just before Christmas or right at the beginning of a school year would not be a good idea. On the other hand, if calm periods of time seem nonexistent, there is no reason not to plunge right in.

Don't Go It Alone

Implementing the program can be a major project. Don't hesitate to share the responsibility with the rest of the family, both children and adults, to the extent of their capabilities, or to call on friends and other supportive people as necessary.

Do One Step at a Time

Without three full-time maids and lots of money, it is probably not a good idea to try to implement a nutritional/environmental program all at once. Having an overall plan and breaking down what needs to be done into steps is a good idea. For example, plan menus in the first week, locate alternative food sources in the second, shop and prepare food in the third, introduce nutritional supplements in the fourth, and institute an exercise program in the fifth. If finding alternatives for both wheat and milk products seems to be too much to handle at the moment, there is no reason not to start by eliminating wheat and wait until life seems a bit more under control before eliminating milk products. Or, concentrate first on instituting healthy breakfasts, then go on to snacks, and leave lunch and suppers till the last.

Find Our Own Best Way of Working

Organizing each room in a house (the kitchen often being the most important as far as a nutritional/environmental approach is concerned) and its contents, and organizing time are two essentials for working efficiently. For example, store the implements and food used most often within easy reach, and follow a schedule.

Any reorganization should be done with a view to making work as easy as possible. Each person has a best way of working, and a method of organizing that is suitable for someone else may, when applied to us, complicate our lives rather than simplify them. It will help considerably to work out our own systems of ensuring that the various aspects of the program can be followed with a minimum of bother.

It was very easy to know what to feed him for meals because all I had to do was consult my list, I had it on the bulletin board so it was always sitting there, what Tyler's meals for the week were. Sunday, Monday, Tuesday, Wednesday. So I knew when to soak beans and when I had to buy something. I would keep the meat frozen in portions in the freezer so that there would be a chicken breast, six chicken breasts in the freezer. I would buy a pound of hamburger and make patties out of it. Which was O.K. as long as he ate it, but if he didn't eat it, that's when it would break down occasionally. —Tyler's mother

Take the Long View

It is almost certain to take longer than we hope to implement the program. When in the throes of impatience and frustration, it sometimes helps to remember that the application of a nutritional/environmental approach, concerned as it is with long-term influences affecting health—such as nutrition, exercise and environmental influences—is, ideally, a lifetime commitment; what doesn't get done today can still get done tomorrow.

The initial period of incorporating the program into daily life is often difficult due to unfamiliarity of procedures and the inevitability of unexpected complications. It is important to recognize that revising, fine-tuning, working out the bugs and experimentation, although slow, is often a necessary process. In other words if children continue to sneak off to the store to gobble down candies, one possibility to consider is a home-made, additive-free, sugar-reduced equivalent. If they refuse to swallow their vitamin pills, either crushing the pills and mixing them in with applesauce or offering a chewy version of the supplement might be more acceptable. If full-spectrum lighting or 100 percent natural, untreated fabric are impossible to find close by, they are probably available through the mail. If children react to the laundry detergent which was substituted for the previous sensitivity-causing detergent, simply go ahead and substitute a third, or a fourth if necessary. And so on. Making the program as workable and effective as possible is an ongoing process and does take time, but usually it is time well spent.

I wanted to get Jen's program going all at once but it was just too much to deal with. However, we have now been working at it for a long time and finally feel that we are getting somewhere. We concentrated on food first—it wasn't easy to figure out but we have come to recognize that Jen can't have any milk products or apples, and only small amounts of sugar and artificial coloring. We have spent hours looking through cookbooks, looking for alternatives to what we used to eat, making up menus, and then changing the menus because some foods we couldn't find in our small city, or were just too expensive for us. As time goes on we are getting better at it, getting a handle on what Jen will or won't eat, remembering to leave enough time to prepare whatever meals we've planned for that day. It takes a lot longer to make a bean dish than a grilled cheese sandwich. We are getting more inventive, too, which is nice, and we are still experimenting. We now know she can't tolerate raw organic apples any better than inorganic; our next step is, after a couple of months off apples completely, we will see if she can tolerate a baked apple once a week.

Jen herself is beginning to accept the necessity for the program, although when we are not around to supervise she is as likely to eat something she knows she shouldn't as not, with noticeable effects on her behavior, I think in time it will get easier for her to say no, and at least now she usually tells us so we have an idea what is going on. It used to be such a problem we decided to let her have a junk day once a week, limiting the junk on that day to one small piece of something, and that seems to be working out quite well.

Recently we have been working on her vitamins and minerals. Finding ones that don't contain anything she is sensitive to and are the right combinations and dosages, especially finding ones that she will actually take, has been hard, and in the beginning we were more often than not forgetting to give them to her, but we are pretty well organized now.

To see if it helps her stuffed nose right now, we are working on removing the carpet from her room, which we delayed for a while because of the work involved—it is glued down—but now that we have started it is going fairly quickly.

Many times I would get discouraged as there always seemed to be so much thinking involved. Sometimes the kids would be such a pain and we would be so tired it just would seem like too much work even to mix up her powdered C and calcium into a bit of juice. And hard, too, to resist her demands, especially for apples; the endurance it took! But I am glad we persevered, much of it is habit now and easier, and Jen is the happiest I've ever seen her—agreeable, humorous, self-reliant—she is doing really well.

—Jen's mother

Even once the program has stabilized, it is likely that occasional changes will still be required as children grow and their circumstances change. In addition, improvements in detection and treatment can be integrated into children's programs as new knowledge is gained.

Maintain a Perspective

Once the program has been incorporated into the daily routine, there will still be the occasional teeth-gnashing times. However, reminding ourselves that teeth-gnashing times are an inevitable part of life will help us survive with our teeth intact. As one parent said:

Going to the class picnic or whatever and seeing red Kool-Aid, there'd be a momentary surge of frustration; but then everything to do with raising kids is little surges of frustration.   —Terry's mother

6

COOPERATING KIDS

*W*e explained to Nick he had allergies; he carried it from there. He just says, "No thank you, I'm allergic to that." He has been extremely cooperative. But he feels so good, I don't think he wants to be sick again. —Nick's mother

She is self-motivated and hates to be hyper. She understands there are substances in food and the environment that make her ill and she must avoid them. —Vanessa's mother

My recovery was by no means spontaneous. I had to work for it. I had to want to get better. It was rough going. The diet was not easy. Unlike crash diets this diet was going to be with me the rest of my life. I had to learn to get used to it, had to learn that candy and cakes and sweets were something that I just could not tolerate. I had to accept the fact that the vitamins had become as necessary a part of my life as the diet had. It became apparent that when I cheated on my diet or forgot my vitamins, I cheated no one but myself. —Suzanne Foster, from *Stoney Lonesome Road*

The cooperation of children with the treatment program is crucial. Children who follow their rotation diet faithfully, refuse sweets, regularly swallow their vitamin pills, exercise without being reminded and avoid places with environmental substances they are sensitive to, not only make life easier but increase the chances that the treatment program will be successful. In addition, cooperative children are much more likely, with our support and encouragement, to eventually take responsibility for their own health.

While it is obvious that the success of the treatment program depends largely on children's attitudes and willingness to exert themselves, a great deal also depends on us: on our own attitudes and willingness to exert ourselves, on how we introduce the program and explain the necessity for the diet and supplements, on what kind of support and encouragement we give, and on how hard or easy we make it for children to cooperate.

For those of us about to initiate a treatment program, following is a discussion of what we can do to make it a cooperative effort.

EXPECTATIONS

Our expectations of children and the attitudes we have toward them are important considerations. For one thing, children are more likely to cooperate with us if we expect them to cooperate than if we expect them to be obstinate, perverse and contrary. For another, it will be very confusing for them if, at the same time as they hear us telling them to give up their Smarties, bubble gum and potato chips, they are receiving the message that if they do give up their treats they couldn't possibly be "real kids," there must be something wrong with them.

In fact, many children are as concerned about their problems as we are and are open to trying anything that might solve those problems. Some children, especially younger ones, like the extra fuss made over them and are envied by their little friends who want to be "allergic" or take vitamins too. As Doug's mother wrote, "They get used to it. (Quite like the importance!)" The wisest course is to start by assuming the best, until proven otherwise; we don't want to end up being more of an obstacle to the treatment than our children are:

Terry's mum phoned and said, "Listen, I made these apple juice popsicles that I was going to give Terry, is it all right for Jen to have one as well?" And though we felt that apples were one of the foods causing some of Jen's problems, I thought, well, she'll be disappointed if Terry can have one and she can't, maybe a little bit won't hurt, so I said to go ahead. Then Terry's mother said, "Oh, what a relief, I got worried because I asked Jen if it was all right for her to have one and she said no, she didn't think so."

When I heard that I sure felt like a prize fool, here was a four-year-old showing more maturity and smarts than me. Not only that, but I felt so bad for having underestimated her.   —Jen's mother

In other words, it is good to remember that children often have more innate good sense than we give them credit for.

Jack, who had rarely had a reasonable day in his life prior to the diet, shocked us completely with his attitude. Unfortunately, he had long been accustomed to drinking cola drinks as he pleased, and we expected a terrible uproar when he learned he couldn't have them. Instead, he accepted this change matter-of-factly. A year later when he had to give up 7-Up due to the sugar, he announced that he didn't really like it anyhow, it didn't make

him grow, and it didn't have any protein in it! —Stevens and Stoner in
How to Improve Your Child's Behavior Through Diet

*He took himself off sugar because he was so fearful—he couldn't stand
himself. He couldn't go downstairs or walk into another room by himself
because he was so frightened of being any place by himself. So I said,
"Look, it could be sugar, Stuart. Let's try it." So he said okay, he was
ready to do anything at that point. . . . He was so unhappy with himself that
he himself decided to stop eating any of these things. It took a month to
recover from that. Now he's fine; he'll go downstairs by himself, upstairs by
himself.* —Stuart's mother

MOTIVATION

Following the treatment program because they "should" or because
we told them to will not ensure the cooperation of most children; the
children who cooperate the best and involve themselves wholeheartedly
in the treatment program are the ones who are the most highly
motivated, the ones who with all their being want to become healthy.

*. . . He desperately wanted to get well. He cooperated in every way, even
though he hated, oh how he hated, ham and pork and stuff for breakfast.
One of the very main reasons that he got well was that he was tremendously
motivated. At no time did you have any problem with him not wanting to
get well. He would sell his soul to get well.* —Jon's mother

To make sure children are fully motivated, following are a few
suggestions:

• EXPLAIN WHAT GETTING BETTER MEANS. Children are more likely to
want to work toward becoming healthy if they recognize that "getting better" means not only the disappearance of stomachaches and
nightmares, it also means they will have less trouble reading, won't
get into as many fights, will be more accepted by others, won't trip
as often playing hockey and will be more likely to wake up in the
morning feeling happy instead of sad. These benefits are not always
obvious to children who have never experienced full health or who
have been unwell for a long time.

• EXPLAIN WHY THE TREATMENT PROGRAM WILL GET THEM BETTER.
Once children have decided that getting better is a worthwhile goal,
the next step is to explain why the treatment program will do this. It
is crucial that they understand the connection between their problems and the cause of their problems, whether this be a sensitivity to

food dyes, excess lead or poor nutrition. For example, we can point out to them that their irritability is linked to their individual requirements for larger-than-average amounts of the B vitamins, their fatigue is related to gas fumes from a neighbor's stove, or their uncontrollable weepiness can be directly traced back to that noontime's corn on the cob.

In general we should explain as much as we can about how nutritional/environmental factors are affecting them (making sure they realize that these factors influence everyone to one degree or another), giving simple explanations to young children and more detailed ones to older children.

For example, Powers and Presley in their book *Food Power* recommend that a hypoglycemic child be shown the blood sugar curve from the glucose tolerance test. They write that this "enables him to see the relationship between how he feels and what has happened inside him. In simple terms, he can be informed of how the blood conveys fuel to the brain in the proper amounts if he eats right and avoids the risky foods and drinks. He can be told that when he eats right, the brain receives a steady supply of fuel that will help him feel full of pep and not 'funny' inside."

Here are two examples of what parents have told their children:

Since my son is only three and a half, I have kept the explanation of his low blood sugar problem very simple—"Sugar makes you sick. Mommy and doctor want you to eat nutritious food so you'll grow big and strong and healthy."   —Michael's mother

We've told him he is "sensitive" to some foods, chemicals and environmental conditions but that some situations he will be able to control and must do so to be the best he can be.   —Bill's mother

We should also know enough to be able to answer children's questions about their health problems and the treatment program, or be willing to look up answers to questions we don't know.

When they understand the reasons why the treatment program will help them, children are much more agreeable to trying it out. A general understanding of the relationship between health, nutrition and the environment will help.

• MAKE SURE CHILDREN KNOW WHAT TO EXPECT. Especially during the testing and beginning parts of the treatment program, children sometimes feel worse before they feel better. This can be very bewildering for children unless they have been forewarned. For example, if not prepared for the withdrawal symptoms that might occur when eliminating from their diets sugar or foods they are sensitive to, many will want to quit the program in disgust. If they have been suitably prepared, however, the withdrawal symptoms may provide them with dramatic confirmation of the effects that nutritional/environmental factors have on them, strengthening their resolve to stay on the program.

They must also know what to expect in terms of how long it will be before any improvement is seen. If for some reason they assume that a week is all it will take to cure every last one of their symptoms and make them completely well, the disappointment when this doesn't happen may make them lose heart.

• ENABLE CHILDREN TO KEEP TRACK OF PROGRESS. Although the improvement of our children may be obvious to us, it may not be so obvious to them, resulting in discouragement; children who don't see any improvement are likely to lose interest. However, working out a concrete way to demonstrate their progress to them will increase their motivation.

To do this it is necessary to realize that what we consider improvement may be completely different from what our children consider to be improvement. To us improvement generally means such visible manifestations of behavior as three screaming fits a day instead of six, while to many children screaming fits are not of much importance. Probably more important to them are, first, symptoms such as an uncomfortable pressure inside their heads or feelings of depression, and second, the consequences of their behavior such as being sent to their rooms, being told off or having privileges suspended. Once we have an inkling of what is important to them, there are a number of things we can do to make their progress concrete:

Either they or we can *fill in a daily chart,* such as the symptoms chart described in Chapter 8. Another possibility is to write a daily log. Children who can't write could try drawing pictures of how they feel instead, dictating to us the explanations.

Repeat at weekly intervals *different "tests"* (such as the ones mentioned starting on page 36 in Chapter 2) and record the results.

Use *weekly progress reports,* either given by us or another adult who is in close touch with our children, or both.

Any of these methods will provide a record for children to refer back to when they feel they aren't getting anywhere. This is very important as it is hard for many children to remember how they were feeling an hour ago, let alone a week or month ago.

• USE A FULL RANGE OF MOTIVATING TECHNIQUES. Besides the wish to achieve full health, there are other ways of increasing children's motivation to cooperate with the program. Some of these include:

• *Using positive reinforcement.* Everyone thrives on praise, and children are bound to try harder with lots of encouragement and praise for cooperating well.

• *Inviting active participation.* Actively involving children in the program gives them a stake in its success. There is a range of possible program-related activities that can be chosen according to a child's age, health, interest, aptitude and willingness. Some children will be able to help cook, plan menus and work out a food schedule. Others are responsible enough to take their own vitamins.

In the morning I set out three bottles. With the vitamin C she takes one an hour until they're gone plus what's in these three bottles. She keeps track—she knows when she's supposed to take them—she takes them. I do not have to oversee—it's no big deal. —Michelle's mother

Part of involvement is allowing children as much control over their lives as is feasible, which for some children is extremely important. This means, for example, not making them eat foods they don't like.

Children who are active participants in the program will work hard for its success, since they won't want to undermine their own efforts.

Attempting bribery. As a last resort, if children don't seem interested in following the treatment program for its own sake, it is sometimes possible to spark their enthusiasm with a material goal to work for, such as money, toys, trips, clothing, records or whatever they would enjoy most that is within our capabilities. Short-term goals will probably work best, for example something specific to look forward to at the end of each week in exchange for following the agreed terms. (It is best to be very specific about these terms: for example, missing their vitamins no more than once in the week, having to be reminded to exercise only twice, or permission required for any diet infractions. Having an irrefutable method of keeping track of adherence to the terms is also a good idea.)

STRESS THE POSITIVE

Although it is important to allow children the freedom to express their frustrations with the treatment program and to show them we understand, it is also important to encourage as positive an attitude as possible.

My child is different from other children because of his diet and hypoglycemia problem, but we believe and try to help him feel that he is different but not less than other children. Our entire family is on the diet and we have

positive self-images and we try to help build positive self-images for both our children. We try to help them see the world as a positive challenge and help them achieve their fullest potential. We see their special diet as one of the aids to them in being better equipped to meet the challenges of their world. My son enjoys taking his vitamins and reminds me if I've forgotten one. I've tried to make it fun for him to take them and the entire family takes them and he tells his friends that they will make him big and strong.

—Michael's mother

As far as diet—my family feels special because of it in a positive way—that there is time and care given to eating more nutritiously.

—Shayna's mother

Part of stressing the positive is showing children that the program can be fun. If we and our children exercise our imaginations a bit, we are likely to come up with some interesting ways of making the program an enjoyable experience instead of a boring necessity. For example, Jason might be surprisingly enthusiastic about experimenting with new recipes, or perhaps he would prefer to make a collage of all the foods he is allowed to eat. Neila might enjoy reading a history of how the different vitamins were discovered. Or the whole family might enjoy making up a game or a crossword puzzle about chemical sensitivities. The possibilities are endless.

Sometimes it is the inessentials (at least from a parent's point of view) that can make the difference—a special container for the vitamins, a new skipping rope to replace the old for exercising with—anything to spark their interest and enthusiasm. Make believe, humor and novelty are often good techniques to use.

Initially she turned up her nose saying, "I hate broccoli" but when I said it was Green Dream Soup because all the vegetables were green it was gone in no time, and she has since asked me when we are having Green Dream Soup again. Another success was Rainbow Delight, with a variety of brightly colored vegetables which she had a good time trying to identify. Making designs out of food, like a mushed up sweet potato face with cashew eyes and mouth has also been successful.

Jen seems to be quite hypoglycemic, but when her blood sugar gets low she also gets particularly unreasonable and often refuses to eat, so we are always developing techniques to avoid out-and-out conflict. The best method we have found is a game Brad made up one day which he calls Mean Pirate, where Jen is the mean pirate who eats up all Brad's food when he isn't looking. Playing restaurant, with me as the waitress, also works. —Jen's mother

Stressing the positive also includes exposing children to films, radio and television programs, books and magazines, meetings and so on which reinforce healthy attitudes.

ENCOURAGE CRITICAL THINKING AND SELF-EDUCATION

Helping children to inform themselves about health-related issues and to learn how to think critically is extremely important. If they have been encouraged to be well-informed and not to accept everything they are told, but to ask searching questions (even when this is uncomfortable for us), they will be better prepared to make wise decisions about their own lives and health. Toward this end, we should try to help them gain an understanding of the political, cultural and commercial factors that affect health, nutrition and environment in modern society. (For more information on this, see the section starting on page 282 in Chapter 19.)

In his *Children's Nutrition,* Lewis A. Coffin has some advice on encouraging critical thinking and on teaching children about the nature of healthful food. "One tactic is to draw your child's attention to the attractiveness of fresh fruits and vegetables displayed in markets, noting, however, where a producer may have used deceptive methods to enhance appearance of produce by, for instance, exposing green tomatoes to a gas to make them red and ripe-looking, or applying green dye to shelled black-eyed peas so they will look fresh and green. Show them what real ripe tomatoes and natural black-eyed peas look, feel and taste like. . . . Read labels on packaged foods to your child so that he will come to recognize the fact that frozen vegetables have chemicals added to prolong shelf life, and that his favorite cereal has artificial coloring added so that his eyes will like it."

Coffin also suggests growing our own fruits and vegetables, even if on a small scale, "so your family can taste the real thing."

Special emphasis must be given to making children aware of the manipulativeness of advertisements, as many ads are aimed directly at children. Concerning advertising, Dr. Coffin writes:

"The advertising agencies use every ploy known to create demand for products they sell to your children. They have staff psychologists who help decide which approach will be the most effective in molding your child's thoughts. . . .

"When faced with the necessity to sell products meant for child consumers, they aim their guns directly at your child with no regard for any possible consequences to health."

This obliges us, Dr. Coffin maintains, to educate our children to "scoff at these commercials and become critics in their own right." He suggests explaining the economics of advertising to them and reminding them of the difference between the toys advertised before Christmas and the actual toys they received. "Teach them contempt," he concludes, "for those who try to cheat their bodies and health."

Brett Silverstein in his book *Fed Up!* gives more information about advertising:

"How do advertisers attempt to persuade us? One way is through outright deception. They substitute shaving cream for whipped cream in ads to make the topping look thicker, or put molasses in coffee to give it the appearance of more body. . . .

"But deception is just the tip of the iceberg. Sometimes ads can mislead by leaving out information rather than by fabricating directly. One ad states that in a survey, kids with a preference picked Peter Pan peanut butter over Jif or Skippy. The ad doesn't say how many kids had a preference. So, as a hypothetical example, out of 100 kids surveyed, fifty-five may have had no preference, eighteen may have preferred Peter Pan, sixteen may have preferred Jif, and eleven may have preferred Skippy. Big deal!"

Silverstein suggests that deception by omission or commission isn't the worst aspect of advertising—that the "bizarre assumptions and crazy attitudes about food and eating" that underlie the all-pervasive ads can come to be unthinkingly accepted.

Both writers underscore how crucial it is that children be as well equipped as they can be to look critically at all information presented to them.

MAKING IT EASY

One way of increasing cooperation that is both self-evident and easily overlooked is to make it as easy as possible for children to cooperate. Making the program a regular part of daily living in the home and being prepared for difficult situations outside the home will go a long way toward preventing both large and small disasters and will help ensure that children stick to their treatment program. Following are a few suggestions on how to "make it easy":

• REMOVE FORBIDDEN FOODS FROM THE HOUSE. It is much easier to resist eating something if it's not there in the first place. If a forbidden food is essential to another family member, it should be kept well out of sight and eaten only when the child is not there.

• HAVE THE WHOLE FAMILY FOLLOW THE TREATMENT PROGRAM. This is the best kind of support and encouragement we can give children. A child's resistance to diet, exercise or other facet of the program will be considerably diminished if everyone in the family is practicing good health (remembering of course to take individual needs into account).

My second child, a little girl, came with none of the ailments that had plagued Theo. While she may be considered "normal," both children eat exactly the same foods. In fact, the whole family follows the Feingold method of nutrition. None of us feel deprived and we are all the healthier for it. —Theo's mother

We all changed and actually all feel better with the diet. —Vanessa's mother

Amazingly all members of my family, including my husband, enjoy this change of eating habit much more than how we used to eat. Brown rice is now a favorite along with a lot of other new foods. —Shayna's mother

At home everyone takes vitamins—so I feel different if I don't. —Albert

My son was an adult, hard to convince, but when I told him I'd take the megavitamins he said he would. I told him I would only take half a dose as I was only half as sick as he was. —Raymond's mother

• DON'T GIVE CHILDREN TOTAL RESPONSIBILITY FOR THE TREATMENT PROGRAM UNLESS THEY ARE READY FOR IT. The amount of supervision required for diet, nutritional supplement intake and other parts of the treatment program will vary according to each child's age, maturity and motivation. With some children the best policy, at least initially, is for us to take care of as many of the details as possible:

What my mum did, she would set [the vitamins] out for me, all the time, which is a lot easier. All I would have to do is take them. I mean it's only two seconds to get them out, but psychologically it's an hour. "Oh, I got to go to school, it's too late," but if they're right in front of you with a glass of water . . . —Albert

I sat with him at first until he took the vitamins. I still set them out for him every day. —Ricardo's mother

• MAKE THE PROGRAM AS SCHEDULED, ROUTINE AND ACCESSIBLE AS POSSIBLE. For example, children who are in the habit of taking their vitamins at the same times every day, at breakfast and supper for example, are less likely to forget them. Children on rotating diets will have a better idea what they can or can't have on any particular day if the food schedule is posted in a prominent spot and outlined in an easily understood manner. Children who get used to exercising first thing in the morning will soon hop out of bed and begin their exercises without even thinking.

To establish a routine, consistency is extremely important. If we forget to get the vitamins out every other meal, frequently relax the diet or decide we're too tired to exercise, children will get the message that the treatment program is not that important anyway. Rather than making it easier for them to follow the program, we will be making it easier for them *not* to follow it.

• NORMALIZE THEIR DIET AND ACTIVITIES AS MUCH AS POSSIBLE. It is very important to find satisfying alternatives to the foods children are no longer allowed. Children who can't have regular crackers because of a wheat sensitivity can often eat rice crackers instead. Children desperate to have milk with their granola or porridge might accept a substitute milk made from soy beans or nuts. Frozen fruit that is blended is one alternative to ice cream.

This same principle applies to activities. If they are unable to go swimming in the pool any more because of a chlorine sensitivity, it is worthwhile making a special effort to take them to the beach or find someone else who can take them. Or, they might enjoy playing soccer or learning to roller skate instead. In the winter they can diversify into tobogganing, skating and cross-country skiing. Finding a friend willing to share new activities will ease the transition immensely.

• DON'T LET THEM FEEL THEY ARE MISSING OUT ON ANYTHING. For the special treats they used to get, and still see other children getting, consider substituting nonfood items. For example, instead of a basket of chocolate Easter eggs, consider a ceramic or fabric bunny. Better yet, encourage them to decorate their own Easter eggs.

We do give him lots of special things that don't involve candy. We try to make celebrations as pleasant as possible with making things, or often I'll make bread at home and let the kids have some dough to knead and fiddle with and they enjoy that. —Stuart's mother

For special school, club or church outings or activities they cannot take part in because of environmental sensitivities, try to plan alternatives.

• TEACH CHILDREN HOW TO SAY "NO" AND HOW TO WITHSTAND PRESSURE. Either for fear of appearing rude, or for fear of appearing "weird," children may end up eating or being exposed to things that are unhealthy for them. That is why helping children learn how to handle awkward social situations politely and with a strong sense of self is an absolute necessity. This means teaching them how to say "no" gracefully when they are offered something that is not on their diet or are asked to enter into a situation where they would be exposed to environmental substances they are sensitive to. It also means teaching them how to remain firm when faced with skepticism or pressure to conform, for example when taking vitamins.

Saying "no" and remaining firm will usually involve explaining why they have a restricted diet, or take vitamins or must avoid certain chemicals. In most cases a short explanation is all that is necessary, such as, "No, thank you I'm allergic to that," "Apples don't make me feel good," "It's not my wheat day," or "Sorry, I'm super-sensitive to paint fumes." If the person is persistent, they can always invoke parental authority: "No, thank you, my mum and dad don't let me eat that" or even medical authority: "My doctor said that I can't eat sugar or I'll get sick." Of course, politeness may not always work, especially with their peers, and some other methods of refusal may be needed. Whatever it takes, children should learn to be firm, as it is their health that is at stake.

The approach that Albert has worked out for himself may help other children with their explanations:

The only time [taking vitamins] would come up was at camp. Normally I said that I'm a werewolf, especially when my hair started to grow long, or I would say something funny. Then if they said, "No, no, seriously," I would say, "Well, I have a vitamin deficiency." Sometimes I would even tell them what they're for, I'd say vitamin C if I have a cold or something. I would try to make it so they were comfortable because I find a lot of people are uncomfortable when someone is taking pills because they don't know what they are for.

This is what I would tell someone, that the body has certain vitamins it needs to live, and vitamins are stuff that you get from food. Now some people can't get it off the food so you have to take it [in a vitamin pill]; if you don't take it you won't feel well.

When Albert is being harassed by other kids (whether about vitamins or other things) he handles it this way:

Normally there is one person who is doing the most bugging. You have to somehow bug that person and just get the others in the group to like you. What I will do is say something about that person that embarrasses him. They won't bug me again because they know that I'll just embarrass them.

It is also a good idea to help children think of other appropriate techniques for handling uncomfortable situations, such as changing the subject, or simply leaving with a quick exit line.

It is important that children receive from us the message that conformity is not necessarily the best policy, that it is a measure of strength to be different when necessary. Being different sometimes requires a thick skin, one of the benefits of a good self-image.

One exercise that will help both us and our children is to role-play a variety of situations where a "no" and a firm refusal may be required. For example, one of us can be a friendly neighbor handing out candies, the other the child, and then roles can be reversed. Next, one of us might be the child and the other a classmate teasing the child about the funny food in the lunch box.

• TEACH OURSELVES HOW TO SAY NO. If we are expecting our children to learn how to decline generous offers graciously, we can't expect any less of ourselves. This is especially the case with younger children, where a more active role is necessary.

It is sometimes hard to refuse a kind offering for fear of offending someone. Generally, however, polite refusals will not result in hurt feelings as most people are sympathetic to others' situations. No blame can be attached to us in the event of the exceptions who do take it personally, or are so insistent that we have to be less polite than we would have wished. By taking offense they are acting inappropriately, as they are not the ones who are going to suffer.

It is our decision to accept or not. The best way to refuse is an explanation of our children's sensitivities or allergies to sugar/food colorings/chocolate/whatever. Chances are the person has a niece or neighbor who has the same problem and will be very understanding. A common reaction is keen interest of the "Oh, I saw a TV program about that, so sugar really does make them wild does it?" variety.

Sometimes, of course, it may not be necessary to say anything:

A couple of times in stores people say, "Oh, isn't he cute," and they give him a candy. What I'll do is I just grab the candy before Tyler gets his hands on it. And he's still young so that's easy, he doesn't know what he's missing. —Tyler's mother

Again, practicing the role-playing technique with another family member or friend will be helpful.

• TRY TO ENLIST EVERYONE'S COOPERATION. The less often children find themselves in the position of having to choose whether to strictly follow the program or not, the better. To ensure children's cooperation, it is helpful to enlist the cooperation of everyone they regularly come in contact with, including relatives, neighbors, the parents of our children's friends, and babysitters, as well as the staff in school, daycare or other childcare situations. Explaining to everyone which foods are harmful to our children and which environmental substances they should avoid, together with the reasons why, will help prevent many situations where children either end up saying "yes" where it would be better for them to say "no," or are presented with no choice at all.

If we give our explanations straightforwardly without being defensive, people are much more likely to respond positively. This is especially so when explanations are made in familiar terms. For example, Pierre's mother explains Pierre's problems as "a biochemical disease that affects the brain as diabetes affects the pancreas." Most people will respect our wishes to avoid exposing children to problem-causing foods or environmental substances, and will either be supportive of our efforts to keep our children as healthy as possible in the way we have decided is best, regardless of what they really think, or at the very least will not interfere.

The people across the street one day were giving the kids these disgusting cookies and they said, "Oh, can Tyler have one?" and I said, "No, he has allergies," but either they didn't know what the word meant or they had no conception so they thought I was really mean and they kept saying, "Oh, just one," but I was very firm, and they just wouldn't do something that I didn't want. —Tyler's mother

Our best bet when starting out is to expect only minimal resistance, if any, of the sort that can easily be solved.

We have been extremely lucky with his teachers, doctors and the majority of the family. Some felt we were being mean by denying him chocolate bars, etc. But once they saw Nick had made that decision for himself, they accepted it. —Nick's mother

It is not unusual to find some people supportive that we thought would be disapproving.

There are people who will never understand nutrition, but we have found them to be rare. When I returned to university and needed a baby-sitter, I was concerned about the foods my children would be given. To my surprise, only one, out of a dozen women I interviewed, showed any resistance to the idea. The others found the Feingold theory rather appealing, and actually began feeding their own children, whether or not they were hyperactive, in a healthier way. —Theo's mother

In enlisting everyone's cooperation, the discussion may include not only a description of the treatment program but an explanation of why our children need it. Whether we attribute the problem to categories like allergies, vitamin dependencies, hypoglycemia, or heavy metal toxicity, or use more traditional labels like schizophrenic, autistic, hyperactive or depressive depends to a large degree on our own individual circumstances, what we are most comfortable with, and our own judgment of the likely effect. There is no right or wrong way and reactions will almost certainly vary.

It's like having leprosy; you can't say to someone in a small town, "My son has schizophrenia." In the first place you're ruining his future because they'll always label him. Because it isn't twenty years from now, it's now. Maybe thirty years from now it will be different. So you have to more or less keep it a secret. To this day we never mention anything but hypoglycemia. People understand low blood sugar but they don't understand the other. You have to do that to protect him . . . —Jon's mother

Friends are very cooperative. Everybody knows somebody who has schizophrenia. —Lyle's mother

As the summer progressed I felt myself growing better and healthier every day. I had even spent an enjoyable evening with my friend Mary. She had changed back into her old self again. It wasn't until I saw her that I realized she had never changed. I had. We talked over dinner and finally I told her I was schizophrenic and was recovering. There were a few moments of startled silence before she spoke incredulously. "I've never had a schizophrenic friend before. What do I say? Congratulations!?" We all laughed. It was such a genuinely warm reaction. It had surprised her for a second but she had overcome it beautifully. It was a relief to see my good friend take the news the way I had hoped she would. Others had reacted as though I had some fatal and contagious disease. Not so Mary. Indeed, not so with any of my close friends. I was a recovered schizophrenic, but to them I was myself again, no more, no less. —Suzanne Foster in *Stoney Lonesome Road*

Once the explanations are done, all that is left are the mechanics. In some cases, when children go visiting it is best to send their snacks along with them. As far as school cafeterias go, some have fairly wide choice; all we have to do then is educate children to choose wisely. When there is no choice, we will have to consider trying to educate the school board, day care staff or nursery school teacher. There will very likely be support from at least a few other parents who are also concerned about their children's health. What many parents do is either prepare lunches and snacks daily, or store a selection in the day-care or school fridge or freezer, making sure the workers are aware of the availability of the substitute food. For example, a bag of wheatless, milk-free cookies does not take up much room and will be welcomed on party days.

• PREPARE FOR SPECIAL EVENTS. Taken all together, special occasions like Hallowe'en, birthday parties, other celebrations such as Christmas, and eating out with friends and at restaurants happen fairly frequently. With a little forethought, ingenuity and preparation we can prevent them from being total disasters.

Before anything else we must decide how rigid about the program we and our children need to be. If children's food sensitivities are under good control and they can tolerate occasionally breaking their diet without the results being too horrendous, we might want to relax a bit for special occasions.

But if eating the forbidden fruit (whether literal or metaphorical) is going to mean a three-hour-long temper tantrum for us to deal with, it is worth it to everyone involved to be inflexible.

We have learned that when we go off the diet it takes about a week to get her settled down again.   —Nadya's mother

Even if the occasional nibble is not a problem, there are a few other variables to consider such as whether the program has just been implemented or is already well established; if a child is old enough to understand why sometimes an exception can be made and other times not; how frequently exceptions might occur; if an occasional exception will be an excuse for constant battles.

Most people will understand if we or our children decline a food item on the basis of health; only we and our children can judge which is the best approach.

Following is a discussion of some of the special events we will have to be prepared for:

Eating out at friends'. It is probably wise whenever children are invited out to eat, whether alone or with us, to briefly mention again our children's food sensitivities at the time the invitation is extended. Most people will be very sympathetic and not mind avoiding the problem foods. Unfortunately, this will not always prevent the occasional surprise. Even people who are warned about a child's sensitivity to milk products, for example, may still serve a meal fried in butter, because they have forgotten, don't connect butter with milk products, or thought only a little bit wouldn't hurt. Two other possible scenarios are that the list of ingredients on the soup can mentioning milk powder will be overlooked, or that a dessert such as ice cream will be served because it is assumed our children must be used to being odd ones out by now.

Most family and friends are highly supportive but don't realize the full impact of labels, etc. . . . —Nadya's mother

What we have to do is outguess our hosts and be as specific as possible, without being too overwhelming, and then hope for the best. "Have I mentioned before that Donnie is allergic to butter, cheese, yogurt, in fact all the milk products?"

Just in case, we should be prepared with some tactful refusals of dishes on our children's behalf, and discuss thoroughly with our children the problems involved.

Eating out at restaurants. First of all the restaurant should be chosen carefully, to ensure there will be food available that our children can safely eat. Read the menu carefully for the tiny print ("with tomato sauce"), and when in doubt ask the waiter or waitress. In any case it is best to specify the foods that are important to avoid, as not all ingredients are mentioned on the menu. Most places are flexible and will omit ingredients such as tomatoes and MSG if asked. However we will never have the same control over restaurant food as we do with home-cooked meals, and there will inevitably be times when we end up either scraping the offending food off or sending the food back and having to wait for a new order. Unfortunately it is not always immediately obvious that an order was mixed up or that we were given incorrect information about the ingredients of a dish; if children are extremely sensitive to even small quantities of certain foods or additives, the safest, easiest, cheapest and healthiest solution is to eat at home.

Birthday parties and other celebrations. It is easy enough to control the food when we are the hosts, as long as we don't let ourselves be trapped by assumptions about what we think children find acceptable. Unbelievable as it may seem, there are children who don't even like sweet stuff till they are older, and will leave most of the cake and ice cream in a gooey mess on their plates. Even if we decide to follow convention and have some goo, we can make sure there are other choices available.

It is a different situation when the party is at someone else's place. Powers and Presley in their book *Food Power* suggest talking to the parent holding the party about making available alternatives that are well tolerated by our children, and hope that our children will cooperate by eating them rather than the other goodies.

Or we can send alternative treats along with our children.

We had phoned and found out that a sour cream vegetable dip would be served at the party so we made Jen a guacamole dip to take with her because of her milk allergy. When she came back she said everyone had wanted her dip!   —Jen's mother

If children do not react too wildly to an occasional exposure to foods they are sensitive to, and if they are capable of restraint, we can try trusting them to restrict themselves to only small amounts of the food served.

Hallowe'en. This is much easier to handle when children are younger. A group of parents can prearrange to give each other's children only healthy treats that the children involved are not sensitive to. Besides safe foods, this could also include items such as balloons, stickers and erasers. We then take our children trick-or-treating to only those places. Hallowe'en parties with only the appropriate foods made available can also be fun. If we are lucky, children will be open to persuasion and will voluntarily eat only the treats that don't bother them.

Trading is another possibility—the Hallowe'en loot in return for something extra special like a trip out of town or a movie. Some parents buy their children's loot from them, and the children in turn buy something that is safe for them.

If children can tolerate junk in small doses, consider rationing. Either let them choose a small number of items from their loot bag and throw the rest away, or let them save it and have a bit once a month or whatever. Letting them eat a bit each day is not a good idea as the junk will be constantly in their systems; it is preferable to let them eat the stuff all at once, let them suffer the bad effects and then no more until next Hallowe'en.

Some children like collecting for UNICEF instead of gathering candies. This way they can still participate by dressing up and trick-or-treating, avoid the junk food problem, and also have the satisfaction of helping children in other countries.

• ENCOURAGE CONTACT WITH OTHER CHILDREN AND FAMILIES WHO ARE FOLLOWING THE TREATMENT PROGRAM. This will provide support and help strengthen our commitment and our children's commitment to better health.

There are many groups listed in Chapter 3 that will give us support and get us in touch with others in similar situations.

NONCOOPERATING CHILDREN

Sometimes, no matter how much effort we have put into gaining the cooperation of our children, we are faced with resistance. We have followed all the suggestions outlined above and still children refuse to follow their diets, or take their vitamins, or avoid the environmental substances they are sensitive to, or exercise. What do we do then?

The first step is to figure out why children are resisting the treatment program. It is important not to make the automatic assumption that they are resisting merely to bother us, but to try to see the situation from their perspectives, as outlined in Chapter 2. Following is a summary of possible reasons for a child's noncooperation:

• THE PRESSURE TO BE "NORMAL." In relation to the treatment program, it can be difficult when children are older and subject to many pressures beyond our control. Societal and peer pressure can be very intense, and it is not surprising that many children are not thrilled about the treatment program when it is sometimes so contrary to prevailing attitudes.

The diet was hard—friends laughed, relatives got mad when I refused to eat desserts fixed especially for me. —Andrea

She just fell apart coming back from playschool and I asked her what she had for a snack and that's when they'd had that pink Care Bears cake . . . they didn't get very good snacks there. I thought, hey, [why not] just inject food coloring right into their veins. —Terry's mother

I think the worst thing is that our environment is so surrounded with children gobbling candy all the time and having all these things that it's too much of a temptation for him never to have any. So we do give him junk days occasionally. But even still, he does get candy and things like that from the children at school and sometimes he'll be in and out of his chair twenty or thirty times during supper. And we'll say, "Now really, what did you have to eat at school today?" Invariably, he will finally admit, "Well, some kid gave me candy." Now often when he comes home he'll say, "Mom, you help control me; so-and-so gave me some candy and you keep reminding me, will you?" It's very hard to control these impulses.

A child comes over and says, "Well, why don't you have Bugles?" Or "I want some popsicles." We have popsicles, but not the kind that are supposedly good, that are just sugar-water and color and flavor. So it's socially very difficult for the child. It's a constant sore point for him. Not only do you

*have those things but when you add milk to the problem it's never ending.
It's always a problem. Everywhere you see the candy canes out, and stuff
like this, in church, school, everywhere you go. It's very difficult to say no
all the time, so we'll say, "Stuart, we'll let you decide." Of course a child
that age, he says, "I can't resist that, I want that, everybody else is having
it."*   —Stuart's mother

In the view of society at large, nutritional supplements are unnecessary and a waste of money, exercise is boring and too much work,
pollution is a small price to pay for "progress" and processed food is
preferable to food that is whole and unadulterated. These attitudes
are reinforced by which foods are most readily available and most
prominently displayed in the stores, what children are taught in
school, messages received from the media, what we are told by
government and industry.

It is hard for children to escape the message that to be happy,
popular, beautiful and successful they have to eat, act and live like
everyone else. Although intellectually they may realize this is not a
true picture, emotional acceptance is quite different. The consequences of a nutritional/environmental program are, unsurprisingly,
occasional resentment, envy and self-pity.

One way of dealing with children's feelings of being left out of the
mainstream and treated unfairly by life is to point out that everyone
is different in one way or another and that they are not unique in
suffering from one or more problems.

*We say, "Look, each of us has our problems." His little friend, who's his
best friend, is an asthmatic child. He said, "Juan can eat anything." And I
said, "Believe me, if you ever had an asthma attack, you wouldn't trade
your problem for his any day." He's heard Juan talk—he knows that he's a
sick child often and he can't do a lot of the things that Stuart does.*

*We've approached it mainly from the point of view that we all have
problems, that there are many other children out there who have terrible
problems, and sometimes don't even know what's the matter. Also, he
should try to be as understanding about his own problems as he is about
Dana's or about his Mom's. So we just approach it from the point of view
that we're all human and we all have problems, and he's just having to learn
a little bit earlier how to cope with these things.*   —Stuart's mother

On the subject of being "different," as some parents have pointed
out, our children are different with or without the diet, with or
without the vitamins. Most children are sensible enough to recognize
that they have the choice to be different because they don't drink
milk, or to be different because they don't have a clue what's going

on half the time, can't sit still for more than ten seconds or are frightened of everything around them.

What I've found with Jen is that when she's on her diet and feeling well she interacts socially a lot better with other kids than when she doesn't [follow her diet]. It's kind of another price to pay, let her feel the same as the other kids, but she won't get along with them, there's a choice there.

—Jen's mother

Some of the peer pressures children will face can be alleviated by:

• *Encouraging friendships* with other children who have dietary or environmental restrictions or must take nutritional supplements.

• Helping children *build their self-esteem* so that what others think is not so important to them.

• Helping them *develop appropriate responses* to teasing.

• Helping them *keep a low profile* on their deviations from the norm.

• THEY MAY LITERALLY BE ADDICTED TO THE FOODS THEY ARE SENSITIVE TO.

I was positively addicted to sugary things, especially sugar-covered donuts and arrowroot cookies. My yearning for them was so powerful that it was nothing for me to consume forty or fifty arrowroots and twelve donuts in one day. I also ate massive amounts of fruit. I'd eat at the very least fifteen mandarin oranges a day during the mandarin season and anywhere from six to fifteen Granny Smith apples a day when they were in season. These were all in addition to my many chocolate bar sprees and my nightly bowl of ice cream. I was in love with sweet things. When I ate them my spirits would soar high and I would feel wonderfully light-headed for a while. But I always got tired and felt very heavy afterwards and the only way to combat the feeling was to eat more cookies or to sleep. When I couldn't eat I generally slept. It was such a frequent occurrence that it soon became a joke among the more lenient teachers.

—Suzanne Foster in *Stoney Lonesome Road*

If children suffering from addictions, particularly caffeine addictions, are having trouble stopping "cold turkey," tapering off their intake gradually is one possibility. Others include keeping them extra busy so they won't have as much time to think about their cravings, and giving them extra incentives such as special presents or increases in their allowances.

• IT MIGHT BE THAT "NEVER" SEEMS TOO LONG. In some cases being a bit more flexible with the diet will mean a better over all adherence to it, whereas in other cases it will mean virtually the end of the diet. One judgment to make is whether the occasional small bite will prevent the regular binge, or will one bite immediately lead to another? We also have to know whether children can tolerate small amounts of the offending foods, or is even a small amount too much. Parents have come up with a variety of solutions, such as once-a-month junk days. Some other ideas follow:

One mother said to me, "I put out all their safe snacks on Monday and tell them that has to last till next Monday. By the second week it is amazing, their whole body feels much better, they don't need that treat." Richard is like that, you know, he can have an apple and then he won't have another one.   —Richard's mother

Usually, if she is allowed one small bite this will satisfy her desire.   —Nadya's mother

When there were situations where it was going to be really stressful for her not to have it, I let her have it. Sometimes she would choose not to have it, she would pick something else. But if she was feeling antsy and cranky and that sort of thing and I could see that it was really going to be a heartbreak for her to watch everybody else have red popsicles and she wasn't going to have one, I'd let her have it, because if I know she's had it, I could be a little bit more patient with her, and we could get through the aftereffects reasonably well and she didn't feel so different from the other kids. I made it pretty clear to her that it was because I was just making an exception and it wasn't that she was going to be allowed to have it all the time, it was for special, it was a treat. She seemed to click to that and she could tell the difference between times when there were twelve kids and they were all having it, like Hallowe'en or a birthday party or whatever, and the rest of the time she just stayed off it as much as she could.   —Terry's mother

When children are on the road to getting better but still creating a fuss about the foods they are missing, letting them stuff themselves full of junk once is sometimes an effective lesson. They often feel so wretched after this that it is a long time before they can even think about repeating the experience:

Last year we let him go Hallowe'en "trick-or-treating." After being miserable and crying, etc. he brought his bag to me three days later and said, "Burn this!"   —Ricardo's mother

He was quite young when he gave up Hallowe'ening and he did because he knew he would just feel lousy after it. We developed a system early on where the kids would go out for Hallowe'en treats and I would buy them all back. They could take a few, because I find it very difficult to be so strict in

this society, but Albert found he could tolerate hardly any of it. I think he was in Grade 5 when he said, "I'm not going to go, what's the point, I don't feel well when I'm finished anyway." —Albert's mother

What works best will vary from child to child, and also depends on what feels best for us. In some situations, calm reasoning may work. In other cases something different might be called for:

Here was a thirteen-year-old boy who spent a lot of time just lying on his bed feeling miserable. It was really frightening and we were starting to have a lot of problems, the two of us fighting and not getting along; no matter what I said it was wrong. One day I found a candy wrapper on his desk and I confronted him with it; there happened to be a drugstore in the vicinity of the school and the kids used to hang out there, and I just simply stated without any great communication skills, that was it; as long as he stayed on his sugar, that he was not to come near me. When we would fight it was sort of like an attention-getter, he needed me to get angry at to feel better, and I said, "That's it, I am not going to do that any more, unless you get off your sugar don't even talk to me." —Albert's mother

• THE PILLS ARE HARD TO SWALLOW. Cutting them in half or crushing them might help. Or buy the equivalent in powdered or liquid form, or in capsules that can be opened up.

• THE TASTE OF THE SUPPLEMENTS IS TERRIBLE. Try mixing them with juice or other food (remembering that some vitamins might be destroyed by heat). If nothing works and children are young, one last alternative that might be considered is to plug their noses and squirt a supplement-juice mixture into their open mouths with a baby medicine squirter from the drugstore.

• SOME OF THE NUTRITIONAL SUPPLEMENTS ARE GIVING THEM UNCOMFORTABLE SIDE EFFECTS.

When I first started taking my megadoses of vitamins, I felt intense discomfort . . . a real high that was uncomfortable. It was almost enough to stop taking them, but I persevered because certain symptoms cleared within the week. I was also desperate for relief from headaches and this lessened dramatically after one week. I had had a very allergic reaction to large doses of sustained-release niacin and felt apprehensive about that happening again. Most helpful was that Dr. D. told me that I would experience discomfort when starting this treatment. —Marilyn

Marilyn's experience illustrates the importance of making sure children know what to expect from the treatment program. Any side

effects from nutritional supplements should of course be checked out
with a doctor. If a supplement is causing side effects, generally an
acceptable alternative can be found.

• THEY HAVE READ AN ARTICLE OR SEEN A TELEVISION PROGRAM WHERE
A NUTRITIONIST OR DOCTOR SAID NO ONE NEEDS EXTRA VITAMINS OR
MINERALS AND THAT ANYONE WHO PRESCRIBES THEM IS A QUACK. The
controversy surrounding the nutritional program has caused at least
one child to abandon the treatment program:

*A four-day rotation diet, vaccine and vitamins were prescribed. Roger had
never been so well as on this routine, which he carried out for almost a year.
I could not get local medical support for this program. My son was aware of
the controversy concerning this approach and as a rebellious teenager, rejected
the whole thing.*   —Roger's mother

In a situation like this, it is extremely important to encourage
children to read the alternative literature. Sometimes the best approach is to line up a few non-family members who agree with our
chosen approach to talk to our children. (Unfortunately, sometimes
the people closest to us will readily believe others before they will
believe us.) Building up an alternative community of people supportive to a nutritional/environmental approach is especially important in
a situation like this. (See chapter 3 for information on getting in
touch with like-minded people.)

• THEY MAY NOT WANT TO GET WELL. Again there are a variety of
possible reasons for this. Children who have been sick for a long
time are sometimes afraid of getting better; they have learned to cope
in some fashion with their problems, and the thought of having to
learn how to deal with a whole new world can be scary. Or, perhaps
they don't want to let go of some of the positive aspects that being
sick has brought them, such as extra attention or extra leniency.
Others are afraid too much will be expected of them when they are
better and they won't be able to deliver. Some like the power they
have to create chaos and get everyone spinning in circles. Occasionally, life has been made too safe and comfortable for them. There are
other reasons for a reluctance to get well, as Suzanne Foster is told
by her mother (quoted in *Stoney Lonesome Road*):

*That's one reason we had such a terrible time getting you on the vitamins
because you were terrified that you'd lose your ability to create the images you
were able to create in your poetry.*

In these situations, it will sometimes be helpful to discuss their fears with them and reassure them, remembering to point out the many new benefits being well will bring.

Sometimes it is not a matter of not wanting to get well, but a matter of not caring or of thinking they won't get well no matter what, so why bother? If they are very depressed, they may have an apathetic attitude toward the whole program, thinking it is all pointless. In this case, we should be as positive and encouraging as we can. Another possibility is that their expectations have not been realized. If they expected a miraculous cure in three days, and three weeks later don't feel any better, they may decide that the program is not worth the effort. It is important to discuss with them what can be reasonably expected from the program and in what kind of time frame.

• THEY MAY FIND THE CHANGES THE TREATMENT PROGRAM BRINGS FRIGHTENING. For example, if they are used to seeing everything in shades of gray and all of a sudden the world is full of bright colors, they may feel threatened or unable to cope with the visual flood of new sensory experiences.

We will have to try to be aware of what is happening and explain what they are experiencing in a reassuring way. Again, children who have been told in advance what might happen are less likely to be put off by such an experience.

• THEY DISLIKE THEIR DOCTOR. In this case, refusing the treatment might be a way of rejecting the doctor. Switching to a doctor who can establish a better rapport with them may help.

• THEY FEEL PRESSURED. Older children in particular will sometimes be resentful if they feel we have given them no choice and are "treating them like children." Organizing everything so they can follow the treatment program if they want to without our intervention and temporarily avoiding any mention of the topic, responding in a brief matter-of-fact manner if they themselves bring it up, is worth a try. Giving them as much choice as possible will also help.

• THEY ARE USING THEIR NONCOOPERATION AS A WEAPON. If we and our children have unresolved conflicts in other areas of our lives, they may choose non-cooperation with the treatment program (because it is important to us) as an effective method of expressing their anger and resentment. This is not always done on a conscious level; sometimes just the awareness (on all our parts) that this is what is happening may ease the situation. The next step is to attempt to resolve the conflicts. In many cases this is easier said than done, but even our acknowledgement that there may be valid grounds for dissatisfaction, and the fact that we are willing to work things out might result in more cooperative children.

• THEY ARE PARANOID. This is probably the hardest situation to deal with. Some children are extremely suspicious and fear that the supplements might harm them, or that the treatment program is part of an attempt to control them, refusing to believe any assurances to the contrary. Being sympathetic and working with their logic as much as possible (no matter how illogical it seems to us) is one approach to try. For example, if they are afraid that someone is poisoning their vitamin pills, we could store the vitamins in a cupboard or drawer with a lock on it, and let them keep the key (as long as we are sure they won't take an excessive amount of pills when we aren't looking). Or, if they decide the food we are giving them is part of a plan to make them weak, taking them shopping with us and letting them decide which of the allowed food in the store is safe may make them feel more secure.

Other children refuse to admit there is anything wrong with them, feeling that anyone who says there is, is out to get them. In this case, an indirect approach might work. One possibility is to say that the treatment program is for the whole family's benefit, explaining that the supplements and diet will help all of us achieve optimum health. Very often children like this feel it is them against the world, and will quite readily agree that they are under stress; mentioning the treatment program as a method of lessening stress will sometimes be at least temporarily acceptable to them. Using words like hypoglycemia and allergies to describe their problems will generally provoke a much less negative reaction than calling them schizophrenic.

As a last resort, we can always try disguising the supplements by mixing them in with food or drink (making sure to put those vitamins destroyed by heat only into cool foods), with the hope that this will get them well enough to make it possible to use a more direct method of treatment.

Whatever a child's reasons for refusing to take vitamins and minerals, persistence on our part may eventually do the trick. Following is Suzanne Foster's reaction to her mother's attempts to get her to take nutritional supplements:

The visit [to a doctor] didn't impress me much since I don't really remember its outcome. However, it was after this visit that the vitamins began to appear. Mother would put them in an egg cup by my place and suggest I take them. The effects of the Moditen had worn off and with them had gone my reasonable attitude. I was back in the fog. The vitamins were a menace to me. I despised them. They were just a lot of pills. Someone claimed they'd help me get better but I laughed and made fun of them. No damn little pills would make me feel better.

As the weeks passed the vitamins became more and more prolific. They were everywhere. They appeared at all my meals, found their way into the bathroom, were left lying on my bed, or on the stairs where I'd see them. Everywhere I went I tripped over an egg cup full of vitamins. They were strategically placed in all my favorite resting places. I couldn't get away from them. I hated them. They could not help me. I knew that. They were a fool's medicine. A sissy's medicine. I would have none of it. However their continuous presence grew on me and eventually I accepted them as having to be there and even took some now and then. When mother chanced upon an empty egg cup she'd check to see if I'd thrown them out. But I'd stopped doing that. The vitamins were getting to me. Their presence was so irksome that I began to take them regularly just to get them out of my sight. It worked. The egg cups stopped appearing, except at meal time and though I still hated them (I'd lost somehow) I managed to swallow and ignore them. Strangely, I began to feel better. My nightmares weren't as horrible, my voices not as menacing, my memory not as bad, and my mind somewhat clearer.

IF ALL ELSE FAILS

If we have tried all the methods we can think of to get our children to cooperate with the treatment program and they remain intransigent, we have four alternatives:

• COMPROMISE. We can always try negotiating with our children to see if they will accept at least part of the treatment program. For example, they might agree to give up caffeine-containing foods and drinks such as cokes, coffee, tea and chocolates, but continue to eat food with sugar. Or they may agree to follow the diet but not take the supplements, or vice versa. They might willingly exercise, but refuse to give up working with model airplane glue. They might give their agreement to a sort-term trial period of the treatment program. While these compromises will make for a less than ideal situation, and we should not expect a great deal of improvement when only half-measures are being taken, these will occasionally help in some cases, and at the very least it is a start.

• TAKE A BREAK. If our children's problems are not too severe, we can always try waiting them out. When they are a bit older or a bit more mature, their attitudes may change.

• FIND A SYMPATHETIC RELATIVE. Particularly if our relationships with our children have deteriorated badly, and if they agree, letting them live for a period of time with a trusted relative or friend may help. In a different situation with different patterns of interaction, some children will be more cooperative.

• FIND A TREATMENT FACILITY. If children have severe problems and refuse to cooperate, an in-patient treatment facility that uses a nutritional/environmental approach is sometimes the best place for them. In an article in the Summer 1987 issue of *Health and Nutrition Update* (Vol. 2 Issue 3, published by the Canadian Schizophrenia Foundation), Dr. Carl C. Pfeiffer mentions that alternatives to hospitalization might include a half-way house (a homelike facility less restrictive than a hospital or other inpatient treatment center, with live-in trained staff who oversee the treatment program and provide care and guidance), or a professional such as a nurse who will either oversee the program in our home or take our children into his or her home.

There are not always easy solutions to the problem of uncooperative children; to a large extent we have to play it by ear and hope for the best. Some of the information in the following chapter on Resistance, although geared more for dealing with resistant adults, will also be useful to apply to resisting children. The section on conflict resolution in particular might be helpful.

Books mentioned in this chapter and further reading:

The Berenstain Bears and Too Much Junk Food, Stan and Jan Berenstain. Random House, New York, 1985. A book emphasizing good nutrition in an entertaining way that some young children might enjoy.

Children's Nutrition, Lewis A. Coffin. Capra Press, Santa Barbara, California, 1984. For a description, see Chapter 10.

Fed Up! Brett Silverstein. South End Press, Boston, 1984. For a description, see Chapter 10.

Food Power, Hugh Powers and James Presley. St. Martin's Press, New York, 1979. For a description, see Chapter 12.

How to Improve Your Child's Behavior Through Diet, Laura J. Stevens and Rosemary B. Stoner. Doubleday, New York, 1979. For a description, see Chapter 14.

7

RESISTANCE

My father [child's grandfather] is the worst to deal with now—slips him gum and apples, then when he's miserable and destructive, I get the blame ("because the child seemed fine till you walked in the door!"). I don't know how to handle this—I just get angry and tell him off. That doesn't do much good.

—Gordon's mother

[My husband Ned] has read everything and he's taken all these psychology classes and he's got a very open mind and all those things, but when it's convenient he can revert right back to "That's all junk anyway, that's silly," you know? He's very suspicious of any kind of really radical attitude and so if it smacks of radicalism he's going to resist it. Ned was very resistant to [a nutritional approach], but finally he said, "I have to agree with you." But he has not taken any initiatives since that time. Once I slacked off he slacked off. One of his failings I suppose is that he tends to follow my lead, he never asked me about it or anything, he just followed my lead. . . .

—Terry's mother

Suddenly, when I'm really getting onto getting this child well, [the school staff] resented it, they were furious, they told me there wasn't anything in the world wrong with Michelle except that I felt guilty that she had problems . . . they retaliated by canceling her out of the annual all-school play and literally broke her heart. If I'm going to be so brazen as to try and get my child well and give her megavitamins, they're going to take her out of everything worthwhile. She was the only one not allowed to be in the school play. . . . They think that treating the allergies and the megavitamins are so much hogwash. Their cafeteria turns out cookies, their behavior mod program is all backed up with candy bars, their food is atrocious—much, much sugar, all refined flours, artificial flavors, artificial colors. . . . They would talk to her and say things like "This is all your mother's fault."

—Michelle's mother

When we are exhausted from the full-time jobs of trying to get our children healthy, looking after the house and worrying about bills, what we need most is a helpful community of friends, family, neighbors, teachers, doctors and others who are supportive of our efforts with the nutritional/environmental approach. What we don't need are people who are negative to the treatment program, at the best draining our energy and at the worst creating unnecessary difficulties.

Unfortunately, some of us will occasionally find ourselves in situations where instead of receiving positive support and cooperation we are met with resistance, sometimes to the actual detriment of our children. For example, the resisters in question may give our children food that is not on their diets, expose them to environmental substances they are sensitive to—such as cigarette smoke—deny us any words of encouragement, continually criticize the nutritional/environmental approach to our children, and abdicate their share of the responsibility for the treatment program. However, as frustrating and disheartening as situations like these can be, there are ways of dealing with resistance.

Following is a discussion of some of the non-supportive people and situations we may come up against, and the sections after this give a general summary of possible actions we can take to minimize resistance.

Doctors

The doctors were certainly not helpful at all and said this was nonsense. It was, as my husband called it, pure stubbornness and curiosity on my part that kept me at it, that kept me going with it. And also desperation . . .
                                                                      —Stuart's mother

We might find it easier dealing with resisting doctors if we understand some of the factors involved in creating their negativity toward a nutritional/environmental approach, such as:

• THE EXPERT/LAYPERSON DICHOTOMY. Many doctors feel that thanks to their hard years of training and experience they have accumulated a wealth of knowledge and expertise, and therefore are in a position to know more and better than we about our children's health problems.

There is of course some truth to this position; but it cannot be denied that as parents we also have a wealth of knowledge and expertise. Doctors have general knowledge, but we have specific knowledge. Luckily, a growing number of doctors are accepting that parents should have the right to question them and have input into the process of getting children well.

• EGO. It may be hard for some doctors to admit they could have done better with the thousands of patients they have previously treated.

• SKEPTICISM. Caution is an important quality in a doctor, and most doctors are legitimately skeptical of treatment methods they don't know much about. There are vast amounts of new information coming out in the medical field all the time, and it is not possible to check out every new method. However, it wouldn't hurt to point out to our doctors that the nutritional/environmental approach is hardly a new method, and although there is opposition to it there is also a large body of evidence indicating its safety and effectiveness. This is of course in contrast to the poor success rates of conventional treatments (psychological and/or drug-oriented in nature) and the dangerous side effects of many drugs that are often given to children with behavioral problems. Both conventional and nutritional/environmental treatments should be fairly and critically evaluated on the basis of actual results.

• TRAINING. The links between health, nutrition and the environment are not emphasized at all in medical school. For the most part, behavioral problems are assumed to be responsive only to a psychological approach of one sort or another, drugs or a combination of both.

• LACK OF TIME. Doctors are generally extremely busy and may feel they don't have time in their hectic schedules to learn a different method of treatment.

• CONFORMITY. In common with the rest of humanity, doctors are susceptible to prevailing attitudes (reinforced by advertising, drug companies, drug salesmen, politicians and the majority of health professionals) and thus feel justified in dismissing anything that goes against commonly accepted views. In addition, many are unwilling to follow an approach that is not yet popularly accepted by the medical establishment for fear of being ostracized by their peers, losing hospital privileges or being punished in other ways.

The path of least resistance, if a doctor refuses to help, is to change doctors. This, however, is not practical for many of us who live in smaller centers where there may not be any doctors who already use a nutritional/environmental approach in their practices. If we can't go to another center, we have to work with what we have.

There are several choices—some of us will try to "convert" our doctors and fully involve them in the treatment program. Some of us will try to "coexist" and use them primarily as backup. A few of us will somehow manage to avoid using doctors at all. Others will find doctors willing to give us guidance by mail or long-distance telephone. (For more information on working with doctors, see Chapter 4.)

Teachers and Child-Care Workers

Teachers and child-care workers are generally overworked and underpaid, often forced to teach or care for too many children with too few resources. Having to cope with so much, in the short term it is sometimes easier for them to ignore nutritional and environmental health issues.

A few situations might arise with a teacher or child-care worker (day-care staff, baby-sitters, etc.). One is where they are merely nonsupportive, for example allowing negative comments about our children's food by other children to go unchallenged. In another situation, they might more directly undermine the treatment program by handing out candies in the class, or pooh-poohing the program to our children.

Our main resistance has been teachers. The Grade 2 teacher was angry that we would diagnose her as hyperactive and seek the type of help we did. She was categorized as "slow" and it took until Grades 4–5 for teachers to be willing to look at her advancements and put her into the regular program. We found this resistance hard to deal with but never gave up trying . . .

Recently, she was chosen to go to the other school to assist Grade 3 children with reading. As she put it, she was anxious to see the look on the faces of the teachers when she walked in to help!   —Dora's mother

We'd tell the school that under no circumstances, in any way, shape or form was he to have anything with artificial coloring or flavoring. If you bring him a cookie from a box you've got artificial coloring. Of course these things kept appearing at school all the time. There was no way around it. I just flipped my lid one day when he came home—it was just unbearable, he was just unbelievable at lunchtime. I asked him what happened. The French teacher had brought in some Pepsi. I said, "There's no excuse for this at school. None at all." I've been quite vocal about it. Fortunately I used to work in special ed in our school system and I knew the right people to contact. So I've not been a very quiet, easy-going parent I'm afraid—I've been very vocal. To the chagrin of some people and the enjoyment of others.   —Stuart's mother

If things do not improve after we have talked to the teacher, we have several options. Some schools have community workers or psychologists associated with them that might have more success in getting the teacher to cooperate. Or, we can work our way up the chain of command in our attempt to get results. The principal is next in line, then the superintendent of schools, members of the school board, and finally the state or provincial Department of Education.

It should be noted that a teacher often has only limited power to change things in the school, and many of our requests should more appropriately go elsewhere in the chain of command. For example, individual teachers will not have authority over which cleaning materials are used in the school, the lunches in the school cafeteria or whether the fluorescent lights can be replaced with incandescent. However, teachers are often good allies and certainly should be our starting point, as generally they will be able to point out to us the most effective method of changing a situation in school that is affecting our children's health.

In a day-care situation, if talking to individual workers does not result in change, we can talk to the director, then the board of directors in the case of non-profit day-care centers or the owners in the case of privately owned ones, and ultimately whatever government departments are responsible for licensing them.

Another approach is to change teachers; in more extreme cases changing schools or day-care centers will sometimes be the only solution. Depending on our own situation, we may even consider pulling our children out of school or day care completely.

One more approach should be mentioned, which is to get together with other parents and interested individuals who are sympathetic, as it is very true that there is strength in numbers. If the problem is fairly broad, say a question of poor quality lunches rather than one specific teacher, we can also try publicizing the problem by sending out statements to the press, writing letters to the editor of the local newspaper and so on.

Friends and Neighbors

One woman friend of mine has been skeptical of the diet and I find that I am dealing with it by establishing more of a distance between myself and her. I feel that I have important supportive people in my life and that it is better for me and my family to enjoy those people and distance those who are not, unless they can show that they can be supportive too. —Michael's mother

The more dependent we are on specific friends or neighbors for support, the harder it is when they are negative toward something important to us. If it doesn't seem likely they will change their attitudes, it is very important that we develop other friendships. We do not necessarily have to give up our old friends, but we should look elsewhere for our support. The danger in not diversifying our friendships is that, without other contacts, we may begin to feel that we are indeed as weird as our friends think we are, and that it is just too much work to follow the program and always be the odd one out.

The best solution is to join up with others in similar situations. We can find them either through word of mouth or by contacting a variety of groups supportive of a nutritional/environmental approach, such as the ones mentioned in Chapter 3. Not only will we not feel so alienated and alone, there is the possibility of making some strong friendships and also learning a lot from the information-sharing that informally occurs between people in similar situations.

Family

I suppose a lot of people had this problem—my husband had done no reading on this. He was very much against the whole deal, had the old theory that if you're strong enough, you'll straighten up and fly right. So we were having very great difficulties at home over this . . . The first year was very bad. Very, very bad. He thought it was absolutely mad. And this was ridiculous. But finally what I actually did was talk him into going back east with me when I took my daughter. And once he went back there and talked to the doctor and saw what was being done then that motivated him to do more reading and since then there's been no trouble. He's totally cooperative. When you have someone who knows nothing about this, it's a tough battle.   —Erica's mother

It is hardest when the people closest to us, such as members of our family, don't give us the support we need. The reasons for their lack of support can be very complex, often rooted in other family conflicts. The children's grandparents may feel that we are rejecting them when we refuse their cookies, cakes and Cokes, or trying to alienate their grandchildren from them. Our children's aunts and uncles may attribute our adoption of a nutritional/environmental approach to our supposed life-long habit of always wanting to be different/difficult/deranged. Our children's other parent may be expressing all his or her frustrations with life or resentments against us through negativity towards the treatment program. Sometimes the real issue is simply power:

It's almost like [my mother-in-law] has used food and snacks and candy as the battleground, and that's where she vents all her desires to be powerful and influential and all that . . . Ned and I have both made such a big deal

about the fact that we want [Terry] to eat nutritious foods and we don't want her to fill up on bread and candy and starch that [my mother-in-law will] go to great lengths, to the point of sneaking candy with Terry in the bedroom and taking her out and buying her treats when we're not there and literally telling her, "Here, don't tell your mum," sitting and making her eat it in the bedroom. So I just decided what I was going to do was I was going to give her carte blanche to feed Terry just about whatever she wanted. And when I did that I discovered that other things became the battleground, that her thing was more to fight than to feed Terry candy. But while other things became the battleground, she still continues to feed her all kinds of junk.
                                                              —Terry's mother.

What action we decide to take to ease a situation will depend on a number of factors. For example, if the children's grandparents live 3,000 miles away and the dietary or environmental transgressions are only a once-a-year occurrence, we may choose to grin and bear it. However, if our relatives live fairly close and are causing us and our children great distress despite valiant attempts to gain their cooperation, we may have to take serious action, such as limiting the number of visits, or requiring that all visiting be done at our place where we will have more control.

Unfortunately, our choices are made more difficult by the strong emotional ties that often exist with family members. It is usually possible to find a different school for children to attend, change doctors or find new friends. But mothers and fathers (ours and our children's) and sisters and brothers are irreplaceable.

However, when it comes time to make a tough decision, we should remind ourselves that we are not required to bear the total burden of maintaining family ties, especially when it is at great cost to ourselves and our children; the responsibility should be a shared one, and if any family members refuse to cooperate to a reasonable degree with us, it is their choice as much as ours to loosen the ties.

Potentially the most serious and distressing situation is when two parents are in disagreement. In this situation, however, often the negative parent will not interfere too much as long as the other one is willing to do all the work and take all the responsibility. The hardest part is likely to be the lack of moral support, making it important for us to develop contacts with others who will give us support. Unfortunately, with one parent so resistant, extra effort may be needed to engage our children's cooperation. (See the previous chapter.)

One possibility that might be tried in difficult situations is mediation by a neutral family member, family friend or professional counselor who is not opposed to the nutritional/environmental approach.

Another possibility that might be successful with resisting family members is introducing them to an outside authority, who is supportive of the nutritional/environmental approach. It is best that this be a personal contact, as it is much harder to dismiss what someone who is actually right there in the flesh is saying than to dismiss a bunch of words in a book or journal. For example, we can introduce the resisters to our children's doctors, who can tell them directly how important it is that our children avoid whatever it is they need to avoid, and discuss how effective the treatment program has been in other cases they have treated. Or, let the resisters talk to other parents whose children have improved on the treatment program. We should definitely use the inclination which often exists among families for relatives to believe someone else before they will believe us.

If we are patient, the more open-minded family members will in time be convinced by the evidence of their own eyes, when they see for themselves the reactions caused by nutritional/environmental factors, and the improvement of our children when they avoid these factors. This is especially so when we make an effort to bring this evidence to our relatives' attention and keep them informed.

If reason and patience don't work, extreme measures are sometimes called for. For example, the following account describes how the cooperation of one resisting grandmother was finally gained by forcing her to deal with the consequences of her actions:

I could never convince my mother-in-law that my five-year-old son was affected by milk. He used to throw up and break out in a rash when he was a baby. Then he outgrew the allergy, but when he began to become hyperactive I remembered reading in Allergy Quarterly *that sometimes food allergies can come back in a new disguise. Sure enough it was milk which was making him so impossible.*

My mother-in-law refused to believe me. I tried to persuade her. My husband tried to convince her. I gave her material to read. All to no avail. She continued to think that I was a terrible mother and over protective, not to mention over reactive, to deprive poor Jason of milk.

My mother-in-law really loves Jason and enjoys looking after him. I have to admit, I enjoy the break, too. But when I left him at her place, although I'd ask her not to give Jason any milk or foods with milk in them, I knew she usually did. Then I'd worry all the time I was out because when she did give him the wrong foods, it was me who reaped the whirlwind when I got him home.

One day I decided to change my tactics. I didn't remind her not to let him have milk. I·just told her that if she gave him milk or anything with milk in it, she could cope with him for a change. That afternoon, when I went to pick him up, I could smell by his breath that he had been given something with milk in it and that his reaction was just beginning, so I refused to take him with me.

An hour later, she called me and begged me to come for him. I said, "No. You fed him the milk. You take the consequences." A few hours later, she called my husband and begged him to come for Jason. My husband supported me. He went over and took one look at his wild son and he too refused to take him. Finally, at 9 o'clock, my tearful mother-in-law showed up at the door with Jason wrapped in a towel, wriggling like an eel. We took Jason then, but it was almost two days before he was back to normal.

That was a year ago. Since then, my mother-in-law, Jason and I have all enjoyed his milk-free visits to his grandmother's.   —Jason's mother
(reprinted from *Allergy Quarterly*,★ Volume 23, Summer 1987)

If it becomes obvious certain family members will never become willing cooperators, sometimes our only choice is to accept the situation as it is and concentrate on minimizing the effects. For example, we can feed children just before a visit so they will be less likely to stuff themselves full of junk food, make sure they get regular breathers away from adamant cigarette smokers, and arrange to be around as much as possible when children are with the resisters so we have an opportunity to counter and mute critical comments regarding the treatment program.

Choosing an Appropriate Action

Whether our difficulties are caused by doctors, teachers, friends, neighbors or family, we should first take the time for a bit of thought and planning before embarking on a course of action. For example, it is important to be clear about what it is we want to accomplish, which alternatives we will find acceptable and who is the appropriate person to approach.

It is also important to take into account the different variables involved, such as the amount of distress the situation is causing us and our children, our children's state of health and how seriously they are affected by deviations from their treatment program, the nature of our and our children's relationships with the resisters and how much we value those relationships, how influenced our children are by the resisters' attitudes, and how mature our children are. We

★Published by Allergy Information Association, 65 Tromley Drive, Suite 10, Islington, Ontario, Canada M9B 5Y7.

also need to consider the resisters' personalities, values and what limitations they are faced with.

Following are a few suggestions for remedying the resistance, related to what might have caused the noncooperation in the first place:

• CLARIFY. Sometimes all that is needed are a few extra words of explanation. What we perceive as resistance is not always that at all, but a simple misunderstanding. For example, the resister may not have realized how strictly we wanted our children to follow the diet either because we weren't clear, they are hard of hearing, our children gave them contradictory information or for any other reason.

Sometimes we need to clarify a situation because we have been giving mixed messages. For example, perhaps we are indirectly indicating that we don't really mind our children being given junk as much as we say we do. One way we may do this is by being inconsistent, sometimes saying it is all right for them to go off their diet and other times not, leading others to assume it must not make all that much difference what they do.

• MAKE THINGS EASY. Sometimes people are overburdened with work or other responsibilities and have little time or energy to accommodate children's special needs. They may feel they are too busy with their own concerns to pay much attention to what they should or shouldn't be doing for our children. In this case a little extra effort on our part will often go a long way towards easing the situation. For example, rather than holding teachers/friends/neighbors/relatives responsible for giving children safe alternative treats, we can supply the acceptable treats ourselves. Or, instead of expecting the baby-sitter to open a multitude of bottles to put together the set of nutritional supplements our children need to take, we can pre-select the vitamins and minerals so that each meal's supplements are together in one container.

• EDUCATE. People who are uninformed about the treatment program are less likely to follow through with it. For example, they may ignore restrictions because they do not realize the full consequences of an ice cream cone to a child with a milk sensitivity or model airplane glue fumes to a child with chemical sensitivities. Or, they may fear that giving children nutritional supplements will harm the children.

Providing resisters with information about the treatment program, including both safety and effectiveness, and about the symptoms children experience if they deviate from it may help in these cases.

We shouldn't be discouraged, however, if people listen politely

but don't really hear. Many people who do not take the time to think
things through will discount what we say no matter what the evidence, if it differs from the claims of those in positions of authority
such as government officials, heads of corporations, university pro-
fessors and doctors.

• CONVEY A TOLERANT AND NONTHREATENING ATTITUDE. We want
to indicate to people that we are not expecting them to conform to
our way of life and neither are we judging the rightness or wrong-
ness of *their* way of life. Unfortunately, some people take even a
simple request for cooperation as an indirect criticism of their diet or
life-style. The resulting resentment and/or guilt will sometimes lead
them to rationalize that our diet/life-style is not really any better than
theirs and therefore they need not pay too much attention to the
nutritional/environmental restrictions as undoubtedly we are taking
it all too seriously anyway.

There is very little we can do to prevent someone from feeling
criticized except to be as tactful as possible, show appreciation when
they are in any way supportive or cooperative, and use other methods of action as applicable.

• DEMONSTRATE. In a number of situations, the most effective
method of engaging the active support of resisters will be to actually
demonstrate to them the cause and effect relationship between nutritional and environmental factors and children's learning and behavior
problems. In practice this means when children are a bit wingy, speedy
or dozy, we must be sure to mention to teachers/relatives/friends/
neighbors/doctors that this reaction is a direct result of eating a
popsicle with red dye, being exposed to fumes from a gas stove or
neglecting to take their supplements for a week. And when they are
free of symptoms for a length of time, we should make sure to
mention what is different in our children's lives to account for this
improvement, whether this be a change in diet, control of environmental sensitivities, exercise and/or the addition of nutritional supplements. Once we point out the connections to people, they are
more likely to start noticing them on their own.

• CONFRONT. If none of the indirect methods of resolving the
situation as listed above work, we should consider using the more
direct method of confrontation.

People working in the area of conflict resolution frequently recommend that when confronting people in order to resolve a conflict,
we take care not to label or accuse them; rather, we should put the
issue in terms of facts and feelings. In other words, we should not
say, "Listen, you jerk, why the hell do you keep giving my kids that
disgusting purple bubble gum? Are you trying to permanently dam-

age them or something?" A more constructive phrasing would be: "I feel really badly that you keep giving my kids bubble gum when I have mentioned several times that we are trying to keep them off sugar and coloring."

There are three main reasons why the second phrasing is more constructive. The first reason is that how we initiate the confrontation will set the tone for what follows. People tend to respond in kind: if we are accusatory they are more likely to be accusatory back; if we are reasonable and low-key they are more likely to be reasonable and low-key. This is partly because they will feel less defensive if they are not directly attacked.

The second reason is that by refraining from personal attacks we maintain the distinction between the people's *behavior* and their *basic identity*. In other words, it is not the people we are criticizing but their behavior.

The third reason the second phrasing is more constructive is that if we are straightforward in presenting the facts and our feelings, the resistors will be forced to discuss the actual issue (from our point of view), and not get into diversionary arguments. In other words, we do not want to argue about whether purple bubble gum does or does not affect our children. Rather, we want the resisters to stop giving our children junk food *because we asked them not to*. (This does not apply in the case of doctors, who must, of course, consider the merits of the nutritional/environmental approach before they agree to use it as a treatment method.)

Taking Action

When we have chosen the action most appropriate to our specific circumstances, the next step is to plan what we want to say and how we want to say it. The chances of success increase when we are friendly, nonthreatening and nonapologetic, or, in other words, pleasant but firm, as people are less likely to want to change if *they* feel defensive or if *we* are defensive. Our attitude should be that the problem is a joint one which can be solved cooperatively.

It is also a good idea to be prepared for different reactions. In many cases we can expect positive responses, but hostility and equivocation are also possibilities. Unfortunately, despite our best efforts some people will react badly. It is important to recognize, however, that how they react to a nonthreatening attempt to improve a child's health is their decision, and nothing to do with us. First and foremost our main priority is our children's health, not protecting feelings that are offended when no offense was meant. Sometimes we will simply have to learn to live with a bit of unpopularity. We can always comfort ourselves with the thought that no trail blazer has an easy time of it.

If a resister launches into an attack on the treatment program, we are not required to argue the pros and cons of the nutritional/ environmental approach with them. Refusing to respond, changing the topic of conversation or stating the subject is not open for discussion at this time are three possible ways of preventing such an argument from getting off the ground. If we wish to be a bit more forthcoming, all we need say is that, after careful consideration of a range of possibilities, we have chosen the treatment best suited to our children's needs. With those who are genuinely interested, non-coercive and open minded, we can go into more detail if we wish.

No matter what the reaction, as much as possible we must try to stick to the issue: what we need from the resisters in the way of cooperation in order to get our children well. As parents we have a responsibility to ensure our children get the help they need to achieve full health and happiness, and others have a responsibility to not interfere with our efforts.

Doing some role-playing with a sympathetic relative or friend will help us prepare for any encounter. There are two other factors that increase the likelihood of success. One is timing, as people are more responsive when not preoccupied with upcoming deadlines, various and assorted demands or personal difficulties. The second is being accompanied by someone sympathetic. This lengthens the odds that the other person will be cooperative, or at least listen more closely, and increases our effectiveness by increasing our confidence. The same effect might be achieved by bringing along a selection of pamphlets, thoroughly researched articles and books that document our position, letters from doctors and test results. (The resisters will not necessarily be swayed by the evidence, but will likely be less vocal in their opposition.)

It doesn't pay to worry too much or too long before attempting to resolve a situation; once a rough plan has taken shape, we should make the plunge. If one method doesn't work, the best idea is to keep plugging away and try another one. Persistence, although tiring, is often effective and a technique worth cultivating:

With resistance, it's survival of the fittest, you just stay with it till they see your point or you wear them out . . . It took a lot of persuasion and talking to convince the school board that the reward was in the deed, with applause, and not the M & M chocolate candy they kept popping into the children's mouths. —Raymond's mother

If Being Reasonable (or Unreasonable) Doesn't Work

Some people will be more resistant to our efforts to gain cooperation than others. Trying to figure out why this is so can be like trying to put a puzzle together when some of the pieces are missing, and is not worth losing any sleep over. The reasons are rarely personal, having little to do with us and much to do with the resisters. They may have a vested interest in not cooperating. For example, some professionals are afraid they will lose their positions or credibility if it is known they are cooperating with a nutritional/environmental treatment approach. They may be excessively concerned with control and authority over others and fear they will be giving up some of their power if they make concessions to us. Or, they may be prejudiced and refuse to take us seriously because of our sex, race, ethnic background and/or perceived status, regardless of our personal qualities.

However, no matter how intransigent these resisters are, there are some possible actions to take which may either change the resister or change the situation.

Following is a summary of some of the options we have when faced with persistent resistance or noncooperation:

• IGNORE THE RESISTERS OR WITHDRAW FROM THE SITUATION. Sometimes it is not worth the effort to try to deal with the resisters. In some cases, attempting to resolve the conflict may end up being the equivalent of beating our heads against a brick wall. In other cases the situation may be annoying but is easily ignored, and does not interfere with our ability to follow the treatment program (though it is often worth dealing with even the merely annoying things of life).

Wherever we can't get through to people we avoid them.
—Bill's mother

Sometimes the best solution, although it is not often an easy solution, is simply to withdraw from the situation and find a more supportive school, doctor, community and so on.

• GO HIGHER ON THE CHAIN OF COMMAND. If the resistors will not change, consider going to someone who has authority to order them to change, such as a boss, supervisor, manager or board of directors.

• COMPROMISE. There are many factors in children's lives requiring our attention, including emotional needs. If children are not in a precarious state of health, it is sometimes in their best interests to compromise on the treatment program when faced with immovable opposition:

[While on] a week's visit here and there, Terry fills up on junk and is a wreck when she comes home—so be it. Because of what was happening, Terry was having a terrible time; she'd be so tense because of all the fighting between two people she loves, and she was just really unhappy, so I decided I wasn't going to push it anymore. I thought it was more damaging to Terry to see her [grandmother] and I at each other's throats over what Terry ate and having Terry have this conflict over who she's going to ally herself with—had she wanted to ally herself with her Grandma [despite the] strong pull towards me—and it's just not fair . . . so I figured, let her eat the stuff . . .   —Terry's mother

• LAY DOWN RULES AND CONSEQUENCES. Sometimes the state of our children's health does not allow for compromise. In the face of adamant opposition, it will occasionally be necessary to make extremely clear which behavior is acceptable to us and which isn't, and what will happen if the resistors behave unacceptably by sabotaging the treatment program in whatever fashion. These consequences may include restricting the number of visits with our children, switching doctors/schools/baby-sitters, or putting in a formal complaint to someone in authority over them.

Light on the Horizon

It is very discouraging to meet with resistance, and this may lower our morale considerably. However, we should keep firmly in mind that we are part of a movement, and there is always resistance to new ideas no matter how obvious and commonsense they seem in retrospect. For example, as Richard A. Passwater writes in *Supernutrition,* "For years no one took Anthony van Leeuwenhoek (1632–1723), a lens maker, seriously when he described what he saw with his invention, the microscope; his observations of life cycles did not end the popular spontaneous-generation theory. Louis Pasteur in 1862 and Robert Koch in 1875 were laughed at for talking of germs, bacteria and disease. Austrian physician Ignaz Philipp Semmelweis was attacked in 1861 by his colleagues for suggesting that physicians should wash their hands before attending women giving birth. Dr. Zabdiel Boylston was almost hanged in Boston in 1721 as he attempted to thwart a smallpox epidemic by giving vaccinations of pox from infected cows. Although physicians in Europe were reporting success, American physicians were helping to pass laws that would imprison both the doctor administering and the patients submitting to vaccinations."

Despite resistance, we can encourage ourselves with the thought that people following the nutritional/environmental approach are part of a movement that is definitely on the upswing, and that this approach is being accepted by more and more people all the time. There is a tremendous difference in terms of levels of acceptance between now and ten years ago, and in another ten or twenty years there will probably not be many around who even question it. Helping to change societal attitudes towards health, which will result in the improved quality of many people's lives, is something we can all feel good about.

Books mentioned in this chapter and further reading:

The Impossible Child, Doris Rapp with Dorothy Bamberg. Practical Allergy Research Foundation, P.O. Box 60, Buffalo, New York, 1986. Subtitled *A Guide for Caring Teachers and Parents,* this is a useful book to pass on to teachers if our children are allergy sufferers. Much of the information it contains is of direct relevance to teachers.

Supernutrition, Richard A. Passwater. Pocket Books, New York, 1976. Nutritional information relating to health; includes a chapter on controversies in nutrition.

8

WHERE TO BEGIN

Some of us have decided to try a nutritional/environmental approach either because it seems logical to us or because there are indications that nutritional or environmental factors are causing our children's problems. Others are interested because it seems safer than some of the more conventional therapies. And still others have already tried a number of other treatment approaches without any success.

Whatever our reasons for wanting to try a nutritional/environmental approach, it is often confusing trying to sort out whether a child's problems are caused by allergies, vitamin dependencies, an overgrowth of yeast or a heavy metal toxicity, and which foods, nutrient deficiencies or environmental substances are causing which problems.

Our very first step should be to rule out or deal with obvious problems such as infections, anemia and hearing loss. (See the section "What the Doctor Will Do" on the next pages.) Once this is done, there are, unfortunately, no simple formulas to follow. Each child is different and what affects one may have either a completely different effect or no effect at all on another. Any particular symptom may be the result of any number of nutritional/environmental factors. Conversely, any specific nutritional/environmental factor may cause any number of symptoms. For example, one child's speediness will be caused by artificial food coloring, while another's will be due to sugar; a sensitivity to milk will make one child hostile and destructive, but cause another to become withdrawn and passive. To complicate matters further, many children's problems will be the result of more than one factor.

However, the situation is simplified when we approach the problem from the perspective of scientists—carefully and methodically researching the nutritional/environmental factors affecting our children. Although our research results will not be applicable to children in general, they will certainly be valid for our own.

The scientific method is very straightforward, and requires neither university degrees nor fancy equipment to be used. The first step is to observe, the second is to form an explanation of what we observe (this explanation is called a hypothesis), and the third is to test this hypothesis by performing an appropriate experiment.

Conducting such a scientific study of a child's problems does not of course exclude working with doctors; on the contrary, forming a research team with our doctors will generally make for faster and better results. Neither should it be thought that having a doctor makes our role as scientists unnecessary. Many doctors would be the first to agree that our active participation in every step of getting a child well is essential, and much of the procedure that will be followed while doing our research will coincide with procedures our doctors suggest.

What the Doctor Will Do

For many parents the first step when investigating the appropriateness of a nutritional/environmental approach for our children is to visit a doctor practicing such an approach. Although doctors vary somewhat in their procedures, the broad outlines are similar.

During the initial visits, the doctor will interview us and our children to learn our concerns and histories (medical, social, personal, nutritional and family), do a physical exam and send our children for lab work (blood, urine and hair) and possibly auditory, visual and psychological testing. The doctor is looking for indications of specific health problems such as impaired hearing and vision, anemia, hypothyroidism, hypoglycemia, diabetes, food and environmental sensitivities, vitamin and mineral deficiencies, heavy metal toxicity, intestinal parasites, organ disorders and infections.

Dr. Abram Hoffer in his examination of children looks for perceptual problems such as night terrors, dyslexia, shadow illusions and hallucinations; problems of thought such as paranoid ideas; problems of mood such as depression; and problems of behavior such as hyperactivity or an extreme of passivity.

It is important to check out all the various possiblities as many problems are easily overlooked. For example, in the past some children were diagnosed and treated as retarded until it was discovered that they were actually deaf. Deafness, however, is not the only type of hearing impairment. Many people are only partially deaf, which, if not recognized, can also cause major problems in learning and relationships. The New York Institute for Child Development in their book *Treating Your Hyperactive and Learning Disabled Child* state that, "The child with an auditory problem may be hyperactive simply for that reason. If all the world of sounds comes in as a buzz, without differentiation, it creates confusion, and the usual defense is

to make your own noise so that there is some contact with reality."
At the Institute, they check both the range of sounds and the difference in sounds such as school/stool/spool. Even a simple ear infection can cause all sorts of behavior problems.

It should always be kept in mind that lab tests are not to be totally
trusted, as there are many factors that can make their results inaccurate. Lab tests should be expected only to help indicate possible
problems or to help confirm suspicions, not to provide definitive
answers. Depending on the information from these initial tests, the
doctor may recommend further testing procedures, such as elimination diets or glucose tolerance tests

On the basis of a child's history, physical exam, test results and the
doctor's personal observations, the doctor will suggest a treatment
program. However, children have to be watched carefully and periodic adjustments made to this treatment program as there is an
element of guesswork involved. As Wunderlich and Kalita write in
Nourishing Your Child, "Follow-up permits the physician to monitor
the individual response of the patient to the treatment. No amount of
expertise will enable the physician to predict the exact response to
the treatment program. Accordingly, general trends can be predicted
fairly reliably, but the specific individual response must always await
the therapeutic trial. Information about the child's response, therefore, is an integral part of the diagnosis and therapeutic plan."

Observations Associated with Specific Causative Factors

The following sections, each relating to a different nutritional/
environmental factor, contain common observations associated with
that particular factor. (Ticking off the statements that apply to a child
will help summarize our observations for us and suggest the possible
cause of the problems.) They also contain outlines of the corresponding hypotheses, experiments and predictions, which can be used as
rough guides when we are ready to make up our own. At the end of
each section, mention is made of the appropriate chapter to read for
more specific details on formulating and testing our hypotheses.

(The rest of the chapter following these sections provides a fuller
discussion of the various steps involved in pinpointing a child's
problems. In the box on page 120–122 is an example of one possible set
of steps.)

INADEQUATE NUTRITION

Observations that if true might be indications of inadequate nutrition:
—A major food group is excluded from our children's diets.

—Our children eat large quantities of junk food (that is, food that is highly refined and/or highly sweetened).
—They eat quantities too small for individual requirements.
—They frequently skip meals.
—They eat few home-cooked meals; most meals are eaten in restaurants, cafeterias, fast food joints, institutions or are from vending machines.
—They are seriously under- or overweight.
Other observations or information relating to inadequate nutrition:

_____

_____

_____

Hypothesis: Our children are suffering from poor nutrition. More specifically, they are eating too much of the following foods:

_____

They are eating too few of the following foods:

_____

Experiment: Institute a high-quality diet and note the results.
Prediction: The following symptoms will diminish significantly in frequency, duration or intensity or clear up completely:

_____

For more information: see Chapter 10.

NEED FOR NUTRITIONAL SUPPLEMENTATION

Observations that if true might be indications of a need for nutritional supplementation:
—Other family members have nutritional dependencies or deficiencies.
—Our children have eaten poorly for a long period of time.
—Problems persist despite a high-quality diet free of additives, sugar and processed food, and avoidance of known sensitivity-causing foods and substances.
—They have received a diagnosis of schizophrenia, autism or mental retardation (including Down's syndrome).
—They are currently under severe physical stress (such as infections or other illness) or mental stress (such as the death of a close friend or relative, an impending separation of their parents or the pressure of exams).

Other observations or information relating to a need for nutritional supplementation:

_____

_____

_____

Hypothesis: Our children are suffering from either a deficiency of, or a higher than average requirement for, specific vitamins, minerals or other nutrients and need the following nutritional supplements:

_____

Experiment: Add nutritional supplements as listed above to their diets and note the results.

Prediction: The following symptoms will diminish significantly in frequency, duration or intensity, or clear up completely:

_____

For more information: see Chapter 11.

HYPOGLYCEMIA (LOW BLOOD SUGAR)

Observations that if true might be indications of hypoglycemia:

—Other family members have hypoglycemia.
—Our children crave sweets and/or starchy foods of all types.
—They eat large amounts of sweet and/or starchy foods (e.g., white bread, rice and pasta, baked goods, candies, chocolate bars, soft drinks, jam, sugar on cereal).
—Their worst symptoms occur two to four hours after eating.
—Their symptoms decrease shortly after eating.
—They have sudden mood swings.

Other observations or information relating to hypoglycemia:

_____

_____

_____

Hypothesis: Our children are suffering from hypoglycemia.

Experiment: Implement an anti-hypoglycemia diet and note the results.

Prediction: The following symptoms will diminish significantly in frequency, duration or intensity or clear up completely:

For more information: see Chapter 12.

YEAST OVERGROWTH

Observations that if true might be indications of yeast overgrowth:
—Our children's problems started after a course of antibiotic treatment.
—Our children have received large amounts of antibiotics.
—They eat large amounts of sweet foods and/or yeast or mold-containing foods (bread, cheese, pickles, fruit juices, mushrooms and so on).
—They have persistent problems with vaginal yeast infections, oral thrush or other yeast or fungal infections (such as of skin or nails).
—They have chronic problems that have not responded to other treatment programs.
Other observations or information relating to yeast overgrowth:

Hypothesis: Our children are suffering from yeast overgrowth.

Experiment: Institute a yeast control program and note the results.

Prediction: The following symptoms will diminish significantly in frequency, duration or intensity or clear up completely:

For more information: see Chapter 13.

FOOD OR FOOD-RELATED SENSITIVITIES (INCLUDING ALLERGIES AND INTOLERANCES)

Observations that if true might be indications of food or food-related sensitivities:

—Other family members have food sensitivities.
—Our children have aversions to certain foods.
—They have cravings for certain foods.
—They eat large amounts of certain foods.
—They have insatiable appetites.
—Certain symptoms consistently appear after they eat particular foods.

—Their behavior improves after not eating for a period of time.

—They have digestive problems such as stomachaches, gas, constipation, diarrhea.

—They have been given a diagnosis of hyperactivity. (In this case special attention should be paid to the Feingold diet.)

—Either parent has an aspirin sensitivity. (Again, pay special attention to the Feingold diet, as this sensitivity increases the chances that children have inherited a sensitivity to salicylates.)

—They have environmental sensitivities. (Food and environmental sensitivities often occur together.)

—They are not of northern European descent. (This would increase their chances of intolerance to lactose, the sugar found in milk).

Other observations or information relating to food and food-related sensitivities:

Hypothesis: Our children are suffering from food or food-related sensitivities. The suspect foods, additives and contaminants are:

Experiment: Eliminate suspect foods, food additives or food contaminants from their diets for a period of time and note the results. Add suspect food items back one at a time and again note the results.

Prediction: The following symptoms will diminish significantly in frequency, duration or intensity or clear up completely:

For more information: see Chapter 14.

ENVIRONMENTAL SENSITIVITIES

Observations that if true might be indications of environmental sensitivities:

—Other family members suffer from environmental sensitivities.

—Our children have food sensitivities. (Food and environmental sensitivities often go hand in hand.)

—They have respiratory and/or skin problems.

—Symptoms occur consistently after exposure to specific physical locations.

—Symptoms occur consistently after specific activities, such as swimming, or after contact with specific substances.

—They are frequently exposed to specific substances, especially strong ones such as glue for model building, paints, pesticides or chemicals for photography.

—Their symptoms decrease after a period of absence from specific locations or substances.

—Their symptoms occur cyclically, for example, at the same time every day, nightly, weekly, monthly or seasonally.

—There is a major source of pollution in the home such as urea formaldehyde insulation.

—They have a keen sense of smell.

—They have a poor sense of smell.

—They find certain odors unusually offensive.

—They find certain odors unusually attractive.

—The onset of their symptoms coincided with exposure to a new location, substance or activity.

Other observations or information relating to environmental sensitivities:

_____

_____

Hypothesis: Our children are suffering from environmental sensitivities. Among the substances which may provoke symptoms are the following:

_____

Experiment: Avoid or minimize contact with all suspect environmental substances for a period of time and note the results. Expose children to one suspect substance at a time and again note the results.

Prediction: The following symptoms will diminish significantly in frequency, duration or intensity or clear up completely:

_____

For more information: see Chapter 15.

HEAVY METAL TOXICITY

Observations that if true might be indications of heavy metal toxicity:
—Other family members suffer from metal toxicity.

—We live near a major source of pollution, such as a busy traffic route, refinery, factory, mine or power plant.

—Our children consume large amounts of fish. (Some fish may contain significant amounts of mercury.)

—Their diet includes large quantities of canned goods, a common lead source.

—Their symptoms started during or after the placement of mercury-containing dental fillings.

—They are exposed to large amounts of cigarette smoke, a major source of cadmium.

—Our water pipes are made of lead or copper.

—We live in an old house or apartment with flaking paint, a prime source of lead.

—We use copper or aluminum cookware.

Other observations or information relating to heavy metal toxicity:

_____

_____

Hypothesis: Our children are suffering from heavy metal toxicity and are being adversely affected by the following metals:

_____

Experiment: Detoxify their bodies, minimize contact with the metals and note the results.

Prediction: The following symptoms will diminish significantly in frequency, duration or intensity or clear up completely:

_____

For more information: see Chapter 16.

MULTIPLE FACTORS

Observations that if true might be indications of multiple factors being responsible for our children's problems:

—Many of the statements in more than one of the above sections seem to apply.

—Our children improved only partially or not at all when the single-factor hypotheses were tested.

—Our children have been diagnosed as schizophrenic or autistic or have other severe problems.

Hypothesis: Our children are suffering from a combination of two or more contributing factors as follows:

_____

_____

Experiment: Follow the procedures as suggested above under the appropriate sections on testing individual hypotheses. For example, implement a program which includes a high-quality diet, nutritional supplements and avoidance of the foods and environmental substances most commonly associated with children's learning and behavior problems, and note the results.

Prediction: The following symptoms will diminish significantly in frequency, duration or intensity or clear up completely:

For more information: see Chapters 10 to 18.

Following is an example of one possible set of steps we might follow to help pinpoint the causes of our children's problems, using the hypothesis that these problems are caused by a combination of common nutritional/environmental factors.

PRELIMINARY OBSERVATION PERIOD: ONE WEEK

1. Making no changes in diet or environment, keep a symptom diary such as the one on page 124. (Once the week is up and changes are instituted, continue to keep the symptom diary.)

ELIMINATION PERIOD: ONE TO THREE WEEKS

2. To minimize the number of environmental contacts children will be exposed to, clear their bedrooms of as many possible sensitivity-causing factors as is feasible, especially those items which give off odors and fumes (for example perfumes, paints, felt pens, chemistry sets, air fresheners, scented paper). Try to remove most synthetic materials such as foam rubber and items made of plastic and polyester, replacing them with natural materials such as cotton. (If the mattress is being removed, folded cotton blankets or camp cots may be used instead.) Seal off the heating ducts, keep out all family pets, and clean (with baking soda or other cleaning agent unlikely to cause a reaction) and air out the room to remove fumes and odors. Keep the room well dusted and ventilated with fresh air, and try to minimize all smells and fumes (from cigarettes, cooking food, furniture polish and so on).

Children should spend as much time as possible in this room or other relatively safe area, and avoid as much as possible places with strong fumes or odors.

3. Eliminate from the diet foods containing any of the following: all forms of sugar (white and brown table sugar, honey, molasses, maple syrup) and artificial sweeteners, refined carbohydrates (white flour, white pasta, refined cereals and grains), caffeine (in coffee, tea, cola drinks, chocolate), yeast and molds (in many baked goods, cheese, fruit juices except those freshly prepared, melons, mushrooms, fermented foods), artificial additives (coloring, flavoring, preservatives), salicylates (see page 215), wheat, rye, corn, milk and milk products.

4. While on this restricted diet children should eat regularly every two hours or so and drink about six glasses of water a day.

5. End the elimination period either when symptoms have cleared up or after three weeks, whichever comes first.

TESTING PERIOD
(IF THERE HAS BEEN SIGNIFICANT IMPROVEMENT)

6. Continuing with the symptom diary, reintroduce foods one at a time and note reactions. (See Chapter 14.)

7. Expose children to environmental substances one at a time and note reactions. (See Chapter 15.)

8. Retest the foods and environmental substances that appear to have caused symptoms to confirm whether these are involved in causing our children's problems.

IF THERE WAS LITTLE OR NO IMPROVEMENT

9. Return children to their previous diets and environmental contacts for a week.

10. Next, eliminate foods containing all sugars and artificial sweeteners, refined carbohydrates, additives.

11. Send off a sample of hair to be analyzed. Indications of mineral imbalances or heavy metal toxicity should be investigated further by a doctor. If confirmed, the doctor will order a course of treatment. (See Chapters 11 and 16.)

12. At the same time, in consultation with a doctor, add to the diet a program of nutritional supplementation. (See Chapter 11.) To give an idea of what such a program might

include, following is an example of a daily schedule of nutritional supplementation as outlined by Allan Cott in his book *Dr. Cott's Help for Your Learning Disabled Child*. As each child is a unique biochemical individual, some children will need higher (or lower) dosages and some will need other nutrients (for example, vitamins A, D and E and the minerals calcium and chromium) in addition to those listed below.

Children weighing less than 35 pounds

niacinamide (vitamin B3):	100 mg.
vitamin C:	100 mg.

Children weighing 35 to 45 pounds

niacinamide (vitamin B3):	100–200 mg.
pyridoxine (vitamin B6):	100–400 mg.
riboflavin (vitamin B2):	100–200 mg.
ascorbic acid (vitamin C):	250–500 mg.
calcium pantothenate:	100–400 mg.
vitamin B-complex:	1 tablet daily
magnesium:	75–200 mg.
zinc:	10–30 mg.

Children weighing more than 45 pounds

niacinamide:	1–2 grams
ascorbic acid:	1–2 grams
pyridoxine:	200–400 mg.
riboflavin:	200–400 mg.

In addition to these nutrients, children weighing more than 45 pounds need one or two tablets of B-complex, 100–300 mg. magnesium and 15–30 mg. zinc.

This program should be followed for three to six months, while at the same time an exercise program is slowly introduced. If children improve significantly, the program should be continued.

If there is little or no improvement, other possibilities to pursue are the existence of sensitivities to foods or environmental substances that were not eliminated, the existence of hypoglycemia and/or yeast overgrowth which needs to be controlled more stringently, or a different program of nutritional supplementation. See Chapters 10 to 18.

Applying the Scientific Method to Children's Problems

Following is a more detailed explanation of the steps involved in discovering which nutritional/environmental factors are affecting our children.

1. The first step is to OBSERVE and GATHER INFORMATION. This is done by itemizing children's symptoms and nutritional/environmental exposures, including when they occur and their measurement. Much of this information can be gained through direct observation, for example by keeping a symptom diary such as the one on the following page. For this period of observation—generally a week is a good period—do not attempt to change anything in the diet or environment; the aim at this point is to produce an accurate record of our children's current circumstances. This record will provide the information needed to form a hypothesis, and provide a standard with which we can compare the results from our experiments.

Following are some suggestions to keep in mind when filling in the symptom diary:

Food columns. The more information included about each food item the better, such as whether the food is canned or frozen, cooked or raw, organically grown or not. The most vital information to include is a complete list of ingredients including all additives, spices, kind of oil or grease that was used for frying and so on.

For amount, put down either the weight of the food item or the volume measure, for example, "one ounce of cheese," "one-half cup of steamed cauliflower."

Location/activity and/or environmental substance column. "Location" in the fourth column refers to any place a child happens to be for any amount of time, whether at home, in the car, at school, at the babysitter's or in the park. "Activity" includes such things as swimming, bike riding, gardening, playing with blocks and sleeping.

Generally, listing the location or activity will imply the environmental substance. "Environmental substances" need only be listed if we would not normally associate the location or activity with the substance. In other words, do mention rare or unusual occurrences related to substances, such as if a child was present when trees were being sprayed with pesticides, had a nap in a room that was freshly painted, played dress-up with a coat that had been mothballed or used a new kind of soap.

If a relationship between any particular location or activity and a child's symptoms is discovered, then we can start working out which specific substances are causing the problems. (For example, a child more lethargic in the kitchen than elsewhere might be sensitive

| Date and time | Food | | Location/activity and/or environmental | | Description of symptoms | | Sample of | Comments | |
	item	amount	substance	us	kids	measure	writing	ours	kids'

to the gas stove; a child most irritable after reading might be sensitive to printer's ink.)

Symptoms columns. The symptoms that will be most obvious to us will be physical (rashes, runny noses, circles under the eyes) and behavioral (temper tantrums, speediness, passivity). The symptoms that will be most obvious to *children* will be physical (headaches, tummyaches, sore muscles), sensory (everything looks blurry and gray, there is a strange smell that won't go away, they hear voices that don't belong to anyone), and mental and emotional (confusion, fear, unhappiness).

Some children, depending on age, level of self-awareness and verbal ability, will be able to help fill in their half of the column by describing symptoms and pinpointing which foods, rooms or activities make them feel strange or uncomfortable. Many children, however, especially younger ones, will find it difficult to itemize their symptoms. They may not be able to identify even to themselves what they are feeling, let alone express these feelings in words. If this is the case, it will be necessary to rely on a combination of observation and discussion to find out what is troubling them. Some of the simple tests mentioned starting on page 36 in Chapter 2 and page 128 in this chapter will be useful for this purpose.

Having their own column will help involve children in their treatment program, with luck resulting in more information for us, plus for them stronger motivation to cooperate. It is often useful to make the distinction between *what we see* (mainly behavioral symptoms) and *what our children feel* (physically, mentally, emotionally) and *experience* (through their senses). (For more information on gaining insight into how children are experiencing the world, see Chapter 2.)

It is a good idea for us and our children each to make a separate list of five or so symptoms that are of particular concern. The more precise a measurement of a symptom is, and the easier it is to make, the more useful it is.

Precise measurement requires, first of all, writing the information down as soon as possible, before details become vague. Secondly, it means recording symptoms in the same way each time, using objective measurements, such as duration of symptoms (how long they lasted); frequency (how often they occurred in any given period of time); and intensity. For example, they can be rated either on a scale of, say, one to three, or, particularly for younger children, as "a little bit" sad/mad/whatever, or "very" sad/mad/whatever. This makes comparison easier when it comes time to judge improvement after testing our hypotheses.

It will simplify matters somewhat if symptoms are translated into concrete terms. For example, if aggression is a problem, observe how it is expressed; in the case of children who express their aggression by bashing things or people, the number of bashes delivered in a given time period can be used as our measure. A runny nose is easy, as the number of times children need their noses wiped can be counted; puffy eyes is harder as a value judgment will be required as to the amount of puffiness (small amount, moderate amount, large amount).

Following is a summary of common symptoms caused by nutritional/environmental factors. (In some cases of course, other factors such as infections may be responsible, and as mentioned previously an investigation of these factors should be our first step.)

Physical: respiratory problems (eye, nose, ear, throat, lungs)
   digestive problems
   skin problems
   pain or discomfort (stomach aches, headaches, muscle aches, itchiness, fatigue)
Perceptual: disturbances of sight, sound, touch, taste, smell
Mental: disturbances of thinking with respect to concentration, logic, content, memory and overall comprehension
Emotional: extremes and/or rapid swings of mood, inappropriateness, flatness, depression, fear, anxiety, irritability
Motor activity: lack of coordination, extremes in amount of activity, developmentally inappropriate for age
Behavioral: aggression, withdrawal, inappropriateness (for either age or situation), lack of judgment, poor social skills
Learning: poor verbal, reading, writing and mathematical skills

These symptoms are discussed in more depth in Chapter 2. It should be remembered that generally behavioral and learning symptoms are the result of disturbances of perception, thinking, emotion, motor ability and physical health, which in turn may be caused by one or more nutritional/environmental factors.

Writing sample column. It is also useful to measure fine motor control of older children (it is not normally well developed in young children) as this is often a good general indicator of how children are doing. This can be done by collecting handwriting samples from children at regular times each day. They should use a fountain pen, as this will show variations better. Dr. Marshall Mandell uses handwriting samples and has noted striking differences depending on what the child has been exposed to.

Comments column. This column is for our and our children's miscellaneous thoughts, impressions and feelings about what is happening. Any relevant physical stresses, colds and flu for example, or psychological stresses that might be affecting children should also be noted here. As much as possible, however, avoid doing observations when extra stresses are present.

In addition to direct observation, children's individual past histories (medical, nutritional, environmental and social) and family history (for inherited characteristics and predispositions) often provide important information. For example, when did symptoms start, and was there any change in diet or environment that coincided with this change? Have there been unusual exposures to chemicals? Was there at one time an allergy that has since apparently disappeared? (Perhaps it has now resurfaced, except this time with different symptoms.) Is there a family history of allergies? (This increases the likelihood that children also have allergies.) The statements summarizing observations relating to individual nutritional/environmental factors, listed earlier in this chapter, starting on page 113, indicate some of the questions to ask.

Obtaining copies of lab test results (together with the interpretations) will also supply us with valuable information.

2. The second step is to FORM A HYPOTHESIS by choosing what seems to be the most logical explanation of the data we have collected. To do this it is necessary to analyze our observations. What we should look for are patterns, relationships and frequencies. Are there more temper tantrums on days our children have drunk a lot of milk? (Possible milk sensitivity?) Do they seem more spaced out after swimming lessons? (Possibly they are affected by the chlorine in the water.) Are they less irritable on weekends or during school holidays? (Perhaps the fluorescent lights in the classroom are the problem.)

Are our children often at the point of exhaustion a couple of hours before mealtime? (The problem could be hypoglycemia.) Is a major food group excluded from their diet? (Possible nutrient deficiencies can be suspected.)

It should be noted that there is not always an immediate time correlation between symptom and causative factor. In some cases reactions do not show up until days later.

When no obvious conclusions can be made from the information we have gathered, then choose a hypothesis using other criteria. For example, we can choose as our hypothesis the simplest and most common reason for children's learning and behavior problems, which is poor nutrition.

Another reasonable choice is to form a hypothesis suggesting that more than one factor is responsible for a child's problems. In fact, the more severe a child's problems are, the more likely it is that multiple nutritional/environmental factors are involved.

When forming a hypothesis it is important not to ignore the role of intuition, which has been responsible for many great scientific discoveries. In other words, we should always pay attention to any strong feelings we or our children have about the causes of their problems, even if initially there is no obvious evidence to support these feelings. (Of course, in testing our suspicions we must be open to the possibility that our intuitions are inaccurate.)

3. The third step is to TEST THE HYPOTHESIS. This means planning an experiment and predicting what results will occur if our hypothesis is correct. Try to make predictions as specific as possible, first of all by deciding exactly which symptoms should be measured (sniffles? temper tantrums? headaches? lethargy? reading ability?), and secondly, by using objective measures of evaluation as mentioned earlier. This makes it easier to gauge improvement. Subjective judgments (both our and our children's gut feelings and intuitions) are also important and should be noted as well.

There are generally two parts to an experiment. The first part involves restricting or eliminating for a period of time a child's exposure to those variables suspected of being detrimental. The more variables eliminated during this initial period, whether these be food items or environmental substances, the more chance there is that the results from the test period will be an accurate reflection of the validity of our hypothesis.

The second part of the experiment is the actual test and involves reintroducing the variables, usually (though not always) one at a time to the child's diet or environment and watching for reactions. These results are then compared to our predictions.

In addition to noting symptoms, children can do simple tests to help us judge the effects of the variables on them. Examples of such tests include those listed on page 36, and those described by Dr. Marshall Mandell in *Dr. Mandell's 5-Day Allergy Relief System:*

"I have children give me writing samples as they are being tested. Changes in penmanship are a concrete evidence that the brain is being affected by a food or chemical test. I have children read as they are being tested. A number of children suddenly become unable to concentrate and to comprehend what they are reading, or they may forget what they have just read by the time they reach the end of a sentence. It is not unusual for visual blurring to develop or to have words misread or to have slower speech or stuttering."

Tests for children who are not yet reading or writing would include drawing circles, squares and triangles, making a tower out of blocks, putting together simple puzzles and so on.

Keeping a written record, such as the symptoms diary used during the observation period (or an adaptation of it), will help ensure accuracy. Writing things down is especially important if a child's improvement occurs over a long period of time and is imperceptible from day to day. When changes are slow and gradual, it is often difficult to remember the exact nature and extent of the original symptoms unless we are able to refer back to our notes.

4. The fourth step is to EVALUATE THE EXPERIMENTAL RESULTS. If the results were what we predicted, this is evidence that our hypothesis is correct.

If there was some improvement in symptoms, but not as much as expected, we have to decide if this improvement is significant or not. For example, say that during the period of observation a child has an average of four screaming fits a day, and at the end of the experiment the daily average number of screaming fits is three. Is this enough of an improvement to at least partially support our hypothesis? Or is the difference in improvement so small that it should be considered meaningless? The possibility that our predictions may have been unrealistic should also be considered.

If the symptoms did not improve, this suggests that our hypothesis is not correct.

Part of our evaluation should include, in the case of partial or no improvement, an attempt to figure out why the results were not better. Do these results indicate that in fact our hypothesis is totally wrong? Some other possibilities, in addition to unrealistic predictions, are as follows:

• *The experiment was inappropriate.* For example, we might have allowed only two weeks for improvement to occur when three or four or five weeks are needed. Or, children might have been given dosages of nutritional supplements that were too low to be effective.

• *Mistakes were made.* For example, perhaps children followed their experimental diet only sporadically. It is just as important that a child cooperate during the experiment as when the treatment program is in full swing. (For more information on gaining children's cooperation, see Chapter 6.)

• *There are other variables affecting our children that were not taken into account.* For example, children may show little or no improvement if only some of the foods they are sensitive to are eliminated. Or, it may be that environmental sensitivities are also causing problems, so that significant improvement will not occur until certain environmental substances are eliminated along with specific foods.

It is tempting to dismiss results that are either contrary to what we think is really happening or for which there seems to be no explanation; but as much as possible, we should remain open-minded and critical. One day the explanation may suddenly occur to us, or we may stumble across it in a book or during a conversation.

5. The fifth step involves either CONFIRMING THE HYPOTHESIS or TESTING A NEW OR REVISED HYPOTHESIS. If the results match our predictions, we should test again to make sure that this was not a matter of chance or coincidence. When results differ significantly from our predictions, then there are three possibilities. One is to test a different hypothesis, another is to design and carry out an experiment that is more appropriate to the hypothesis, and the third is to do the same test again but either more carefully or for a longer period of time.

We may be lucky and discover the solution to our children's problems right away, but more likely we will end up testing a few hypotheses, learning more each time, before being satisfied with our results.

6. The sixth and last step is to MAKE A CONCLUSION and IMPLEMENT OUR FINDINGS. Once we feel confident of having found the hypothesis that correctly explains our children's problems, this hypothesis can be used as the basis of a treatment program.

In addition to implementing the specific findings of our experiments, it is extremely important to incorporate into children's treatment programs a high quality diet (see Chapter 10 for more information) and regular exercise (see pages 263–265, in Chapter 18). Both good nutrition and regular exercise are not only essential to children's overall health and well-being, they also increase the likelihood that other parts of the treatment program will be effective. In addition, they are good preventive measures.

Books referred to in this chapter and other suggested reading:
Allergies and the Hyperactive Child, Doris J. Rapp. Cornerstone Books, New York, 1980. A wonderful book for anyone suffering from food or environmental sensitivities, whether hyperactive or not. Contains lots of useful information. Highly recommended.

Dr. Cott's Help for Your Learning Disabled Child, The Orthomolecular Treatment, Allan Cott, J. Agel, E. Boe. Times Books, New York, 1985. Interesting and informative.

Dr. Mandell's 5-Day Allergy Relief System, Dr. Marshall Mandell and Lynne Waller Scanlon. Thomas Y. Crowell, New York, 1979. For a description, see Chapter 14.

The Hyperactive Child, What the Family Can Do, Belinda Barnes and Irene Colquhoun. Thorsons Publishers Limited, Wellingborough Northants, England, 1984. This useful book, "a self-help manual written by parents for parents," includes information on nutrition, allergies and heavy metal toxicity.

Nourishing Your Child, A Bioecologic Approach, Ray C. Wunderlich, Jr. and Dwight K. Kalita. Keats Publishing, New Canaan, Connecticut, 1984. An extremely well-written, helpful and informative book, well worth reading.

Solving the Puzzle of Your Hard-to-Raise Child, William G. Crook and Laura Stevens. Random House, New York, 1987. As is to be expected from such a winning combination of authors, this provides a comprehensive and highly readable overview of factors that may be involved in children's behavior problems.

Treating Your Hyperactive and Learning Disabled Child, The New York Institute for Child Development, Inc. with Richard J. Walsh. Anchor Press/Doubleday, New York, 1979. For a descripton, see Chapter 10.

9

GETTING BETTER

My son, now thirty-nine, is doing very well. In the past he's been in and out of the hospital, but with the megavitamins he stays well longer and is better than the time before. Nothing is all up hill. If you prepare yourselves for the ups and downs and bend with the breeze, it's not so bad, as you must realize there will be setbacks. But once they have had good days for months you know they will again.
—Raymond's mother

The road to recovery is variable. Some children improve dramatically within days of starting on a nutritional/environmental program, while others show few signs of improvement until months have gone by. The rate of improvement depends partly on the age of the child (younger children tend to get better more quickly than older children), partly on the severity of the problem, and partly how long the problem has existed. Also involved are how quickly the cause or causes of the problem can be pinpointed, how appropriate all parts of the treatment program are (for example, vitamin and mineral dosages may need to be readjusted), how quickly all aspects of the program are instituted and how rigorously the treatment program is followed.

Getting better is often a long, slow process and we should try not to become too discouraged if if takes longer than we expect. Progress will not necessarily be steady, as relapses may occur due to infections or other illness, emotional upsets, deviations from the program, growth spurts and so on.

Some children, despite major improvement, will not reach the point where we consider them completely well. However, new information concerning diagnosis and treatment does come up from time to time; by keeping ourselves informed in the areas of health and behavior and continuing to work with our children's doctors, we may eventually discover some missing answers.

Sometimes complete improvement will not occur until patterns of behavior have time to change; once a child is used to reacting in a certain way, it may be hard to break the habit. It is not unusual for there to be other remnants of long-term illness requiring attention:

I know these kids—after a while they hang their head, and they don't talk, they don't look you straight in the eye, they feel less. Our society makes them less. If in achievement you're always at the bottom, you're never a winner. Everybody should be programmed somewhere to win at something. But there are some kids like Michelle—she's been psychotic for ten years— there's no way that she could be programmed to win anything. She's a loser. So she has lack of confidence. This is where your counseling comes in; after she's well through the megavitamins, treating the allergies, then we will have several years of counseling to help her understand what she's been through. And help her look at how bright her future can be.

—Michelle's mother

It is important to note that getting better can be a scary experience, particularly when children have been unwell for a long time. In some cases they will be faced with an unfamiliar world where everything looks and sounds different. They will often have to get used to changed relationships and new self-images. This can be very bewildering and unsettling, making some children prefer the security of their illness. For this reason it is crucial that we extend a great deal of support and encouragement at this time.

Difficulties sometimes occur at the beginning of a treatment program for two reasons. One is that children's bodies need time to adjust to changes, such as new diets or the addition of nutritional supplements. For example, withdrawal symptoms may occur if the new diet eliminates items a child is addicted to.

The second possible reason for difficulties is that changing long-term patterns of living such as eating habits and leisure activities can be very stressful. It is not easy to avoid favorite foods, drop a hobby or have familiar routines disrupted. Lisa Brownstone, an occupational therapist who has worked with children and has a strong interest in nutrition, mentions that parents should not be surprised if symptoms worsen and children act out more during the initiation of the treatment program because of this stress. She emphasizes the importance of persevering with the program long enough for children to get used to the changes in their lives; this will give the program a better chance to work, and its effectiveness can be more fairly judged. (See pages 268–274 for more information on the effects of stress and how to deal with them.)

Once children have adjusted physically and mentally and all necessary corrections have been made to the treatment program, they should start feeling better. As mentioned previously, this improvement may take anywhere from days to months to occur, so patience is necessary.

Following are some descriptions of the ups and downs of children's recoveries:

It was very strange being back at school. I was afraid that I might not be able to handle it. Yet it was a challenge and I needed a challenge. I lived at home that year and saw a lot of [my boyfriend] John. I kept having relapses but longer and longer periods would elapse between each bout. I had different kinds depending upon which part of my treatment I had ignored. What scared me most were the relapses that occurred when I was strictly following both diet and vitamins. When I investigated I found a pattern which corresponded to my menstrual cycle. Each time I relapsed I could trace the cause to my period, a cold, bad diet—in short anything that altered my body chemistry.

Mum: We noticed a change within three weeks [after starting the vitamins]. You weren't quite so bad. You could still be pretty nasty, but your hallucinations and nightmares weren't as bad and you had the hope of handling them better because they were getting less intense. You realized that the vitamins were having an effect.

Suzanne: Was my recovery fast? Slow?

Dad: I would say that it wasn't fast, but it was steady. You'd be better for maybe a week and then you'd have a relapse, and then you'd be better for two weeks and have a slight relapse and then four weeks and then there wasn't a relapse. It's when you really persuaded yourself that the diet and vitamins you were using were going to help you that there were very few additional problems.

Suzanne: Did you ever think I was completely better and then realize two months later that I was still getting better?

Mum: I did but your father kept saying, "No, not yet" and I'd say, "Of course she's okay, she's completely better." "No, not yet." And this went on for months and I kept realizing he was right.

—Suzanne Foster in *Stoney Lonesome Road*

When he was thirteen he did have a small sort of relapse and I remember phoning [the doctor] just before his final exams. He was very tense and very depressed and I phoned and asked him about it, [he] asked me if he was growing rapidly; the questions were as if he could see him right in front of him. Albert wasn't growing, he was exploding, it was literally as if you could see the change in front of your eyes. I said, "yes." "Well, look at his fingernails and see if he has white spots." Sure enough he did. "Put him on zinc." Within two or three weeks it made a difference. —Albert's mother

[The doctor] doubled the niacinamide to six grams a day where she'd been on three. He doubled the C and he quadrupled the B6. . . . We did run

into a problem because Michelle became very nauseated. It didn't happen instantly. If it happened instantly we would have picked it up. Then when she started getting really nauseated and she was losing weight and she complained about abdominal pains and she was obviously really sick, I thought of hepatitis, mononucleosis, appendicitis, maybe an ulcer, because this kid was really sick, so I took her in, and the doctor had the same problem, went through the same four things I had gone through. She stayed sick a month and I kept saying I believe it's the vitamins, how about the niacinamide. Her doctor said, "I've never seen it cause a side reaction. It should be within the safe level." I didn't think so and I took her to her orthomolecular doctor and he said, "No, that couldn't possibly be it." He dropped her niacinamide down to three grams for a week but by that time her vomiting had taken such a hold that she couldn't stop. I thought she was going to die. But anyway we did find out through the orthomolecular convention talking to Dr. C. that her niacinamide was twice too high and that was the problem and the minute we cut it back, she's gaining weight and doing fine now.
—Michelle's mother

I put my child on Feingold diet with vitamin and mineral supplements added later. Change was apparent within a couple of days—calmer, longer attention span, no whining, obeyed instructions at home—school situation took much longer to improve—results good at present time.—Bill's mother

We were told by one doctor here he was suffering from schizophrenia and by another that he did not know. One of them suggested we put him on welfare and let him wander around the country, and the other doctor said we should lock him up and forget about him as there was no hope for him . . . He was given four hospitalizations using electroshock treatments, and given Mellaril. These would help for a few days but never very long. He couldn't function. He couldn't work or go to school . . . He is twenty-six now. He is on the orthomolecular maintenance program . . . He is not completely well, but slowly improving. He has completed two years of a program as an X-ray technician and is studying for his boards now in hopes he will find a job.
—Pierre's mother

She was different from birth, cried often when awake, only slept six out of twenty-four hours from birth onwards . . . At eight months our family doctor confirmed what we already suspected, that she was hyperactive. She would scream in any new situation and this included visits to the doctor's office. By fourteen months . . . she was easily irritated and frustrated, and had no patience, had emotional outbursts and temper tantrums for no apparent reason, could rarely concentrate and play. By twenty months we found she was worse after eating wieners, Smarties, Jell-o and drinking Kool-Aid so we stopped giving her those. She is six and a half now and since twenty-

three months has been on the Feingold diet. She is now completely well, has no problems at all, but must *keep to her diet.*   —Vanessa's mother

By the time he started school, he didn't speak well, couldn't sit still when checked up on, temper started showing up. By the age of eight he was put into a special clinic, one-to-one basis, for uncontrollable outbursts and rages. He wanted to destroy himself, a lot of self hatred. Finally he was placed in a clinic, but by this time that didn't help. At that time after a year one of the counselors suggested a Dr. E. in P. By this time we were desperate, so I called and made an appointment. Our appointment was in July of 1979. Nick was given allergy tests. Then a vitamin treatment. Also put on allergy shots. He started back in the clinic in September 1979. By watching his diet and taking his injections he did very well. In February 1980 he was placed back in a regular classroom, 30 students. By this point he was two full years behind. He had a very hard time reading, short attention span. From Feburary to June of 1980 he progressed so rapidly that at the end of June he received an award for the most achievement academically and in behavior. He is doing extremely well. Has picked up one full year.

He is now eleven and a half. He is very careful about what he eats. He is on vitamins, and also still taking his injections for allergies. Nick seems to be completely well, behaves like a very normal boy. Nick is doing very well in a regular classroom.

In closing, all I have to say is that if two years ago someone would have told us that Nick would be doing so well, I wouldn't have believed it.

—Nick's mother

In third grade he became suicidal and we placed him in a private school for "L.D." [learning disabled] and "E.D." [emotionally disturbed] children, and under psychiatric care. Over the years he was diagnosed as having psychomotor seizures, learning disabilities and associated neuroses.

However, this past year his psychiatrist diagnosed him as having paranoid schizophrenia with a future prognosis as "poor." Most tranquilizers had a horrendous effect on Ian, but he certainly needed something to just cope with his daily routine.

Several months ago we took him to a doctor in N., who started him on "megavitamins." Now he doesn't experience auditory or visual hallucinations with the frequency or intensity as before. He hasn't experienced the deep depressions, and no longer feels that people don't like him as much as before. He also feels less isolated from his surroundings and feels his memory and reading comprehension has improved. (It was extremely low.)

He is more outgoing and is beginning to take an interest in gardening, people, TV and reading. Before his only interests were eating and music, if at all. Sometimes even those were difficult for him to become involved in.

We still saw very bizarre behavior, particularly after meals, when fatigued or under stress.

More recently the doctor treated him for food allergies—Ian was very ill as a preschool child—and many foods such as milk, soy, peanuts, oranges, yeast and molds aggravated his mental symptoms; however, wheat made him completely psychotic. It was comparable to a "bad LSD trip." It was totally surprising to see this happen under such circumstances, with wheat being the responsible agent.

Very impressed and rather frightened, we kept Ian off all wheat for four days. We then figured a plate of spaghetti wouldn't hurt. We were wrong. Not only did he have a violent emotional reaction, he also broke out in many hives . . . Needless to say we no longer give him wheat products and he is presently taking sublingual drops to desensitize his other allergies. His present improvement is amazing. We feel we are at the beginning of a road to his cure at last . . . —Ian's parents

Our family's exposure to hyperactivity began at the time of our first child's birth. Like many expectant parents, we had read volumes about infant and child care, thinking that the prenatal research would result in the perfect baby.

Our nine-pound son did not live up to our naive expectations. He drove us to the edge of insanity with constant diarrhea, diaper rash that refused to heal and one cold after another. He cried day and night. Often, in desperation, we would wearily drag Theo into the pediatrician's office, praying and pleading for a solution to our exhausting trials. The doctor's advice never varied: "You have a colicky baby and you're a nervous new mother. Try to relax."

I was nursing then, totally convinced that there was no other method for a dedicated mother to feed her child. But one day when Theo was two months old, and I was physically and emotionally worn out, a friend came to me with a can of infant formula. I felt beaten by that time, and didn't have the energy to refuse her suggestion. Twelve hours after the first bottle of formula, I began to think that Theo might recover.

Though the manufactured food certainly helped, I suspected, as Theo grew older, that he was not a contented baby. At the age of ten months he still had not slept through the night, and it was unusual for him to take a daytime nap, even though he routinely awoke at 6:00 a.m. He whined continually for no apparent reason and he was never satisfied to amuse himself. He demanded constant attention. Many of our friends delicately suggested that we might try discipline. That failed to improve the situation, and I wondered how I would cope with him and the new baby I was expecting in two months.

After forty-eight hours of eating the Feingold way [after hearing about the

Feingold association on a radio program and contacting them], Theo slept all night. The next day he slept all afternoon. Miracles happened one after the other that first week. He played by himself and stopped whimpering. The minor accidents that I had believed to be an inescapable part of childhood abruptly stopped, and Theo became the happy, cuddly baby I had always wanted.

Theo is now two-and-a-half years old, and I believe many of his difficulties in infancy were probably caused by his inability to tolerate artificial foods. His reaction to breast-feeding may have been caused by my own intake of additives and preservatives, although I had been trying, at the time to eat sensibly. —Theo's mother

When we received him for adoption at three-and-a-half months, he wouldn't cuddle. When we picked him up, he would just balance himself away from us, and refuse to cuddle. I had had a lot of training in special education, and this was one of the symptoms of childhood autism to come later—often autistic children didn't cuddle as babies. Then we'd had a lot of problems with him. Many, many infections, he had no sense of danger, he would just dive off the changing table—once he just dove off and broke his arm. He just paddled out into the air at the top of the stairs—would just have no concept of the necessity of stopping. We spent a lot of time in emergency. Later on he became hyperactive. He would just ride his tricycle out into the sides of cars, and fall out of trees, and any old thing.

He had a lot of earaches, and many, many bouts of gastroenteritis. He was sick all of the time; he would turn blue on us. We never knew what was the matter.

He always seemed to be just in a fog. Never knowing what was going on where. School was a complete disaster. At first he just huddled in the corner I guess, and didn't have anything to do with anybody. Then he became extremely hyperactive. He was put in a learning disabilities class to meet children, and even in that class he had to have one volunteer parent on him at all times to keep him from going over tables and under chairs and essentially disrupting the whole place.

And yet he was not a nasty child at all. He seemed to want to please so much. He seemed to be a very burdened, anxious human being and we just didn't know what to do with him . . . We dragged him from doctor to doctor and finally heard about the Feingold diet and I thought, well I'll try this.

The teachers had always told me he was so much worse right after lunch. This clued me in that it was food of some sort. Then I realized that I was giving him a colored vitamin, one of these children's chewable preparations, at lunch time and I stopped that. The worst behavior after lunch ended.

Once I put him on the Feingold diet [at age six], to us there was an improvement. For years, maybe four or five years, he had us up every night

five or six times with horrible nightmares. It was very, very hard on us, just not getting any night's sleep. There were very few nights that we ever slept through, because of his nightmares.

With the Feingold diet then, the nightmares disappeared. With the Feingold diet, we realized that oranges were the worst problem of good food, and all the colorings and flavorings we eliminated and behavior improved but it certainly wasn't normal.

Then in the fall of 1977, my son's teacher went to hear the Canadian Association for Children with Learning Disabilities. There, Dr. L. spoke. She came back and said, "You've got to get a tape and listen to this man." So I did and he said that milk and chocolate were the worst, so I thought, "I've got nothing to lose, I'll try this. So I removed milk from his diet, and within two days I had almost a normal child. The leg pains stopped, the hyperactivity stopped, the ceaseless chatter stopped, he could look at us directly in the eye, which he wasn't able to do before, the severe reaction to sunlight stopped, and the digestive problems stopped, the tummy-aches stopped and he was just like a new being.

What he did—in fact he realized this himself—he felt so different that he went around introducing himself to people as the new Stuart. So it was really quite a dramatic thing for him too. He is a very normal, mischievous child now. He still has a lot of problems—especially, every May we go through a very bad period with him, we don't know why. We assume it's some sort of allergy. He's still in a learning disabilities class to try to catch up in math. He's still very disoriented spatially, which seems to be a long-term thing to outgrow. But he will work now on his own and enjoy things and read and talk to us, and play without being excessively irritable, and things like that. He's not out of the woods—I don't think you ever are with such a child, but it's enjoyable living with him now.

—Stuart's mother

He knew he was sick and he didn't know what was wrong with him, and without telling us went to a psychiatrist. The psychiatrist apparently told him that he must really hate his parents or something and the thing to do is to break off all ties. So I phoned him not too long after that and he said, well, he was really sorry Mom, but he didn't want me to write to him any more. And he didn't want us to phone and he wasn't going to phone in any case.

Of course, that was a really bad blow. But I said, "Okay, I'll do this if you promise to let us know if you leave so we'll know where you are." This is what we did; it was a very long winter. We did not hear from him. But in the summer, he hitchhiked home. We were just tickled to see him, we couldn't hardly stand it. He looked terrible . . . I remember I put my arms around him and he sort of pushed them away. Which really broke my heart when he first came in the door. But, anyway, after a few days, he asked me if I'd ever read the book I Never Promised You a Rose Garden. And I had—I had been reading everything I could get my hands on for years as a matter of fact . . . I had read it and I said "Yes," and he said, "Well then, if I tell you that I feel somewhat like that girl will you accept the fact that I've got to have some help?" Of course we did.

Now he was finding that he couldn't read. This was of course very distressing, so our first step was we started with an eye doctor, on some eye exercises [using special] machinery. But the girl called me down in about three weeks and she said, "It isn't going to work." She said, "There's something more wrong with his eyes." and she suggested a doctor in S., an M.D. that was in the megavitamin field.

We took him to this doctor and he gave him the HOD test and started him on megavitamins and Stelazine. We came back to our smaller town eighty miles away and started him on this Stelazine and very shortly, within four days, he was having a dreadful reaction from it. I was walking miles with him. Just pace, pace, pacing. We called the doctor and he said keep giving him more and we were frantic, we didn't know what to do, so we kept giving him more, and of course with the end result, we ended up having to call our hometown doctor and we rushed him to the hospital that night because he was suicidal and everything else. He had a terrible reaction to that tranquilizer . . . He wanted to get well so desperately, so he wanted to go back to this doctor. We went back and the doctor said, "Well then, you'll have to stay here and live in the city and we will try these other antipsychotic drugs." The two of us went up and stayed in a motel near the doctor and he tried these different drugs. None of them worked. One of them made him so dopey that he couldn't move for three or four days. We stayed there three weeks; we tried the whole bit. The doctor didn't know what else to do. Finally the last night he started going into a reaction, I think it was from Haldol if I recall—we tried about four drugs—anyway, he started getting jumpy like he did with the Stelazine so we called it quits. We decided to go home in the depths of depression. I decided the only thing to do was to get back to Dr. N.'s clinic in M.—so we took him back, they put him through the HOD test again, the psychiatric questioning. We were there three days. And they put him through the whole routine they do back there and we were very, very pleased—that was the first time they ever started him on the road to recovery. And then they gave him again different megavitamins and in large dosage. It's awfully hard being three thousand miles away from your doctor. He broke into a rash all over his body from, as I recall, the niacin. We couldn't get a hold of the doctor naturally, so we switched to niacinamide.

The weeks went by and he slowly, slowly got better, so slowly that it was imperceptible. He was very discouraged. He couldn't get out of bed in mornings. In the testing he was badly hypoglycemic. We did a very fine job *on the diet. Oh, did we eat—you never saw so many proteins in your life! He slowly, very carefully, started getting better. He started back to school in the fall. It was very slow. He was able to see, his perceptions started clearing up, his pep started coming back, gradually I taught him how to care for his hair.*

He went back once a year always to M., and it seemed like he was getting better but he was just not over the hump somehow. He still had his ups and his downs so much. He went to the U. of W. Then we sent him back to the Brain Bio Center, because we felt that was a closer monitoring of the chemical balance. Lord, he has a sheet that high of all these perfectly balanced vitamins, but meanwhile he went ahead and graduated as an engineer, and has a very fine job in the company; he's been there two years, he's functioning, he's happy, he's well, he's managing his money well. He went through a stage I might add where he wasn't doing so well, he was so sick, but he's doing beautifully. He phones us a lot, he's happy, he's bought himself a car, he's painting, he's writing a book, and he's so far very successful in his job.   *—Jon's mother*

As these experiences show, the path to recovery is not always easy or straightforward. Although patience and persistence are required in many cases, the results are more than often worth it.

10

BASIC NUTRITION

Food and water supply the materials for the growth, renewal, repair and overall functioning of the human body, with the quality of this food and water determining to a large extent the quality of a child's life. When children eat well they are better able to cope with physical and emotional stresses.

Unfortunately, many children eat poorly. They consume large quantities of sugar, refined carbohydrates, caffeine and food additives and contaminants, while avoiding more nutritious foods such as vegetables and whole grains. The possible consequences of such an inadequate diet include increased susceptibility to infections, slow growth, fatigue, the start of degenerative diseases (cancer, arthritis, heart disease), as well as a host of learning and behavior problems.

Following is a short description, summarized mostly from the *Nutrition Almanac* (see book list for this Chapter, page 167), of the nutrients that must be supplied by diet in order for children to enjoy good health.

PROTEINS are the body's major source of building material. They are also a necessary ingredient in the production of hormones, enzymes and antibodies.

CARBOHYDRATES are the body's main energy source. Fiber is a constituent of some carbohydrate foods and is important in aiding elimination of wastes.

FATS provide energy, protect the body's organs, act as insulation and are essential for the body's use of the fat soluble vitamins A, D, E and K. The three essential fatty acids (linoleic, arachidonic and linolenic) are crucial for normal growth, and for healthy blood, arteries, nerves, skin and other tissues.

VITAMINS are constituents of enzymes, which means that they are important in regulating metabolism, converting fats and carbohydrates into energy, and making bone and tissue. The functions of some individual vitamins are discussed in Chapter 11.

MINERALS are important in the maintenance of the body's physiological processes, and contribute to the health of the skeleton, heart, brain and muscle and nerve systems. The functions of some individual minerals are discussed in Chapter 11.

WATER, according to the *Nutrition Almanac*, "is by far the most important nutrient. Responsible for and involved in nearly every body process, including digestion, absorption, circulation and excretion, water is the primary transporter of nutrients throughout the body and is necessary for all building functions in the body. Water helps maintain a normal body temperature and is essential for carrying waste material out of the body."

Because of the intricate working relationships of these nutrients, a deficiency of even one nutrient can have severe effects on the functioning of other nutrients and the overall health of children. Ray C. Wunderlich, Jr. and Dwight K. Kalita in *Nourishing Your Child* describe the interrelationship of nutrients and the consequences of any deficiency this way:

> Because you and your child are human beings, you have a body whose structure is both elegant and complex. It is a highly complicated, dynamic, superbly organized system consisting of over sixty trillion cells. Each of these sixty trillion cells has a unique structure, and each requires just the right amounts of a chain of chemical substances called nutrients. If the cells receive the proper amounts of these nutrients, then and only then can they sustain themselves in an optimum fashion. This chain of about forty nutrients is composed of links (e.g., vitamin C, calcium, folic acid, magnesium, methionine, valine, zinc, to mention just a few); all the links are essential for optimum health. If one or more of these nutrient links is weak or missing, the whole chain is weak and the cellular structure, depending on the strength of the chain, begins to fail. Severe malnutrition, such as that found in many of Africa's suffering children and adults, is a state in which a prolonged deficiency of one or more nutrient links actually retards physical, mental and emotional development or causes such specific clinical conditions as goiter, rickets or anemia to appear. Marginal malnutrition, a more subtle form of malnutrition that is found in a growing number of America's suffering children and adults, is a state in which "marginal" deficiencies of one or more nutrient links can cause such "modern" disorders as minimal brain dysfunction, attention deficit disorders, learning and language disorders, hyperactivity . . . diabetes, poor resistance to infectious invasion, etc.

Many of the marginal deficiencies that Wunderlich and Kalita mention can be traced directly to the large quantities of sugar, caffeine and refined carbohydrates that some children consume. Their inclusion in a child's diet actually increases nutrient requirements; this is because sugar, caffeine and refined carbohydrates are unable to supply most of the nutrients needed for their digestion and waste disposal. Although not nutritious, they are temporarily filling and very addictive with the result that often more nutritious foods remain uneaten.

Additives (preservatives, flavoring, coloring) and contaminants (pesticides, antibiotics, metals) found in many food items are also often harmful to children's health. Many of them are toxic and are particularly dangerous because in some people their effects may not be felt for years. In a number of children, however, the effects are more immediate.

The reason for the nutrient-deficient, sugared and additive-rich diet of many children is not hard to find, given the scarcity of whole, unadulterated foods, the lack of nutrition education, the proliferation of nutritional misinformation, and manipulative advertising. All of these factors combine to shape and reinforce an attitude that regards food for children as reward (the sweeter and stickier the better), entertainment (junk food gluts at home or at fast-food joints) and convenience. (In an age of multiple time pressures and responsibilities, it is only too tempting to heat up the canned stew and pass the cookies when children are hungry.)

What Is a Good Diet?

Although a good diet is not a guarantee of good health, eating nutritiously will increase children's general health and well-being even when the basic problem is unrelated to food. It follows then that a good diet is an essential component of any program to improve children's learning ability and behavior, as well as an extremely important preventive measure.

There are two aspects to a good diet, the first being what should be eaten and the second what should not be eaten. In brief, a good diet should include a balanced variety of high-quality fresh, whole, unadulterated foods in the quantities required to supply each child's unique nutritional needs. It should *not* include food that is nutrient-poor, sweetened and chemically polluted (either with contaminants or inessential additives). Of course, foods that children are sensitive to should also be excluded.

In practical terms this means children should eat a variety of fresh vegetables and fruits, whole grains (for example, whole wheat, brown rice, pot barley), additive-free sources of protein (meat, fish, poultry, eggs, dairy products, legumes, nuts and seeds), and unpolluted water. They should eat only limited amounts of highly processed foods (white bread, white rice, refined cereal and pasta, canned goods, sausages, frozen dinners) and restrict their intake of highly sweetened or caffeinated foods and drinks.

Balance and Variety

Including a balanced variety of foods in a diet requires that children should eat a variety of food items from each food group, unless they have food sensitivities or are vegetarian. (The major food groups are generally considered to be protein sources such as red meat, fish, poultry, eggs, legumes and nuts and seeds; dairy products; grains; and fruits and vegetables.) Also, no one food should be eaten to excess. During the course of a day foods containing protein (whether of plant or animal origin is immaterial), fat and carbohydrates should be eaten. If the foods used to provide the fat, protein and carbohydrates are from varied and high-quality sources and prepared in a nutrient-conscious way, they will supply many of the minerals and vitamins that are necessary for a good diet, plus fiber, which is also extremely important. And of course, water must not be neglected as an essential part of a balanced diet.

If due to food sensitivities or for any other reason a major food group is omitted from the diet, great care must be taken to supply the missing nutrients from the remaining groups.

The reasons that balance and variety are important are:

• TO ENSURE THAT A CHILD'S DIET INCLUDES ALL THE NECESSARY NUTRIENTS. This is because nutrients are not evenly distributed throughout all the food groups.

• TO ENSURE THAT A CHILD DOESN'T CONSUME LARGE AMOUNTS OF POTENTIALLY HARMFUL SUBSTANCES. Some substances (either natural constituents of food which interfere with the availability of certain nutrients to the body or contaminants such as lead and pesticides) are concentrated in certain foods. Obviously this does not mean that children should completely avoid foods like spinach, which even though it contains oxalic acid, an inhibitor of calcium absorption, also contains important nutrients such as vitamin A. It only means they should not eat spinach in huge quantities to the exclusion of all other vegetables.

• TO ENSURE THAT ALL NUTRIENTS ARE PRESENT IN THE DIET IN THE RIGHT PROPORTIONS. For example, eating too much protein might lower a child's calcium, phosphorus, zinc and iron levels. One consequence of eating too few foods containing pyridoxine (vitamin B6) is that carbohydrate, fat and protein metabolism will be negatively affected. And so it goes with all the nutrients; because of their intricate interrelationships, they do not work as effectively when their ratios are out of kilter.

• TO PREVENT THE START OF FOOD SENSITIVITIES. Some children have a tendency to become sensitive to the foods they eat most frequently. If sensitivities exist among family members, a rotation diet might be the best idea (see the section starting on page 220 in Chapter 14).

The Quality of Food

High-quality foods are those that are nutrient-rich and as close to their natural state as possible; they are fresh, whole and unadulterated. Unfortunately, it is not always obvious from the way a food item looks, smells, feels or tastes what the nutritional quality of that food actually is. To judge nutritional quality requires some knowledge of the background of a food, such as the conditions it was grown under and the subsequent processes it was subjected to. Following is a discussion of some of the factors affecting the quality of a food:

• THE SEED. High-quality food cannot grow from nutrient-poor seeds. There has been a switch in modern agriculture to using hybrid seeds which, according to Brett Silverstein in his book *Fed Up!*, may produce crops with lower nutrient content. Also, seeds may be treated with pesticides before they are planted.

• GROWING CONDITIONS FOR PLANTS. A food crop can only be as good as the soil it is grown in. Plants grown in soil depleted of any minerals will not contain those minerals. That is why the mineral content of a food crop can vary so widely from one region to the next, depending on the nature of the soil it was grown in. Unfortunately, modern agricultural practices have caused mineral-deficient soil to become more widespread, partly because of soil erosion, non-rotation of crops and the use of synthetic fertilizers, which do not replace the soil nutrients (but do sadly add nitrates).

Also, some plants will take up toxic metals that are in the soil. The more acid the soil is, the easier it is for a plant to absorb the metal. Some plants are more likely to be contaminated than others.

Food crops can also be contaminated with toxic metals through air and water pollution.

Modern agriculture uses large amounts of pesticides (which include insecticides, fungicides, herbicides and rodenticides) on crops and this also affects the quality of our food. With better agricultural methods, pesticides would rarely be needed; if the criterion of health were used rather than a criterion of expediency, a program of phasing them out would be instituted immediately. Despite claims of safety, a large number of these are toxic, as can be testified by many farmers who have suffered from weight loss, nausea, neurological disorders, reproductive disorders and cancer as a result of pesticides. While it is true that many highly toxic chemicals are now prohibited, there is no guarantee that the ones remaining are safe. There is in fact a great deal of evidence to show that they are unsafe.

Another aspect of growing conditions that should be mentioned is the length of growth time a crop is allowed. Unfortunately, many fruits and vegetables are picked before they are ripe and are instead ripened artificially. This results in a lower nutrient content than if they had been left to ripen naturally.

Some crops (usually grains and nuts) can also be infected by mycotoxins, a product of certain molds.

• GROWING CONDITIONS FOR ANIMALS. Most animals destined to end up on our children's plates are raised in what have been called factory farms, where the animals are subject to unnatural conditions such as crowding, restrictions of movement, artificial lights and forced feeding. Because these unhealthy conditions encourage disease, the heavy use of antibiotics (both as a preventive and treatment) is an integral part of the current methods of raising animals, resulting in drug residues in our children's food.

In addition to the danger of some children being allergic or sensitive to even minute quantities of antibiotics, antibiotics deplete the body of some vitamins, destroy some of the good intestinal bacteria, and encourage the creation and proliferation of drug-resistant disease-causing bacteria. It has been speculated that this indiscriminate use of antibiotics in the raising of animals is responsible at least in part for yeast overgrowth in some people. (See Chapter 13.)

Food from animals also contains pesticides, as a result of the animals eating plants containing pesticides, and sometimes because of direct applications to keep away certain insects. Pesticides are more concentrated in animals than they are in plants, which is one argument for consuming more plant protein and less animal protein.

Hormones, given to animals to increase their growth, are another possible contaminant of food.

Animals are also subject to pollution, with the result that their tissues sometimes contain metals such as lead and cadmium (metals accumulate particularly well in organ meats such as liver and kidney) and mercury (mostly found in fish). Chemicals such as PCBs are also found in animals.

The quality of the food from animals will of course be affected by the quality of the feed they are given, plus the general state of their health.

• SOURCES AND TREATMENT OF WATER. The water we drink from the tap comes either from wells or, more commonly, from a commercial or governmental water supply. This is usually surface water— reservoirs, lakes, and in some cases rivers and streams. Surface water can be, and far too often is, contaminated by a variety of pollutants, from insecticides and fertilizers that wash off treated land to airborne toxins like lead from auto exhaust.

Factory runoff and toxic-waste dumping are widely deplored sources of chemical pollution of our water sources. There is also considerable doubt about the usefulness and safety of many substances, including chlorine and alum, which are often added to water for supposedly beneficial purposes such as purification. Many municipalities add fluorides to the water supply to reduce dental decay in children; there is a strong minority opinion that this may be harmful.

Well water, drawn from the subsurface water table, is free of some of these problems, but is subject to contamination through seepage, especially where septic sewage-treatment fields have been overloaded, and in any case has a highly variable mineral content. It may have high levels of nitrates, a particularly dangerous situation in the case of babies up to six months of age. It is imperative to test the nitrate levels of any well water before it is used for babies. (If the levels are high, alternative water sources must be found.)

In addition to contamination of water from pollution and purification measures, water may contain lead due to lead piping or lead seams in copper piping, or contribute excess copper to children due to copper piping.

Unfortunately, there is one more thing to worry about in connection with food quality in addition to nutrient-deficient soil, mycotoxins, pesticides, toxic metals and stray chemical pollutants. This is the appearance of radioactive material in plants, animals and water (and ultimately, of course, our children), thanks to nuclear industry. Radioactive material can travel large distances, carried by the wind and rain, so that even non-nuclear countries suffer from radioactive pollution. Two examples are the Chernobyl disaster in the U.S.S.R. and the Three Mile Island disaster in the U.S.

• FRESHNESS. The sooner a food is eaten once it has been picked or slaughtered, the higher its quality will be. The longer it remains uneaten, the more the levels of the nutrients decrease. Unfortunately, much of our food today is not very fresh, first of all having traveled long distances before it reaches the grocery store, and then perhaps sitting awhile before it is bought. During transportation and storage, food may be subjected to various conditions that will increase the rate of deterioration, such as exposure to air, light and heat. (Nutrients vary in what they are affected by.)

• PROCESSING. Despite the fact that whole, unadulterated foods are generally the best for children, many foods are not allowed to go straight from farm to store to our kitchens, but undergo a large number of processes in between, further lowering their quality. Here is a brief description of some of these processes:

In *refining*, part of a food is removed, with the resultant loss not only of many nutrients but of fiber, which is also essential for children's health. For example, when wheat is refined to make white flour, the parts that are removed are the germ of the grain, which contains most of the nutrients, and the bran which is the fibrous part. According to Wunderlich and Kalita in *Nourishing Your Child*, "The milling of wheat into white flour removes 40 percent of the chromium, 86 percent of the manganese, 76 percent of the iron, 89 percent of the cobalt, 68 percent of the copper, 78 percent of the zinc and 48 percent of the molybdenum. All of these trace elements are essential for good health. Likewise, 60 percent of the calcium, 71 percent of the phosphorus, 85 percent of the magnesium, 77 percent of the potassium, and 78 percent of the sodium are removed by refining whole wheat into white bread. Only iron, and that in a form poorly absorbed, is later added to the white flour. By the same milling process, eight vitamins are removed from wheat, but only three or four (depending on the baker) are then returned to the 'enriched white bread'."

Fruit and vegetable juices are highly refined as well, much of their nutrient value thrown away with their peel and pulp. Oils are also generally highly refined, losing many valuable nutrients in the process.

Other processes include *drying, freezing* and *canning* with a consequent decrease in nutrients in each method used.

Irradiation is a process now being used on some foods, despite possible dangers. According to David I. Poch in *Radiation Alert*:

> While food irradiation is presently quite restricted in both Canada and the U.S., broader licensing is imminent and the technique is already widely used in the Netherlands, Israel and South Africa.

In North America, the irradiation of potatoes to inhibit sprouting has been permitted for many years but has not proven to be useful due to problems of contamination after treatment.

Vitamins A, B1, B6, B12, C and E are sensitive to irradiation although alternative preservation techniques such as canning and precooking also destroy them to some degree. Very high doses of radiation can reduce the nutritional value and in some cases even produce toxic substances—a factor one hopes regulators will consider in determining permissible limits.

Animals fed irradiated food have been found to have some cells with abnormal chromosome counts, a condition known as polyploidy. Questions about the likelihood and seriousness of polyploidy in humans have yet to be laid to rest . . .

Unfortunately, as in the case of chemical additives, there is very little understanding of the subtle long-term effects on human health due to food irradiation, and we may all become experimental guinea pigs. Foods which have been irradiated will likely bear a euphemistic notice such as "TREATED WITH IONIZING ENERGY" if current proposals become law. This will allow you to identify these products if you wish to avoid them until more is known about their effects.

Unfortunately not only do we have to contend with a loss of nutrients, which is bad enough, but with the deliberate addition of substances to our food which in many cases are not only unnecessary but actually harmful.

There are three main reasons that food manufacturers use *additives*, none of which have much to do with the nutritional quality of our food: for cosmetic purposes (to improve the appearance, taste and texture of foods that would have been perfectly fine if they had been left alone in the first place), for the prevention of oxidation (to increase the shelf life of foods so they can be transported longer distances and hang around the supermarket for greater lengths of time) and for convenience (to make dough more manageable, and so on). Following is a short summary of additives:

Preservatives: these can be added either to the food or the packaging. BHT and BHA are two common preservatives causing hyperactivity in some children. Sodium nitrite, added to some meats, when combined with amino acids forms nitrosamines which are carcinogenic.

Flavoring and flavor enhancers: Linda Pim in *Additive Alert* writes, "At present there are no controls on the quantities of flavour enhancers [for example, monosodium glutamate] used in Canadian food. Similarly, permitted levels for flavourings are absent from the

Food and Drug Regulations and most flavourings are not even listed
at all."

Coloring: many of the dyes used are coal-tar derivatives and may
be carcinogenic. Food dyes cause hyperactivity in some children.

Salt and sugar: these are added to foods in vast quantities, and are
implicated in many health problems. Excess salt may lead to high
blood pressure, and sugar, in addition to its negative effects on
children's behavior (not to mention their teeth), may also be a factor
in degenerative diseases such as cancer and heart disease. Sugar, as
mentioned previously, has little nutritional value and depletes the
body of many nutrients not only directly but also indirectly; in
common with refined foods, foods that contain sugar often displace
nutritious food from our children's diets. Both salt and sugar are
highly addictive for some people.

All the reasons for limiting sugar intake apply to other sweeteners
such as corn syrup and honey, as their nutrient content, although not
as low as white table sugar, is still generally insignificant. Commenting on sorbitol, made from mountain ash berries and found in diet
drinks and sugarless chewing gums, Powers and Presley write in
Food Power, "It has caused irritability and fatigue in some of my
patients." It is best to minimize the use of all sweeteners, whether
natural or artificial.

Others: there are a variety of other additives including those used
to polish, bleach, thicken, keep firm and prevent lumps in the food
we buy. A few lonely nutrients that have been refined out of foods are
sometimes added back, but the vast majority of nutrients lost due to
refining are not replaced. The metal aluminum in its various manifestations is an additive with many different functions, from helping
to bleach flour to acting as a preservative. Unfortunately aluminum
may be a factor in the learning and behavior problems of some
children.

It should be noted that additives from natural sources are not
always safer than additives made artificially. As Linda Pim writes in
Additive Alert, "Would you trust an all-natural extract of wild mushrooms? If not, then there is no reason to trust carrageenan in 'all-
natural' ice cream simply because the additive is extracted from
seaweed instead of being concocted in a laboratory. The source of a
food additive is not nearly as important as whether or not it is
actually necessary in the product and whether or not it has harmful
effects."

In addition to all the substances which are deliberately added to
our food, there are those which inadvertently contaminate our food
and which can sometimes be even more harmful. Some of these,

mentioned previously, are incorporated into our food sources while they are growing as a result either of farming techniques (application of pesticides, antibiotics and hormones) or of pollution (heavy metals such as lead, mercury and cadmium, radioactive materials and chemicals such as PCBs).

However, food can also be contaminated during processing and packaging, depending on what the equipment used is made of and what material is used in packaging.

For example, regarding canning, Linda Pim comments in *Invisible Additives* that ". . . poisoning from lead in tin cans is like an accident waiting to happen." This is due to the lead solder.

The most important factor determining the degree of lead contamination in canned food, she writes, is the food's pH level: "Metals dissolve more easily when the acidity is high . . . So, lead can be expected to be particularly high in canned fruit, fruit juices, and tomatoes. The longer a canned food is stored before opening and eating it, the higher the lead in it will be."

Other factors increasing the likelihood of lead contamination mentioned by Pim are the presence of oxygen (for example, leftover food stored in an open can in the refrigerator) and the food's nitrate content: "High-nitrate fertilizers often used in agriculture give rise to the high nitrate levels in foods. Nitrate causes 'detinning' in canned foods, an effect which increases with time in storage."

The phenolic resins in cans also migrate into foods, causing reactions in some children. Food that is wrapped or stored in plastic can absorb plastic molecules, some of which may be carcinogenic. Some plastics are treated with preservatives. Food can be contaminated with benzene which is in styrofoam.

Food products that are filtered, including sugar, lard and soft drinks, can be contaminated with asbestos. Linda Pim in *Invisible Additives* writes that asbestos can be carcinogenic not only when inhaled but also when ingested.

• STORAGE. As mentioned previously, foods may be contaminated by contact with plastic, aluminum or tin cans. Many nutrients are destroyed by exposure to light, heat and air. The longer a food is stored, the more likely it is to lose nutrients.

• PREPARATION. Nutrients may be lost by soaking foods in water, cooking at high heats for long periods of time (especially without the lid), and adding baking soda to the cooking water. Cooking with aluminum and copper pots and pans can unfortunately transfer these elements to food. Iron also migrates into food, which in some cases is beneficial if it helps children meet their iron requirements and does not cause an excess.

Nutritional Requirements

The quantities of nutrients required to supply each child's unique nutritional needs vary depending on stage of development, weight, state of health, level of activity, weather conditions, stress levels (both physical and emotional) and individual biochemical makeup. Needs of children even within the same age group or the same family can vary widely. In fact, a child's needs sometimes vary from day to day depending on many variables, and can be expected to change as the child gets older or as circumstances change.

For a rough guide to children's nutrient requirements, see the *Nutrition Almanac* chart below. This chart is largely based on the Recommended Dietary Allowances, and it is important to keep firmly in mind the following point: the suggested levels for RDAs are absolutely minimum requirements, and although these amounts may prevent severe deficiencies, they are set too low for the needs of most children, especially if the goal is optimum health.

Following is an abbreviated form of *Nutrition Almanac's* Nutrient Allowance Chart:

Children (Boys and Girls)

	0–6 mo	6 mo– 1 yr	1–3 yr	4–6 yr	7–10 yr
Carbohydrates, g	115		165	240	330
Fats, g	28		38	58	80
Protein, g	14	14	23	30	34
MINERALS					
Calcium, mg	360	540	800	800	800
Iodine, mcg	40	50	70	90	120
Iron, mg	10	15	15	10	10
Magnesium, mg	50	70	150	200	250
Phosphorus, mg	240	360	800	800	800
Potassium, mg	350– 925	425– 1275	550– 1650	775– 2325	1000– 3000
Sodium, mg	115– 350	250– 750	325– 975	450– 1350	600– 1800

Children (Boys and Girls)

	0–6 mo	6 mo– 1 yr	1–3 yr	4–6 yr	7–10 yr
VITAMINS					
Vitamin A, IU	1400	2000	2000	2500	3300
Vitamin B complex					
Thiamine (B1), mg	0.3	0.5	0.7	0.9	1.2
Riboflavin (B2), mg	0.4	0.6	0.8	1.0	1.4
Pyridoxine (B6), mg	0.3	0.6	0.9	1.3	1.6
Cyanocobalamin (B12), mcg	0.5	1.5	2.0	2.5	3.0
Biotin, mcg	35	50	65	85	120
Choline, mg*	Average daily intake 500–900 mg				
Folic acid, mg	.03	.045	0.1	0.2	0.3
Inositol, mg*					
Niacin, mg	6.0	8.0	9.0	11.0	16.0
Para-aminobenzoic acid (PABA), mg	No Recommended Dietary Allowance				
Pantothenic acid, mg	2.0	3.0	3.0	3.0–4.0	4.0–5.0
Vitamin C (ascorbic acid), mg	35.0	35.0	45.0	45.0	45.0
Vitamin D, IU	400.0	400.0	400.0	400.0	400.0
Vitamin E, IU	4.0	6.0	7.0	9.0	10.0
Vitamin K, mcg	12.0	10.0–20.0	15.0–30.0	20.0–40.0	30.0–60.0
TRACE MINERALS					
Chromium, mg	.01–.04	.02–.06	.02–.08	.03–.1	.05–.2
Copper, mg	.5–.7	.7–1.0	1–1.5	1.5–2	2–2.5
Fluoride, mg	.1–.5	.2–1.0	.5–1.5	1–2.5	1.5–2.5
Manganese, mg	.5–.7	.7–1.0	1.0–1.5	1.5–2	2–3
Molybdenum, mg	.03–.06	.04–.08	.05–.1	.06–.15	.1–.3
Selenium, mg	.01–.04	.02–.06	.02–.08	.03–.12	.05–2
Zinc, mg	3.0	5.0	10.0	10.0	10.0

	Girls		Boys	
	11–14 yr	15–18 yr	11–14 yr	15–18 yr
Carbohydrates, g	345	345	——	——
Fats, g	80	78		
Protein, g	46	46	45	56
MINERALS				
Calcium, mg	1200	1200	1200	1200
Iodine, mcg	150	150	150	150

	Girls		Boys	
	11–14 yr	*15–18 yr*	*11–14 yr*	*15–18 yr*
Iron, mg	18	18	18	18
Magnesium, mg	300	300	350	400
Phosphorus, mg	1200	1200	1200	1200
Potassium, mg	1525–4575	Adequate daily intake 1875–5625 mg	1525–4575	Average daily intake 1875–5625 mg
Sodium, mg	900–2700	Adequate daily intake 1100–3300 mg	900–2700	Average daily intake 1100–3300 mg

VITAMINS

Vitamin A, IU	4000	4000	5000	5000
Vitamin B complex				
Thiamine (B1), mg	1.1	1.1	1.4	1.4
Riboflavin (B2), mg	1.3	1.3	1.6	1.7
Pyridoxine (B6), mg	1.8	2.0	1.8	2.0
Cyanocobalamin (B12), mcg	3.0	3.0	3.0	3.0
Biotin, mcg	100–200	Adequate daily intake 150–300 mcg	100–200	Adequate daily intake 150–300 mcg
Choline, mg*	Average daily intake 500–900 mg			
Folic acid, mg	0.4	0.4	0.4	0.4
Inositol, mg*	Average daily intake 1,000 mg			
Niacin, mg	15	14	18	18
Para-aminobenzoic acid (PABA), mg	No Recommended Dietary Allowance			
Pantothenic acid, mg	4–7	Adequate daily intake 5–10 mg		
Vitamin C (ascorbic acid), mg	50	60	50	60
Vitamin D, IU	Adequate daily intake 400 IU			
Vitamin E, IU	12	12	12	15
Vitamin K, mcg	50–100	Adequate daily intake 300–500 mcg	50–100	Adequate daily intake 300–500 mcg

	Girls		Boys	
	11–14 yr	*15–18 yr*	*11–14 yr*	*15–18 yr*
TRACE MINERALS				
Chromium, mg	.05–.2	Adequate daily intake .05–.2 mg	.05–.2	Adequate daily intake .05–.2 mg
Copper, mg	2.0–3.0	Adequate daily intake 2–3 mg	2–3	Adequate daily intake 2–3 mg
Fluoride, mg	1.5–2.5	Adequate daily intake 1.5–4 mg	1.5–2.5	Adequate daily intake 1.5–4 mg
Manganese, mg	2.5–5.0	Adequate daily intake 2.5–5 mg	2.5–5	Adequate daily intake 2.5–5 mg
Molybdenum, mg	.15–.5	Adequate daily intake .15–.5 mg	.15–.5	Adequate daily intake .15–.5 mg
Selenium, mg	.05–.2	Adequate daily intake .05–.2 mg	.05–.2	Adequate daily intake .05–.2 mg
Zinc, mg	15	15	15	15

*Robert S. Goodhart and Maurice E. Shils, *Modern Nutrition in Health and Disease*, 5th ed. (Philadelphia: Lea and Febiger, 1973), p. 263.

It should be noted that children need a steady supply of nutrients throughout the day; for this reason, they should not skip meals, particularly breakfast. For many children, five or so small but nutritious feedings a day are best, to keep blood sugar levels normal.

It should also be noted that although ideally children's diets should provide all their nutrient needs, due to a combination of the scarcity of high-quality food and some children's particularly high nutrient requirements, this is not always possible. (For information on nutritional supplements see Chapter 11.)

IS POOR NUTRITION CAUSING OUR CHILDREN'S PROBLEMS?

Poor nutrition is probably the major cause of learning and behavior problems. Some of the clues suggesting that children's diets need improving were mentioned in Chapter 8. These included the consumption of large quantities of processed foods (refined, sweetened, colored and flavored), the avoidance of major food groups (for example, a refusal to eat vegetables), excessive thinness, obesity, meals often skipped or extremely small amounts eaten, few home-cooked meals (for example, replaced by food from restaurants and fast-food joints or by institutional eating such as at school cafeterias or in hospital).

It is important to note that the nutrient most commonly deficient in children is iron, and that there is some evidence linking iron deficiency with learning problems.

The foods most incriminated in children's learning and behavior problems (in addition to nutritionally sound foods which may cause food sensitivities in some children as described in Chapter 14) are foods that are highly refined, highly sweetened, colored with food dyes, preserved with BHA or BHT, contaminated with metals such as lead, mercury and aluminum, and contain caffeine. Other additives and contaminants may also cause problems, as each child reacts individually to each substance.

The first step in evaluating a child's diet is to keep a symptom diary for a week as outlined in Chapter 8. This will give us an overall picture of the strengths and weaknesses of the diet. A fast but imprecise method of evaluation is to pick a nutritionally representative day from the week (or alternatively, tally up the totals for the week and divide by seven to get an average day) and use the information to fill out the chart on page 124.

Beside each food category on the chart simply write in the number of servings of food or liquid eaten or drunk that day. (Suggested serving sizes are given in each section but are best used as a guide only, as nutritional needs vary from child to child depending on age, size and other variables.) No food portion should be counted more than once. That is, the choice is ours whether to enter a portion of steamed broccoli into the vegetable category, vitamin C-sources category or calcium-sources category, as long as it is listed in only one of these categories.

FRESH WHOLE FOODS
—green vegetables
—yellow vegetables
—other vegetables
—vitamin C-rich fruits or vegetables (citrus fruits, melons, tomatoes, broccoli, green peppers)
suggested: 4 servings vegetables and fruits per day minimum, preferably raw or steamed and at least two of them yellow or green. One serving is approximately ½ cup (125 ml) raw or cooked or the equivalent of 1 medium apple or potato.

—whole grains (in bread, cereals, pasta)
suggested: 4 servings daily. One serving is approximately 1 slice of bread or ½ cup (125 ml) of cereal or pasta.

—calcium sources (dairy products, soy, sesame seeds, almonds, dark green, leafy vegetables)
suggested: 3-4 servings daily. One serving is approximately 1 cup (250 ml) milk, yogurt or cottage cheese, 1 ounce cheddar cheese, 2 cups cooked soybeans or 8 ounces tofu, 2 tablespoons unhulled sesame seeds or ¼ cup sesame meal, 1 cup almonds, 1 cup cooked collard leaves, bok choy or kale or 1½ stalks cooked broccoli.

It is important to note that children not receiving their calcium from milk must be extra careful to ensure that vitamin D intake is adequate, especially when exposure to the sun is limited. Particularly in cold climates supplements such as halibut liver oil may be necessary.

—protein sources (meat, fish, poultry, eggs, dairy products, legumes, nuts and seeds)
suggested: minimum 2 (2–3 ounce) servings daily.

—water
suggested: minimum of 6 servings. One serving is 1 cup (250 ml), perhaps somewhat smaller for younger children.

PROCESSED AND SWEETENED FOODS
—Sweet treats (candies, chocolate bars, gum, baked goods, ice cream, sugared cereals, fruit canned in syrup, etc.)
—Sugar and/or caffeine drinks (soft drinks, chocolate milk, fruit drinks, Kool-Aid, coffee, tea, etc.)
—Refined foods (white bread, white rice, refined cereals and pasta, etc.)

___Fast food items/convenience foods (hamburgers, pizzas, french fries, prepared meats, TV dinners, etc.)

suggested: that the amount of processed and sweetened foods consumed be restricted.

If large amounts of processed and sweetened foods are being consumed, children's diets may be nutritionally deficient and need to be improved.

A longer but much more accurate and informative method of judging the nutritional status of a child's diet is to compare the exact daily nutrient intake with the *Nutrition Almanac* table of minimum daily nutrient requirements on pages 153–156. (Books such as *Nutrition Almanac* and *Laurel's Kitchen* contain tables giving nutrient values for different foods.) This will give us some idea of the child's dietary nutrient deficiencies, indicating which foods should be increased in the diet.

Two alternatives to doing a diet analysis ourselves are either to consult a nutritionist or to find a place that uses a computer program to analyze diets.

Once we know what areas of a diet need improvement, we can put our knowledge into practice and see what effect this has.

Implementing the Diet Program

When ready to implement the diet program, keep in mind that our aim is to feed children meals that include all the essential nutrients and restrict foods that are either nutritionally valueless or harmful. The recipe for a good diet is: lots of fresh vegetables, fruits, whole grains, dairy products, nuts and seeds, protein sources and water, and a minimum of food that is refined, processed, sweetened or contaminated. An important point to remember is that children should avoid foods they are sensitive to, making sure of course to supply the missed nutrients from other sources.

Following is an outline of the steps involved in implementing a diet program:

1. PLANNING. The first step is to sit down for a few minutes to plan a week's menus, and from this make up a shopping list.

In planning children's meals, it is worthwhile considering the approach taken by the New York Institute for Child Development as mentioned in their book *Treating Your Hyperactive and Learning Disabled Child:* "*Appetite and feeding habits* are considered before we recommend a diet. Diet recommendations must be realistic and take texture and taste into consideration. A child who does not eat foods with a mushy consistency may go hungry on a regimen of boiled chicken, brown rice, and squash." Even a preschooler can participate in menu planning by contributing likes and dislikes.

When making menus, take into account the following points concerning various nutrients:

• *Proteins* are made up of amino acids. Although the majority of these can be made by the body, there are eight which can only be supplied from food. Foods which contain all eight essential amino acids are called complete proteins, and include fish, meat, poultry and dairy products. Foods missing or containing low levels of one or more of these eight amino acids are called incomplete proteins and include most vegetables, fruits, grains and legumes. However, it is possible to make a complete protein meal by combining two (or more) incomplete protein foods that contain the essential amino acids missing in the other. For example, grains and legumes generally complement each other to make up complete proteins. In *Diet for a Small Planet*, a vegetarian cookbook, Frances Moore Lappé gives more specific information on combining proteins. It is important that during the course of a day (not necessarily at each meal, though complete protein meals are probably a good habit to get into to ensure a child's adequate protein intake) all the essential amino acids be present in the diet so the body's cells can work more effectively.

(With a bit of care a child's protein needs can easily be met on a meatless diet, but it should be noted that a strictly vegetarian diet excluding all meat, eggs and dairy products is deficient in vitamin B12, making it important for vegan children to be supplemented with this vitamin.)

Because children are still growing and developing, their protein needs are comparatively higher than those of adults. The consequences of a low-protein diet are much more serious for them, possibly resulting in, among other things, inhibited growth and mental retardation. On the other hand, eating too much protein can cause water imbalance, malabsorption and increased loss of calcium, phosphorus, iron and zinc.

• The best *carbohydrates* to include in a child's diet are complex carbohydrates, such as those found in whole grains, vegetables, dairy products, legumes, and nuts and seeds. As with other nutrients, carbohydrate requirements are variable.

The possible dangers of eating too many refined carbohydrates are the disruption of glucose levels which will affect the functioning of the brain and obesity. Excessive carbohydrate intake increases the need for the B vitamins, as these are necessary for carbohydrate metabolism.

The possible dangers of eating too few carbohydrates are the use of protein for energy purposes rather than for its other main functions, the accumulation of poisonous acids in the body which can negatively affect a child's growth, and depression and weakness.

• The melting points, flavors and textures of fats are determined by acids they contain, called fatty acids. *Saturated* fatty acids are usually solid at room temperature, like butter and congealed meat fat, and are usually derived from animal sources—meat or dairy products; coconut oil is the chief plant source. *Unsaturated* fatty acids are liquid at room temperature; most of us are familiar with them in the form of cooking and salad oils produced from plants such as safflower, sunflower and corn. Unsaturated fats can be forced into a form that will stay hard at room temperature by hydrogenating them—adding hydrogen to the fatty acid molecules—which is how we get margarine and vegetable shortenings.

The human body produces many fatty acids, but not three important ones, which must be supplied by the diet and are therefore called "essential." The essential fatty acids are linoleic, linolenic and arachidonic. They are of the unsaturated type and are vital to our health. Because the brain does most of its growing and developing in the early years of life, children up to the age of three or so have relatively greater needs for the essential fatty acids; arachidonic acid in particular is necessary for this brain spurt.

Too much fat can cause obesity. A high-fat intake (of both saturated and polyunsaturated fats) has been implicated in heart disease and some cancers (although fish oils in moderate amounts appear to have a role in preventing heart disease).

The more polyunsaturated fats in the diet, the greater the vitamin E and vitamin A requirements. Polyunsaturated fats when heated at high temperatures may form harmful byproducts.

• Some foods contain substances which can hinder the effectiveness of certain nutrients in the body. For example: Foods such as uncooked legumes (dried beans and peanuts) contain enzyme inhibitors which interfere with the digestion of *protein*. The absorption of *thiamine* (vitamin B1) is interfered with by the antivitamin thiaminase, which occurs in raw fish, shellfish, some berries, Brussels sprouts and red cabbage. *Biotin*'s absorption is interfered with by the antivitamin avidin, which occurs in raw eggs. (The avidin is destroyed when the eggs are cooked.) Substances that may interfere with the absorption of *calcium* are oxalic acid (found in beet greens, chard, rhubarb and spinach), excess fiber, and phytic acid (found in bran and some whole grains). *Iron* and *zinc* may also be affected by phytic acid. Members of the cabbage family contain goitrogens which interfere with *iodine* in the body.

As mentioned in a previous section, this does not mean these foods should be avoided; on the contrary, most of them have a great deal to contribute to a healthy diet. The only caution is that they not be eaten in large quantities to the exclusion of other foods.

• Sunlight in reasonable amounts is a nutrient booster, enabling children to synthesize *Vitamin D* in their bodies.

• Some vitamins and minerals are depleted in the body by the use of medicines such as antacids, antibiotics, aspirin, alcohol-containing cough syrups, milk of magnesia, mineral oil and phenobarbital.

• The most familiar method of purifying water is boiling it, but this is not a good idea if done for a long time. Even though hostile microorganisms will be killed, in the process pollutants such as toxic metals and nitrates become more concentrated. A combination of distilling—boiling the water but capturing the steam and then cooling it back to water again—and reverse osmosis is probably the most effective way of purifying water, especially in removing nonliving toxins. This method, though, also eliminates many important minerals, which means that we have to obtain them from food or from supplements.

Our best choice is unpolluted and untreated fresh well water containing a healthy mineral content. If we do not have access to well water such as this or a home purifier, it is important to run our drinking water for a few minutes every morning before use, as water that has been standing for a length of time is more likely to be contaminated.

2. FOOD SHOPPING. How we shop for food is a major factor in our ability to provide nutritious meals. The widespread use of additives and inadvertent contamination of food requires that we all become critical shoppers. This means actively informing ourselves about the foods we buy by asking the following questions:

• *Under what conditions did the food grow?* For example, fish from waters free of mercury will be safer to eat than those from waters containing mercury, and farmers who use organic methods of farming will generally produce food less chemically contaminated than those who use the more common agricultural methods.

Unfortunately, however, it is impossible to produce food that is completely pure in this polluted world (even an unsprayed crop may be contaminated with pesticides if the soil it is grown in contains pesticides or if pesticides are blown over by the wind from a sprayed crop). For this reason it is important to find out what the maximum allowed level of contamination is for any food that is labeled organic, as standards may vary. Standards for food that is not labeled organic also vary, as food imported from other countries may contain chemicals that have been banned in our own countries.

• *How far has the food traveled?* Food is more likely to be fresh if it is in season and locally grown.

• *How long has it been sitting on the shelf, and in what conditions?* If a store does not have a high turnover, food may tend to be stale. Proper coolers for perishables are also important.

• *Which processing method has the food been subjected to?* Appearances can deceive. For example, a loaf of bread that looks like whole wheat may only be 60 percent, with food coloring added to make it look darker.

If the food item does not have a label, we should not hesitate to check the food out with the store manager, food manufacturer or farmer. If the food item does have a label, we should be aware that the information may be incomplete or misleading; it is important to understand both the importance of reading the small print on labels and the limitations of labels. In this regard Brett Silverstein in *Fed Up!* has some useful comments.

He points out that while to most people "natural" means "without anything artificial," the food industry doesn't see it that way. He notes that while a product labeled "natural" will contain at least one natural ingredient, it may also contain artificial ingredients such as BHA and artificial colors and flavors. He makes a further point:

> The labeling laws allow the manufacturers to leave hundreds of ingredients off the labels. If in the official food standards of the FDA an ingredient is listed as "optional," it must be mentioned on the label. But if the ingredient is listed as "permissible" for a particular kind of food, it need not be mentioned.
> As a result, there is no way, short of doing a chemical analysis, for anyone but the manufacturer to know exactly what ingredients are included in most foods. Sometimes the laws mandate that an ingredient be listed on the labels of some foods but not others. Emulsifying agents, for example, must be listed on pasteurized, processed food but not on pasteurized, processed cheese. In addition, some ingredients are included on labels only in vague, general categories like "batter and breading ingredients" mentioned on breaded shrimp labels.

Even an accurate and complete list can be used misleadingly, Silverstein adds. Sugar can be listed in several different ways—for one product, a variety of canned baked beans, he gives six: invert sugar, molasses, brown sugar, corn syrup, sugar and apple concentrate— concealing the fact that the product may be predominantly sugar.

(Concerning labels and sugar, see also page 196 in chapter 12 on hypoglycemia.)

According to Linda Pim in *Additive Alert*, there are some ingredients which do not have to be listed in descending order of weight on the label. "Those ingredients which may be shown at the end of the list in any order are: spices, seasonings, herbs (except salt); natural and artificial flavors; flavor enhancers; food additives; vitamins and their salts or derivatives; minerals and their salts. You therefore never really know how much azodicarbonamide is in that loaf of bread. . . ."

Linda Pim also gives examples of some of the ingredients that are not required by law to be listed on labels, such as mineral oil used to grease bread pans, preservatives which are added to cereal boxes and migrate into the cereal, anti-caking agents (to prevent clumping) in table salt and baking powder, and some substances which have been added to an ingredient used to make a food item. (For example, butter may be listed on the label of a food product, but the coloring that the butter may contain might not be listed.)

3. STORAGE. In order to prevent nutrient loss, most food should be stored in a cool dark place (often a refrigerator is the best place) in air-tight containers, as some nutrients are destroyed by exposure to air, light and heat. Storing food in containers that are least likely to react with the food, such as glass or stainless steel, is preferable to storing food in plastic (containers, bags or wraps), aluminum (pots or foil), or in tin cans (especially open ones). Food should be stored the least amount of time possible.

4. PREPARATION. Food should be washed before eating to remove surface pollutants, but not soaked, which might remove some of the nutrients. It is a toss-up whether it is best to peel or not to peel. On the one hand, many nutrients are lost when the outer leaves and peel of vegetables and fruits are removed, while on the other hand, these parts are more likely to contain contaminants such as pesticides. (Then again, in some cases the whole fruit or vegetable is permeated with pesticides.) Contaminants tend to concentrate in animal fat, which should for this reason alone be cut away before cooking. Nutrient loss can be kept to a minimum by cooking food in the shortest time necessary at low heats with the pots covered; a large proportion of food in the diet should be raw (except when cooking

for very young children). Steaming is generally better than boiling or frying. The water used in cooking contains many of the nutrients lost from the food, and can be recycled into soups, as the liquid for the cooking of grains, and so on. Care should be taken not to use pots and pans that may react with food. Unfortunately, aluminum cookware is common, but it should be avoided so as not to contaminate children's food, as should copper cookware which destroys vitamin C (and may also help increase copper to excessive levels in some children). Iron also leaches into food; however this may be acceptable depending on the individual child's iron requirements.

5. MEALTIME. Meals should be regular, and as calm and pleasant as possible; tension can interfere with digestion.

6. EXERCISE. Regular exercise is an extremely important factor in healthy digestion and absorption and should be automatically included in any diet program (see pages 263–265 in Chapter 18).

7. EXPERIMENTATION. The only way to find the optimum diet for each child is by giving careful thought to individual needs, and, ultimately, by trial and error. Some children will do better with more calories and some with less, and so on; we will have to experiment and observe.

8. EDUCATION. The more children understand about nutrition and the effect that food has on them, the more likely they are to actually eat the food we prepare. (See Chapter 6 for more information on cooperating children.) Part of education is simply getting used to different tasting foods.

9. ATTITUDE. A sense of fun and adventure will go a long way in encouraging acceptance of a new diet. The sooner we and our children reassign food values—let's hear it for vegetables, down with sugar—the less resistance we will face.

One important ingredient of attitude is the recognition that it is nearly impossible to attain a perfect diet. Lack of time and money, not to mention the difficulties in finding high quality food, are only a few of the obstacles that conspire against our best efforts. There are ways to minimize these obstacles (see Chapters 3, 5, 6 and 7), but inevitably some compromises will be forced on us. It is important not to fret too much about any dietary imperfections or we may find ourselves giving up on the diet before barely getting started. All we can do is try our best.

Testing the Hypothesis that Diet Is a Factor in Our Children's Problems

Many learning and behavior problems will disappear, or at least diminish, with an improvement in diet. Sometimes changes will be noticeable in four or five days; other times three weeks or a month will pass before children show signs of getting better. If significant improvement does occur, this supports the hypothesis that diet was the cause of our children's problems.

If after a month of nutritious eating there is either no improvement or only moderate improvement, we can suspect other factors are involved in our children's problems besides diet. Unfortunately, sometimes children's nutritional needs are not met despite excellent diets. This can happen in cases of faulty digestion or absorption, or when children have above normal requirements for certain nutrients due to individual biochemical makeup or other factors. (See Chapter 11.) In addition, children on high-quality diets may not improve due to hypoglycemia (Chapter 12), food and environmental sensitivities (Chapters 14 and 15), heavy metal toxicity (Chapter 16), stress (page 268 in Chapter 18) or illness. Or the effectiveness of the diet might be lessened due to lack of exercise.

It is crucial to remember that even when diet seems to make no difference, it is still essential that children continue to eat nutritiously. Children on good diets are more likely to respond to other parts of the treatment program, and nutritious eating is the best method there is of preventing current problems from worsening and future problems from starting.

Books referred to in this chapter and other suggested reading:

Additive Alert: A Guide to Food Additives for the Canadian Consumer, Linda Pim. Doubleday, New York, 1979. A handy informative book including explanations of the different types of additives, their dangers and misuses, and material on federal laws, labeling and who to contact about concerns.

Children's Nutrition, A Consumer's Guide, Lewis A. Coffin, Capra Press, Santa Barbara, California, 1984. A useful, well-written book which covers a lot of areas including weight control for children, exercise, healthy vs. non-healthy food, vitamins and minerals, etc.

The Complete Eater's Digest and Nutrition Scoreboard, The Consumer's Factbook of Food Additives and Healthful Eating, Michael F. Jacobson. Anchor Press/Doubleday, New York, 1985. This is a very helpful, informative book covering various aspects of nutrition. The section which describes common food additives and their relative safety is extremely useful.

The Cook's Book, Howard Hillman, Avon Books, New York, 1981. Fascinating reading: starts at abalone and ends at yogurt, with information about each entry's background, availability, how to choose, storage, preparation, cooking.

Diet for a Small Planet, Frances Moore Lappé. Ballantine Books, New York, 1976. A vegetarian cookbook with delicious recipes and helpful information.

Fed Up! The Food Forces That Make You Fat, Sick and Poor, Brett Silverstein. South End Press, Boston, 1984. An excellent description and analysis of the U.S. food system (much of which will apply to other countries), with chapters on farming, technology, processing, marketing, food preparation and the family, advertising, education, health, eating disorders, government and world hunger.

Feeding Your Child, From Infancy to Six Years Old, Louise Lambert-Lagace. Stoddart Publishing Co. Limited, Toronto, 1982. A helpful book, including information on prenatal eating, breast-feeding and different diets for each age group, as well as recipes.

Food Power: Nutrition and Your Child's Behavior, Hugh Powers and James Presley. St. Martin's Press, New York, 1978. For a further description, see Chapter 12.

The Invisible Additives: Environmental Contaminants in Our Food. Linda R. Pim, Doubleday, New York, 1981. An excellent book containing a thorough and informative discussion of the additives that inadvertently find their way into the food chain due to industrial wastes, the use of antibiotics and pesticides, etc.

Laurel's Kitchen, Laurel Robertson, Carol Flinders, and Bronwen Godfrey. Bantam Books, New York, 1978. A wonderful vegetarian cookbook containing not only lots of excellent recipes but a wealth of information about food and nutrition.

Nourishing Your Child, A Bioecologic Approach, Ray C. Wunderlich, Jr. and Dwight K. Kalita, Keats Publishing, Inc., New Canaan, Connecticut, 1984. For a descripton, see Chapter 8.

Nutrition Almanac, Nutrition Search, Inc., McGraw-Hill Book Company, New York, 1984. An excellent book with extremely useful and complete information on vitamins, minerals and other nutrients and their relation to health. Includes an extensive table of food composition.

Radiation Alert, A Consumer's Guide to Radiation, David I. Poch. Doubleday, New York, 1985. For a description, see Chapter 17.

Treating Your Hyperactive and Learning Disabled Child, What You Can Do, The New York Institute for Child Development, Inc. with Richard J. Walsh. Anchor Press/Doubleday, New York, 1979. Discusses nutrition and motor skills and gives exercises for developing sensorimotor abilities.

11 A NEED FOR
NUTRITIONAL SUPPLEMENTS

S ome children with learning and behavior problems have a
need for larger amounts of nutrients than can be supplied from
food alone, and improve satisfactorily only when nutritional
supplements such as vitamins, minerals, enzymes and amino acids
are introduced into their diet.

There are a number of reasons why food may not provide children
with an adequate supply of nutrients, making nutritional supplements a necessity for optimum health. For example:

• Children eating a poor quality diet for a long period of time may
suffer from nutritional deficiencies. In such cases, larger amounts of
nutrients than are normally found in food are often required for the
correction of these deficiencies.

Unfortunately, it cannot be safely assumed that children whose
diets exclude junk food are necessarily eating well; even food that is
whole and unsweetened is not always abundant in nutrients. For
example, no matter how nutritious the vegetables in the produce
section may look, chances are they have been grown in nutrient-poor
soil, sprayed several times and transported over long distances. (For
more information on the nutritional quality of food, see Chapter 10.)

• Deficiencies can also result from the use of certain drugs and
medicines.

• A diet excluding major food groups due to food sensitivities
may make nutritional supplementation necessary.

• A faulty digestive system may mean that larger amounts of
certain nutrients than found in food are required to ensure the availability of those nutrients to the body. In some cases poor digestion
not only contributes to a state of nutritional deficiency but has in fact
been caused by a lack of certain nutrients.

• In the case of nutritional dependencies, some children are born
with a greater than normal requirement for certain nutrients because
of their genetic makeup, so that even a diet of the highest quality will
be unable to meet those needs.

• Excess stress (due to illness, environmental toxins, sensitivities
or psychological pressures) can also increase nutrient requirements.

If nutrient requirements are not fulfilled, children may suffer both physically and mentally. Deficiencies and dependencies can have devastating effects on the development and health of children, including impaired growth, retardation, psychosis and diseases such as scurvy, pellagra, beriberi and rickets. Some children suffer from fatigue, irritability and lack of concentration, others from hallucinations, violent outbursts and refusal or inability to speak. Although many children have relatively mild symptoms and get along fairly well in their daily lives, in extreme cases some children are barely able to function on a day-to-day level.

Do our Children Need Nutritional Supplementation?

Some of the clues suggesting that children might benefit from nutritional supplementation were mentioned in Chapter 8. These included the existence of nutritional dependencies or deficiencies among other family members, poor dietary habits over a long period of time, problems that persist despite a high quality diet and the avoidance of known sensitivity-causing foods and substances, a diagnosis of schizophrenia, autism or mental retardation (including Down's syndrome) and the existence of excess physical and/or mental stress.

In addition, nutritional supplementation is sometimes helpful for children suffering from food and environmental sensitivities, hypoglycemia, drug-related problems and heavy metal toxicity.

There are some physical indicators of a need for extra nutrients, such as white spots on the nails, possibly due to a lack of pyridoxine (vitamin B6) and/or zinc, but since most physical manifestations are not so specific they could be caused by many things. It is important to note that a need for extra nutrients may exist even when there are no obvious physical signs. (Possible symptoms of deficiencies are mentioned in the description of individual nutrients starting on page 181.)

Tests involving blood, urine and hair can be useful in helping to pinpoint which if any nutrients children are lacking.

It is important to remember, however, that these tests are, for the most part, simply *indicators* of possible problems. Mistakes may happen during the collecting of the specimen, in the lab, in the bureaucracy (for example a mix-up in names or a lost report), or in the interpretation of the test results. Any of these errors, all of which do happen, may result in incorrect information.

Error aside, there is the intrinsic nature of the material being worked with that may lead to misleading results. For example, the nutrient values that appear in blood, urine or hair may not correspond to the amounts that are in various body tissues. Blood and urine may indicate only that day's nutritional status (that is, what was eaten or not eaten for a short period of time before the test), rather than long-term excesses or deficiencies. Hair analysis is most useful in providing information concerning minerals and toxic metals rather than vitamins or amino acids. The results must be interpreted by someone familiar with the field of hair analysis. For example, high zinc levels may actually indicate a deficiency of zinc; and often it is the ratio between two minerals that is important rather than the actual values of each individual mineral. (See pages 248–249 in Chapter 16 for a further discussion of hair analysis.)

A "therapeutic trial"—designing a supplement program, trying it out for a period of time and then noting the results—is also a valid testing method and one which many of us will end up using either alone or in conjunction with other tests such as hair analysis. Its main drawback is the length of time needed to get results. Ultimately, however, a series of therapeutic trials is the only way to find out precisely and definitively what a child's nutritional needs are. This method of testing should be done in cooperation with a doctor. In the next section is a more detailed description of the supplementation program, which will give information useful in designing a therapeutic trial.

The Supplementation Program

Designing an effective supplementation program involves many considerations. Following are brief discussions of some of these considerations.

Which Nutrients Should Be Included
in the Supplement Program?

A supplementation program for children with learning and behavior problems as suggested by most nutritional/environmental doctors centers on the B-complex vitamins—especially thiamine (B1), riboflavin (B2), niacin or niacinamide (B3), pyridoxine (B6), cyanocobalamin (B12) and pantothenic acid, with special emphasis on niacin/niacinamide and pyridoxine—as well as vitamin C and minerals magnesium and zinc.

(The supplementation program is of course meant to be used in conjunction with a junk-free, high quality diet and control of other nutritional/environmental factors such as hypoglycemia, sensitivities and heavy metal toxicities.)

Other nutrients are added according to the needs of the individual child. In addition to the nutrients already mentioned, other nutrients commonly included in a supplementation program are vitamins A, D and E, the essential fatty acids, minerals calcium, chromium, iron, manganese and selenium, and amino acids such as tryptophan.

Below is a summary of which nutrients may help control specific problems. Please note that the categories are not necessarily as distinct as they may appear in black and white; a great deal of overlap can be expected as many children fall into more than one category. For example, a child who has been diagnosed as schizophrenic may have hypoglycemia and various food and environmental sensitivities as well as an inborn requirement for higher than average amounts of nutrients. Or the hypoglycemic symptoms of some children may be caused by sensitivities, which in turn are related to digestive problems, and their digestive problems may be caused by a lack of certain nutrients. Unfortunately, it is not yet always possible to clearly define the precise origins of a specific problem. For this reason it is best to use whichever combination of supplements and other aspects of the nutritional/environmental program works, even when it is not known why that combination works.

It should be mentioned that terms like schizophrenia, autism, hyperactivity and retardation are used in this book purely as a shorthand method of describing certain sets of symptoms and in no way imply that there is one specific cause to that symptom cluster. Some children exhibit schizophrenia-like symptoms due to food or environmental sensitivities, others due to hypgolycemia, others in absence of nutritional supplementation. The same applies to other diagnoses. However, the more severe the symptoms, the more likely it is that more than one factor is involved and that nutritional supplementation will help ameliorate the symptoms. Nutrients often have a role to play in the control of a variety of problems, such as the following:

• Children suffering from NUTRITIONAL DEFICIENCIES will benefit from the supplementation of the nutrients they are deficient in plus associated support nutrients.

• Children suffering from NUTRITIONAL DEPENDENCIES associated with mental, emotional and behavioral symptoms (often resulting in diagnoses of schizophrenia, autism, hyperactivity and mental retardation) may benefit from taking supplements of vitamins niacin/niacinamide, pyridoxine and C, and minerals magnesium and zinc.

As will be mentioned further on, it is best to give these in combination with a number of other related nutrients.

(Parents of children with Down's syndrome should note the work of Dr. Henry Turkel, whose book *Medical Treatment of Down Syndrome and Genetic Disease* is mentioned at the end of this chapter. Dr. Turkel appears to have good success treating Down's syndrome with the "U" series, which includes a combination of vitamins, minerals, unsaturated fatty acids, digestive enzymes and thyroid supplements, plus a few medications.)

• Children suffering from FOOD AND/OR ENVIRONMENTAL SENSITIVITIES may benefit from taking vitamins A, B-complex (especially pantothenic acid), C, D and E, the essential fatty acids, and minerals calcium, magnesium and selenium. (See Chapters 14 and 15 for information on food and environmental sensitivities.)

• Children suffering from HYPOGLYCEMIA may benefit from taking the B-complex vitamins (pyridoxine, cyanocobalamin and pantothenic acid in particular), vitamin C, the essential fatty acids, and the mineral chromium. (See Chapter 12 for information on hypoglycemia.)

• Children suffering from HEAVY METAL TOXICITY may benefit from taking vitamins C and E and minerals calcium and zinc. Selenium is also helpful in some cases but should be used only in small doses and with great caution due to its potential toxicity. (See Chapter 16 for information on heavy metal toxicities.)

• Children suffering from YEAST OVERGROWTH may benefit from taking supplements of garlic, *Lactobacillus acidophilus*, caprylic acid (a short chain fatty acid), as well as vitamins A, B-complex, C and E, minerals calcium, magnesium, zinc and essential fatty acids. (See Chapter 13 for information on yeast overgrowth.)

• Children suffering from SLEEP PROBLEMS may benefit from taking niacinamide, inositol, vitamin C, calcium, magnesium and the amino acids tryptophan, phenylalanine and tyrosine.

• Children born to addicted parents or who are or who have been DRUG ABUSERS themselves may benefit from B-complex vitamins (especially choline, niacin/niacinamide, pyridoxine, cyanocobalamin and pantothenic acid), vitamin C (usually in the form of sodium ascorbate) and vitamin E.

Bernard Green, in his book *Getting Over Getting High*, writes that large doses of choline will help minimize symptoms when withdrawing from stimulants (caffeine, amphetamines, marijuana, hashish and hallucinogens). The minimum amount of choline that he suggests for an *adult* is 500 mg. three times a day.

• Children who have DIGESTIVE PROBLEMS may benefit from taking digestive enzymes, *Lactobacillus acidophilus* (there are some types available not derived from milk), and the B vitamin complex (especially thiamine, niacin/niacinamide and pyridoxine). In some cases an acid/alkaline imbalance may be present, and supplements such as glutamic acid hydrochloride or sodium bicarbonate may be helpful, but only under strict medical supervision. (See page 177 further on in this chapter and page 266 in Chapter 18 for more information on digestion.)

• Children undergoing a period of EMOTIONAL STRESS may benefit from a general program of nutrient supplementation, with special emphasis on the B-complex vitamins, vitamin C, calcium, magnesium and zinc. (See pages 268–274 in Chapter 18 for more information on control of stress.)

When deciding which nutrients to include in a supplement program, it is crucial to remember that nutrients work best when balanced with each other. In other words, nutrients do not work in isolation in the body and should not be supplemented in isolation, or this may cause a depletion of other vitamins or minerals. For example, the B vitamins should generally be taken together, calcium should not be supplemented without magnesium and large doses of vitamin C can cause the body to lose some minerals.

It is not only a question of depletion, however, as many nutrients simply do their jobs better when adequate amounts of specific other nutrients are present, such as selenium increasing the effectiveness of vitamin E.

Following is an example of what a nutritional schedule might include. The actual nutrients and dosages will of course vary from child to child, depending on such factors as physical and mental symptoms and their severity, age and weight of the child and the tolerance level of the child for each nutrient. Some children will need either higher or lower dosages, some will need only a few of the nutrients listed below, and some will need totally different combinations. It is important to work out the specifics of any individual nutritional supplementation program with a doctor knowledgeable in nutrition.

Vitamin A: 5,000–15,000 I.U. (International Units)
    Vitamin B2: 100–200 mg. (mg. stands for milligrams)
    Vitamin B3: 100–3,000 mg.
    Vitamin B6: 100–300 mg.
    Pantothenic acid: 10–300 mg.
    Vitamin C: 100–3,000 mg.
    Bioflavonoids: 50–600 mg.
    Vitamin D: 400 I.U.

Vitamin E: 50–400 I.U.
Calcium: 250–1,000 mg.
Magnesium 75–350 mg.
Zinc: 10–30 mg.
Iron: 7.5–15 mg.
Selenium: 100–200 micrograms
Chromium: 100–200 micrograms
B-complex: 25–100 mg. of each B vitamin except folic acid
     (30–400 micrograms), biotin (10–25 mcg.) and B12 (5–10
     micrograms)
Amino acids such as tryptophan, cysteine and tyrosine:
     400–1,000 mg. each

Which Dosage of Each Nutrient Should Be Chosen?

Most doctors using a nutritional/environmental approach treat children with behavioral problems with nutrients in dosages higher than would ordinarily be found in food, as these higher dosages often seem to be required before improvement will occur.

Finding the most effective nutrient dosage for each child is at this point in time (in common with much of medical practice) a combination of educated guesswork and trial and error. Taking into account the child's weight and age (in general, very young children should receive dosages only in the lowest ranges), the results of lab tests, and severity and nature of the problem, an optimum dosage is postulated. The dosage of the nutrient is then gradually increased, watching carefully for any adverse effects, until the proposed optimum dosage is reached. (Of course, if there are any adverse effects stop immediately and check with the doctor.) If there is no improvement when children have been on the proposed optimum dosage for a good length of time, a higher dosage may be indicated (taking care to stay within safe guidelines). However, if children seem to be steadily improving on a specific dosage, increasing the dosage will not necessarily make the improvement more rapid and may in some cases affect children adversely.

The vitamins to be most concerned about in terms of taking excessive amounts are vitamins A and D, as these are fat-soluble; this means they are stored in the body and can be toxic if too much is taken. The other vitamins, being water-soluble (except for vitamin E which is also fat-soluble but appears to have a low toxicity, and vitamin K which is rarely supplemented) are not as dangerous as A and D can be, but may have unpleasant side effects. Some of the minerals can be toxic and should be dealt with cautiously.

Read dosage information on labels carefully; generally information is given in terms of nutrient quantities for *one* capsule or tablet, but sometimes the amounts given refer to the total quantities of *three or more* capsules or tablets.

Because many supplement preparations contain several nutrients (which is often convenient and limits the amount of fillers a child must take), it is important to add up the total combined quantity of each individual nutrient being taken in supplement form. For example, vitamin D might be included in a liquid calcium preparation, halibut liver oil capsule *and* multivitamin tablet for a total exceeding a child's daily requirements.

Should Supplements Be Natural or Synthetic?

Synthetic vitamins are the same in molecular structure as natural vitamins, and as Dr. Doris Rapp observes in *Allergies and the Hyperactive Child*, synthetic vitamins have been particularly useful in short-term acute diseases or severe cases of deficiency. But vitamin preparations from natural sources contain substances such as the bioflavonoids in natural vitamin C—absent in the final product—which many nutritional authorities feel are necessary for maximum effectiveness in promoting health. "In short," Dr. Rapp sums up, "both seem helpful but the natural appears to have a possible edge in superiority."

However, nutrients derived synthetically are generally less costly than nutrients from natural sources, which is a major consideration for many. It is also important to note that some vitamins labeled "natural" aren't completely natural. It is legally permissible to use the word on a label if even some of the product comes from a natural source. Dr. Marshall Mandell in his *5-Day Allergy Relief System* also reminds us that toxic pesticides and other chemicals used in raising the plants the vitamins are derived from can contaminate otherwise unexceptionably natural vitamins.

When deciding, the most important criterion is which form of the nutrient, natural or synthetic, a child tolerates best. This will vary from child to child.

Is Chelation Helpful?

Many minerals are available in a chelated form. This means that they are attached to protein molecules in order to increase their assimilation in the body. Because of this increased assimilation, chelated minerals are a good choice for most, with the possible exception of those sensitive to milk or soy, who may have problems if the protein used is from dairy sources or soy.

What Is Each Nutrient Derived From?

This is especially important to know in the case of children who suffer from food or chemical sensitivities. For example, most vitamin C is derived from corn, making vitamin C derived from an alternative source such as sago palm a better choice for corn-sensitive children (unless of course they are also sensitive to sago palm).

What Other Ingredients Are Included in the Supplement?

In addition to the actual nutrient, supplements often have many other ingredients such as fillers, binders, sugar and other sweeteners, preservatives, coloring and flavoring. Again it is important to know what these ingredients are in the case of children with sensitivities. If a nutrient supplement contains, for example, wheat, yeast and salicylates, children who happen to be sensitive to these may be affected adversely, despite their need for the particular nutrient. It is generally best to choose supplements without sugar and artificial additives for all children, whether they have sensitivities or not.

Remember to read supplement labels carefully. Some vitamin and mineral companies include complete lists of contents on their labels, others list only a few items they do *not* contain, and some mention neither. If sensitivities are a concern, contact the company directly for a full description of ingredients.

Which Form of the Supplement Should Be Chosen?

Supplements come in powdered, liquid, tablet or capsule form. (Vitamins can also be given through injection.) Often our choice will be determined by what is available, what is affordable and what we can get our children to take. Older children are generally able to swallow tablets or capsules while powdered or liquid supplements are easier for younger children. Of course, tablets can always be crushed and some capsules can either be pulled apart and their powdered contents poured out, or pricked (as with halibut liver oil capsules) and their contents squirted out. Tablets that can be chewed may be necessary for children who can't swallow or are resisting the idea of taking supplements, but unfortunately are often sweetened and flavored. Also the acid in vitamin C tablets may be harmful to teeth, requiring careful brushing. Powdered supplements, easy to give mixed into juice, are most likely to contain the least amount of extra ingredients.

Which Supplements Are Most Easily Digested or Assimilated?

One point to consider if children have poor digestion is made by Nan Kathryn Fuchs in *The Nutrition Detective*: "Poor digestion often means a difficulty in absorbing fat-soluble vitamins [A, D, E and K]. For this reason, be certain the supplement you take is in water-soluble tablet or an emulsified liquid, rather than an oil-based capsule, for easier, more complete assimilation."

Another point to be aware of is that nutrients exist in different forms, some of which are better assimilated or digested in the body than others. For example, calcium carbonate, calcium gluconate and calcium lactate (except for those with a milk sensitivity if it is derived from milk) are better tolerated than calcium chloride. The sodium ascorbate form of vitamin C may be better tolerated than ascorbic acid if fairly large doses are being taken. An organic form of iron such as ferrous gluconate or ferrous fumerate is better than the inorganic ferrous sulfate, and zinc gluconate is usually better tolerated than zinc sulfate.

A third point is made by Dr. Philip Zimmerman in the Spring 1987 issue of *Health and Nutrition Update*: "Tablets, whether medicinal or nutritional, are only beneficial if they dissolve properly in the system. If a nutritional tablet passes through the body without dissolving, then the body has not benefited from the product. If the tablet passes the initial parts of the digestive system and remains in the lower stomach or in the intestines, then problems can occur. The tablet can become putrified or irritate the digestive tract. Enzymes and stomach fluids needed to dissolve the tablet are not available in the final part of the digestive tract."

Zimmerman describes a simple test which will indicate whether tablets are dissolving properly or not: "Place the tablet in a glass of lukewarm water to which a little bit of vinegar has been added. Stir the water with a spoon (without touching the tablet) preferably at short intervals. Under these conditions the tablet should dissolve in approximately one half to one hour."

Should Time-Release Supplements Be Chosen?

To ensure that children receive a constant supply of the nutrients they need, especially the water-soluble ones—such as vitamins C and

B-complex—which leave the body quite quickly, time-release supplements can be both more convenient (for example, in some cases necessitating only one dose during a day rather than three) and more effective (ensuring the nutrient is available to the body at all times). However, they do tend to be more expensive.

In addition, there are indications that time-release supplements of certain nutrients may be less well absorbed by the body than supplements that dissolve more quickly.

Implementing the Program

It is probably best to add supplements one at a time, so that if any do cause a reaction, it will be simpler to figure out which one. It is a good idea to keep a symptom diary as outlined in Chapter 8. It is also best to raise the dosage slowly up to the desired amount, again watching carefully for any adverse reactions.

If children are on drugs or other medication, it is important to withdraw the drugs gradually and only under the guidance of a doctor. Dr. Rimland writes (in *Orthomolecular Psychiatry*, edited by Drs. David Hawkins and Linus Pauling):

"Although our instructions advised the parents to continue for a time whatever medication the child was taking, then try to taper it off, many parents removed the tranquilizers abruptly, with ensuing problems. These problems could usually be resolved over a few weeks time by adjusting dosages of the drugs or vitamins."

It should be noted that tranquilizers may be made more active by niacin and niacinamide, and their dosage may have to be reduced accordingly when these vitamins are given.

Best results are obtained when supplements are taken with meals, two or three times a day, rather than all at once.

To make sure supplements maintain their potency as long as possible, they should be stored in an air-tight container in a dark, cool place and not used past the expiration date marked on their container.

Testing the Hypothesis

The therapeutic trial should last for a period of one to six months. Three months is generally considered an adequate amount of time, although longer is often better when problems are particularly severe. Children who improve rapidly need a correspondingly shorter trial period.

If children improve significantly and stay improved, most of us will feel this is enough evidence to confirm that they do indeed have a need for nutritional supplementation. In general, when a definite improvement occurs and we and our children are satisfied with the way things are going, the wisest course is to leave well enough alone.

For those interested in confirming a need for nutritional supplementation beyond a doubt, the best procedure is, in consultation with our children's doctors, to stop the supplements (in the case of vitamin C, taper off gradually) and watch to see if symptoms return. It is important to note that some children's symptoms will return rapidly, while the symptoms of other children will not reappear until up to one or two months after the cessation of the nutritional supplements.

If symptoms return quickly and dramatically after the supplements have been stopped, this will likely help reinforce our and our children's motivation for continuing the supplementation program.

On the other hand, Dr. Abram Hoffer writes in a personal communication that "one must be careful with discontinuing the program because I have seen some severe setbacks when this is done, and it has taken much longer to get the child back to the same condition they were in. I think the best time to try discontinuing the program is right after school stops in summer, so that if the child relapses in July, it is possible to get him back on the program again before school starts once more in the fall. Also, the longer the child has been well, the safer it is to try this experiment."

In addition to the possibility of improvement being slower and harder to achieve the second time around, there are two other possible dangers involved with stopping the supplements. One is that it may be difficult to get children to restart the supplementation program. The second is that if symptoms return very slowly and gradually (which is not a rare occurrence), any cause and effect relationship between stopping the supplements and the return of the symptoms will be much less noticeable.

If this should happen, it is extremely important that we restart the supplements for another therapeutic trial despite the lack of a clear-cut relationship. If the symptoms clear up again after a minimum trial period of 90 days, we can be confident that the supplements are in fact helping.

If children do not improve, or improve only slightly, before deciding that our hypothesis is not correct and our children do not need nutritional supplementation, we should explore some other possibilities. One is that other factors such as diet (Chapter 10), hypoglycemia (Chapter 12), yeast overgrowth (Chapter 13), poor digestion (page 266 in Chapter 18), heavy metal toxicity (Chapter 16) or food and environmental sensitivities (Chapters 14 and 15) are involved and affecting children adversely. If the program was not followed regularly this would also affect results. Another possibility is that the nutritional supplementation program our children were on was not the right one for their needs. It is possible that they have a need for nutrients that were not supplied, the dosages of some of the nutrients were too low, or the nutritional supplements were of low quality. Or, perhaps, more time than we allowed was needed before improvement could occur.

Unfortunately, until more knowledge is gained through continuing research, not all children will be able to gain complete normality. We should expect there will be varying amounts of improvement depending on the child. This is especially so in the case of retardation, although this does not in any way detract from the joy of an increase in learning ability or decrease of behavioral symptoms occurring in a retarded child.

Especially if there is at least some improvement, it may be a good idea to redesign the therapeutic trial and try again, as well as investigating other possibilities, such as heavy metal toxicity.

The Maintenance Program

Those of us who find that our children have benefited from nutritional supplements should be aware of two dangers. The first is that once their symptoms have disappeared we will feel it is safe to discontinue the supplements. For some children this may well be safe to do, especially if their problems were caused primarily by poor diet. Others, however, may have lifelong requirements to supplement their diets with extra nutrients. In some cases it may be possible to lower nutrient dosages to maintenance levels, but this should be done cautiously, with extreme vigilance for the return of symptoms. It may be found after experimentation that a lower dose of one form of a nutrient can do the same job as a higher dose of another form of the same nutrient. (For example, natural B-complex vitamins might be more effective for some children than synthetic, and vice versa.) Or, if previously unrecognized problems, such as food sensitivities, are brought under control lower dosages may also be sufficient.

The second danger is being unaware of changing needs. As circumstances change due to illness, psychological stress, physical activity or physical growth, children's nutrient requirements also change. What fulfilled nutritional needs at the age of five will probably not be suitable when children are twelve. What is perfectly adequate when they are enjoying good health may be completely inadequate when they are sick with the flu. (In fact it is quite common for relapses to occur after the onset of infections.) And of course allergies or sensitivities can develop at any time.

It is extremely important to keep in mind that all nutritional supplements should be treated with respect and kept out of reach of young children. Children should be warned of the possibly serious consequences of randomly swallowing pills, capsules, powders or liquid preparations, no matter how good (or foul) they taste. For example, children have died from taking too many iron-containing multivitamin tablets.

The Nutrients Themselves

Following is a brief description of the nutrients most often supplemented in children with learning and behavior problems. (Much of this section is summarized from *Nutrition Almanac*, although many other sources were used as well, such as *Earl Mindell's Vitamin Bible for Your Kids* and *Nourishing Your Child* by Wunderlich and Kalita.)

VITAMIN A is important for healthy eyes, skin, bones and teeth, resistance to infections, the protection of the mucous membranes of mouth, nose, throat and lungs and of the linings of the digestive tract, kidneys and bladder, the digestion of proteins, and overall growth and repair. It is sometimes used in the control of food and environmental sensitivities.

Symptoms of a lack of vitamin A include eye and vision problems and rough, dry skin.

Because it is a fat-soluble vitamin and stored in the body, overdoses are possible and extra care must be taken to make sure children do not take too much. Bone pain, hair loss, headaches and nausea are some of the symptoms that might indicate an excess of vitamin A is being taken. Symptoms usually disappear once the vitamin A is stopped.

Vitamin A itself or beta-carotene, a substance that the body can convert into vitamin A, can be found in liver, dairy products, eggs and yellow and green vegetables. Beta-carotene is generally used by the body only when needed and thus may be the best form of supplementation for children.

Antacids, mineral oil and polyunsaturated fats (unless sufficient vitamin E is present) decrease the amount of vitamin A available to the body.

Vitamin A works best when vitamin D and zinc are present in sufficient quantities.

B-COMPLEX VITAMINS are necessary to convert carbohydrates into glucose, metabolize fats and proteins, for a healthy nervous system, and for healthy skin, hair, eyes, mouth, blood and digestion. The B-complex vitamins may be helpful in the control or treatment of hypoglycemia, food and environmental sensitivities and drug-related problems. Although they each have their specific functions in the body many of them are interdependent on each other and they work closely together. The B-complex vitamins include thiamine (B1), riboflavin (B2), niacin or niacinamide (B3), pyridoxine (B6), cyano-cobalamin (B12), biotin, and folic acid; substances which, though not actually vitamins, are associated with the B family are orotic acid, choline, inositol, pangamic acid, para-aminobenzoic acid (PABA) and carnitine.

Niacin (and niacinamide) and pyridoxine appear to be the B-complex vitamins playing the major role in combatting symptoms associated with hyperactivity, schizophrenia and autism, although the others are usually necessary in at least a supporting role. Depending on the individual child, in some instances the remaining members of the B-complex assume importance equal to, and occasionally greater than, niacin/niacinamide and pyridoxine. For example, pantothenic acid seems to be particularly important for those suffering from food and environmental sensitivities. Dr. Allan Cott writes in his book *Help for Your Learning Disabled Child* that he uses up to 200 mg. daily of pangamic acid (a special nutrient related to the B complex) for children who don't talk, or who have asthma and allergies.

Symptoms of a need for vitamin B-complex supplementation include cracks at the corner of children's mouths, tongues that are grooved, cracked or bright red, oily or itchy skin, or an inability to remember dreams.

B-complex vitamins are relatively safe to take in that they are water-soluble and excess amounts leave the body through the urine. However, because of the close relationships of the B-complex vita-mins to each other, taking a large dose of one may cause a deficiency in another; they should be taken together. It is often recommended that riboflavin and pyridoxine be taken in equal doses.

Possible side effects include the following (all of which will disap-pear when the vitamin intake is stopped or the dosage is lowered):

Thiamine. According to Earl Mindell in his *Vitamin Bible for Your Kids*, "Rare excess symptoms include tremors, nervousness, rapid heartbeat, and allergies."

Riboflavin. Yellow urine is a consequence of taking riboflavin, but a consequence that can be safely ignored.

Itching and tingling of extremities may also occur and should not be ignored.

Niacin. A hot, itchy flush may occur during the first week or so of its introduction. (Niacinamide often does not cause the flush.) Infrequently, it may elevate blood glucose and uric acid levels. Nausea may occur. Problems are usually lessened by taking the vitamins on a full stomach.

Niacinamide. Nausea is again a possible side effect, as are headaches.

If both niacin and niacinamide cause side effects, Dr. Abram Hoffer in *Medical Applications of Clinical Nutrition* suggests as an alternative "inositol niacinate (Linodil) which is not available in the U.S.A. but can be obtained over the counter in Canada. It is an excellent nicotinic acid derivative which releases the nicotinic acid slowly in the body. Inositol also has useful centrally active relaxing properties."

Pyridoxine. This may cause restless sleep. (Giving it to children early in the day may reduce this side effect.) In some cases, its diuretic effect may result in the loss of trace minerals. Diarrhea and nausea can also occur. Larger doses may induce neurological problems. Parents of diabetic children should note that it may decrease insulin requirements, sometimes making it necessary to adjust insulin intake.

Pantothenic Acid. This may cause irritability in some children. According to Dr. Bernard Rimland (describing a study using vitamins in *Orthomolecular Psychiatry*, edited by David Hawkins and Linus Pauling), "A few children showed deterioration of behavior when the last vitamin, pantothenic acid, was added. A few others, who showed no behavioral response to the earlier vitamins, appeared to improve dramatically when the pantothenic acid was added. Parents of children showing problems on the initiation of pantothenic acid were advised to discontinue giving it, since the first several children showing the pantothenate-induced irritability did not improve until the vitamin was withdrawn." Wunderlich and Kalita suggest that when an increase in hyperactivity is caused by a dose of 50 mg. or more of pantothenic acid, a dose of 10 to 50 mg. may be tolerated with no problems.

Most of the B-complex vitamins are found in brewer's yeast, liver and whole grains.

Some of the B vitamins are produced by intestinal bacteria which may grow poorly on a milk-free diet and be destroyed by antibiotics. A strictly vegetarian diet which excludes all meat, eggs and dairy products is generally deficient in cyanocobalamin (B12). Physical stress such as infections, emotional stress, and excessive carbohydrate intake increase the need for the B vitamins.

VITAMIN C plays an important role in the formation and maintenance of all body tissues (including bones and teeth) and red blood cells, increases resistance to infections, helps metabolize some of the amino acids and helps the body use some of the other vitamins and minerals. It often plays a major role in the control of mental, emotional and behavioral symptoms such as hyperactivity and hallucinations. It is a detoxifier and has anti-allergy properties.

Bleeding gums, bruising easily and constant infections may indicate a need for extra vitamin C.

Vitamin C is another water-soluble vitamin, making its use, as with the B-complex vitamins, relatively safe. The main side effects that may occur due to vitamin C supplementation are increased frequency of urination and diarrhea, both of which will disappear when the supplementation is reduced or stopped. Vitamin C buffered with minerals will reduce the likelihood of stomach problems. It is important when using vitamin C not to decrease its dosage suddenly, as this may make children more vulnerable to infections than they would otherwise have been. A gradual tapering off is much preferable. Large doses of vitamin C may lower mineral levels in the body.

It is found in most fresh fruits and vegetables, especially citrus fruits, Brussels sprouts, broccoli, green and red peppers and kale.

Vitamin C requirements may be increased by stress, illness and injury, the use of certain medications and baking soda, and the inhalation of smoke, DDT and petroleum fumes.

BIOFLAVONOIDS (VITAMIN P) supplement the function of vitamin C and include citrin, hesperidin, rutin, flavones and flavonals. Vitamin C and the bioflavonoids are sometimes called vitamin C-complex.

According to *Nutrition Almanac* bioflavonoids are found in lemons, grapes, plums, black currants, grapefruit, apricots, buckwheat, cherries, blackberries and rose hips.

VITAMIN D helps the body use calcium and phosphorus, thus aiding in the development of bones and teeth, the clotting of blood and the healthy functioning of the heart and nervous system.

Symptoms of vitamin D deficiency include bow legs or spinal curvature due to soft bones.

As with vitamin A, it is important not to take too much as there can be serious side effects. Indications that too much vitamin D is being taken include appetite loss, nausea, vomiting, frequent urination and dizziness.

It is found in fish, milk and eggs and can be synthesized in the body when the skin is exposed to sunlight.

Vitamin D works best with vitamin A.

VITAMIN E is made up of tocopherols which include alpha, beta, delta, epsilon, eta, gamma and zeta. It protects nutrients from the harmful effects of oxidation, protects the body against toxins, makes the body's use of oxygen more efficient and aids circulation.

Symptoms of a deficiency in infants include anemia and hemorrhaging.

Although Vitamin E is a fat-soluble vitamin, it appears to have a very low toxicity when used orally. However, people with high blood pressure and rheumatic heart disease should take care when using it. Excessive amounts may depress the immune system.

To avoid the problem of rancidity, it may be preferable to use a water-soluble dry E for supplementation rather than vitamin E from wheat germ oil. There is also some evidence that this water-soluble dry E is better assimilated by the body than vitamin E that is oil based.

It is found in whole grains, nuts, seeds and soybeans.

Vitamin E can be destroyed or depleted in the body by chlorine, ferric chloride, rancid oil or fat, inorganic iron and polyunsaturated fats.

Vitamin E is most effective when selenium is present in adequate amounts.

The essential UNSATURATED FATTY ACIDS are linoleic, linolenic and arachidonic acids. They are important in the health of the glands, cells, mucous membranes and nerves.

Belinda Barnes and Irene Colquhoun write in *The Hyperactive Child* that along with vitamins such as niacinamide, pyridoxine and C, and the mineral zinc, supplements of evening primrose oil, which contains gamma linolenic acid, have been found helpful to some hyperactive and allergic children. They warn that evening primrose oil should not be given to children who are epileptic without expert advice. They suggest that goat's milk or safflower oil taken with vitamin C, E and the B-complex and zinc may be adequate instead of evening primrose oil.

Earl Mindell in his children's *Vitamin Bible* lists as possible symptoms of a developing deficiency of the unsaturated fatty acids "brittle hair, dandruff, dry skin, brittle nails."

They are found in whole grains, seeds (and their oils) and most nuts.

CALCIUM is necessary for healthy bones, teeth, muscles, blood and nerve transmission. It lowers histamine levels, helps in the utilization of iron, the activation of some enzymes and the regulation of nutrients passing through cell walls. Children who have low body amounts of calcium may be more susceptible to the accumulation of lead and other toxic metals in their bodies.

Muscle cramps, insomnia and excessive nervousness may indicate a lack of calcium.

Calcium lactate and calcium gluconate are the easiest forms of calcium to absorb, although calcium carbonate may also be a good choice for some. Calcium lactate derived from dairy sources should not be taken by those who have a milk sensitivity. Bone meal and dolomite, both of which are calcium sources, may sometimes be contaminated with lead or other heavy metals (although usually to no greater extent than is food). Calcium chloride may irritate the stomach lining. It is important to remember that calcium should never be taken without magnesium. The optimum ratio is thought to be 2:1, although this is questioned by some who feel that the ratio should be closer to 1:1, due to magnesium being less available in food and more easily lost to the body than calcium.

As necessary as calcium is, it should be noted that excessive amounts may cause side effects.

Calcium is found in milk and milk products, sesame seeds, legumes and dark green, leafy vegetables.

Substances that may interfere with the absorption of calcium are oxalic acid (found in beet greens, chard, rhubarb and spinach), excess fiber, and phytic acid (found in bran and whole grains). In addition, calcium may be lost to the body through urine if the diet contains excess protein.

Calcium needs the vitamins A, C and D, the minerals magnesium and phosphorus, and acid in order to be absorbed and work effectively. Exercise aids the absorption of calcium.

CHROMIUM is important in the metabolism of glucose, the synthesis of fatty acids and cholesterol and helps insulin work more effectively.

The existence of hypoglycemia or diabetes may indicate a need for chromium.

It is found in brewer's yeast, clams, whole grains and meats.

IRON is necessary for healthy blood and muscles, and helps in protein metabolism and respiration.

Symptoms of a lack of iron, according to Wunderlich and Kalita, include "constipation; lack of appetite; difficulty swallowing; weakness; irritability; lusterless, brittle and spoon-shaped nails; and difficulty in breathing," in addition to paleness and fatigue.

It is only the inorganic form of iron, ferrous sulfate, which destroys vitamin E. Acute poisoning can occur if children take too many iron tablets, even in the organic form.

Iron is found in organ meats, oysters, eggs and leafy green vegetables.

Its absorption in the body can be decreased by the presence of excess fiber and by phytic acid in bran and whole grains.

Its absorption is aided by the presence of vitamin C, and it functions best with copper and calcium.

MAGNESIUM works closely with calcium and phosphorus and is important in the metabolism of carbohydrates, amino acids, many minerals and vitamin C, and is necessary for healthy bones, teeth, nerves and muscles.

Some of the symptoms of a magnesium deficiency listed by Wunderlich and Kalita in *Nourishing Your Child* are "apprehensiveness, nervous irritability, muscle twitch, tremors, noise sensitivity, confusion and disorientation."

Earl Mindell writes about magnesium that "large amounts, over an extended period of time, can be toxic—especially if a child's calcium intake is low and his phosphorus intake is high. In children with kidney problems, there is a greater danger of toxicity because the rate of excretion will be slower."

It is found in green vegetables, corn, soybeans, apples, nuts and seeds and figs.

High calcium and protein intakes in the diet increase the requirements for magnesium.

MANGANESE is necessary for the activation of many enzymes, for healthy bones, nerves and brain, helps the body utilize choline, proteins, carbohydrates and fats, and is important in the synthesis of fatty acids and cholesterol.

Excess manganese can result in the loss of iron to the body.

It is found in green vegetables, eggs and whole-grain cereals.

Manganese requirements increase in the presence of large amounts of calcium and phosphorus.

PHOSPHORUS generally works with calcium in the body and is involved in almost every body process, being found in all body cells. It is needed for healthy bones, teeth, kidneys and nerves, the utilization of carbohydrates, fats and proteins and the contraction of muscles.

Signs of phosphorus deficiency are loss of appetite, irregular breathing, fatigue and nervous problems.

Excess phosphorus increases calcium requirements.

It is found in eggs, fish, meat, poultry, nuts and seeds and whole grains.

Excess iron, aluminum and magnesium increases phosphorus requirements.

Vitamin D and calcium are necessary for its absorption.

POTASSIUM is important for growth, muscle contractions, the correct acid/alkaline balance of body fluids, healthy skin, cell metabolism, enzyme reactions, protein synthesis and kidney function. With sodium it is important in regulating the body's water balance and for a healthy heart and muscular system.

"Deficiency symptoms," write Wunderlich and Kalita, "include: acne, continuous thirst, dry skin, general weakness, abdominal bloating, constipation, kidney dysfunction, insomnia, poor muscle tone, muscle damage, nervousness and a slow irregular heartbeat."

It is found in vegetables (potatoes and green leafy ones in particular), bananas, oranges, whole grains and sunflower seeds.

SELENIUM is an antioxidant like vitamin E and increases vitamin E's effectiveness. It is antagonistic to mercury.

Only small amounts are necessary. It is very toxic, so it should be used with caution.

It is found in broccoli, onions, tomatoes, whole grains and tuna.

ZINC is vital to the body's use of vitamins, particularly the B family, and is a component of more than a score of enzymes important to the major body processes of metabolism and digestion. Zinc is found in insulin, and is important in the digestion of carbohydrates, the metabolism of phosphorus, the formation of proteins, general growth and healing, and the health of the reproductive organs. It often seems to play an important role in the alleviation of symptoms of behavioral problems in children.

Symptoms of a zinc deficiency include fatigue, increased susceptibility to infection, decrease in appetite or loss of taste, white spots on fingernails, wounds that take a long time to heal and eczema.

Excess zinc may increase copper, iron and vitamin A requirements.

It is found in whole grains, brewer's yeast, pumpkin seeds and some meat.

Excess copper (often due to copper water pipes or copper cookware) may lower zinc levels. High amounts of calcium, pyridoxine and phytic acid (in some whole grains) may also increase zinc requirements.

Following is a letter originally printed in the *Huxley Institute-CSF Newsletter*, January 1981.

To the Editor
REGARDING MEGAVITAMIN THERAPY FOR AUTISM
AND RELATED DISORDERS

Much of the current interest in megavitamin therapy stems from the publication of our report on a double-blind evaluation of vitamin B6 in a group of autistic children, which appeared in the *American Journal of Psychiatry*. The results of this study, like the results of our original study were positive. Following the publication of our two successful studies, several additional studies have been completed by other investigators which have confirmed our research results: a substantial proportion of children variously described as autistic, psychotic, schizophrenic, etc. show very marked and worthwhile benefits when given a large daily supplement of vitamin B6 (pyridoxine). There are now nine published reports in the world literature showing that vitamin B6 is helpful to the majority of autistic and autistic-type children. There are no studies showing vitamin B6 to have been unsuccessful, nor are there any reports showing any children to have been harmed by the administration of megadose vitamin B6.

Further, a recent report of a double-blind study by Dr. Mary Coleman and her associates showed that vitamin B6 was significantly more effective than Ritalin in controlling the hyperactivity in a group of hyperactive children.

While a single vitamin (or mineral) may sometimes produce favorable results, good results are most likely to occur when certain other nutrients are also provided. Nutrients must form compounds in the body to be effective, and their effectiveness is limited when the other constituents of the compounds are in short supply. (Vitamins differ from drugs in this respect. Drugs operate as blocking agents, and can thus function alone. Vitamins act as facilitating or enabling agents, and this requires the presence of other nutrients. Vitamins are immeasurably safer than drugs for the same reason.)

Magnesium is the most important supplemental nutrient, inasmuch as the body cannot properly utilize B6 without a sufficient supply of magnesium. If the child's diet does not provide him/her with a good supply of this mineral, and it often does not, magnesium must be provided as a supplement. Vitamin C, the B vitamins and zinc are among the nutrients which should be given if the B6 is to be most useful.

There are several other points I would like to make:

1) It is wise to eliminate sugar, soft drinks and other junk foods from the child's diet. There is ample evidence that these are harmful for all children, whether or not on a megavitamin therapy.

2) In most cases behavioral improvement is seen after a few days on megavitamins. In other cases behavior improves gradually so little change is seen for two or three months. In perhaps 40 percent of the children, the vitamins seem to be of no help, but I would not conclude that any given child will not be helped until there has been at least a 90-day trial.

3) If a child is on drugs, most physicians who use megavitamins recommend that they continue the drugs for several weeks after vitamins have been started. If improvement is observed, a process of weaning the child from the drugs may be initiated. It is often possible for the drug dosage to be cut in half, and in many cases the drugs could be discontinued. (This should be discussed with the child's physician.)

4) The vitamins should be administered with meals in two or three divided doses per day. This provides the vitamins and minerals the optimum opportunity to form proper compounds with other nutrients in the digestive system and blood stream.

5) The benefits which have been most often observed in autistic children with the use of B6 and the accompanying nutrients are: increased use of sounds, words or speech;

improved sleeping habits; decrease in irritability; better attention span; increase in interest in learning; in some cases, self-injurious behavior has decreased.

6) The only side effects observed have been in children who were not getting a sufficient supply of magnesium in their diets. These side effects have quickly been reversed with the addition of magnesium: irritability, sound sensitivity, enuresis.

Bernard Rimland, Ph.D.
Institute for Child Behavior Research

Books referred to in this chapter and other suggested reading:

Dr. Cott's Help for Your Learning Disabled Child. Allan Cott, J. Agel, E. Boe. Times Books, New York, 1985. For a description, see Chapter 8.

Dr. Mandell's 5-Day Allergy Relief System, Marshall Mandell and Lynne Waller Scanlon. Thomas Y. Crowell, New York, 1979. For a description, see Chapter 14.

Earl Mindell's Vitamin Bible for Your Kids, Earl Mindell. Rawson, Wade Publishers, New York, 1981. In addition to useful information about each vitamin and mineral, contains more general nutritional information.

Getting over Getting High: How to Overcome Dependency on Cocaine, Caffeine, Hallucinogens, Speed and other Stimulants the Natural and Permanent Way, Bernard Green. William Morrow, New York, 1985. The approach described in this book uses vitamins to help withdraw from stimulants and stresses the value of good nutrition; it talks about natural ways of "getting high" using exercise, meditation, relaxation, etc. and has advice for the parents of teenagers.

The Hyperactive Child, Belinda Barnes and Irene Colquhoun. Thorsons Publishers, Wellingborough, Northants., England, 1984. For a description, see Chapter 8.

Medical Applications of Clinical Nutrition, Jeffrey Bland, editor. Keats Publishing, New Canaan, Connecticut, 1983. Somewhat technical, but interesting and informative.

Medical Treatment of Down Syndrome and Genetic Diseases, Henry Turkel and Ilse Nusbaum. Ubiotica, 19145 West Nine Mile Road, Southfield, Michigan, 48075, 1985. Discusses Down's syndrome and its treatment using the "U" series (mainly composed of a variety of nutritional supplements, plus a few medications). The book includes many first-hand accounts written by parents whose children have been helped by the "U" series.

Nourishing Your Child, Ray C. Wunderlich, Jr. and Dwight K. Kalita, Keats Publishing, New Canaan, Connecticut, 1984. For a description, see Chapter 8.

Nutrition Almanac, Nutrition Search, Inc. McGraw-Hill, New York, 1984. For a description, see Chapter 10.

Orthomolecular Psychiatry, David Hawkins and Linus Pauling, editors. W.H. Freeman, San Francisco, 1973. For a further description, see Chapter 4.

12

HYPOGLYCEMIA

According to Jeraldine Saunders and Harvey M. Ross, M.D., in *Hypoglycemia: The Disease Your Doctor Won't Treat*, hypoglycemia (also called low blood sugar) "occurs when the body can no longer regulate the amount of sugar in the blood, which . . . causes the sugar level to fall to lower than an optimum level, or for it to fall too quickly." It can be caused or made more severe by certain diseases, malfunctioning of organs or glands, poor eating habits, food and environmental allergies or sensitivities and physical and emotional stress. Although it is not a condition that is generally recognized by the medical profession, many nutritionally oriented doctors estimate that it is fairly common.

Symptoms vary widely from one hypoglycemic to another, but the feature common to all hypoglycemics is their bodies' difficulties in managing sugars and refined carbohydrates, which convert extremely quickly to glucose (blood sugar) in the body. When people who are hypoglycemic eat foods highly concentrated in sugar (white and brown sugars, honey, molasses, maple syrup) or foods containing refined carbohydrates (for example white flour, white rice, white pasta) their blood sugar levels shoot up, then fall dramatically. Hypoglycemics may feel energetic and pleasantly high immediately after eating a chocolate bar or a piece of white toast with jam, but all too soon their blood sugar will drop, resulting in a return of familiar but unwelcome symptoms. For this reason, diet is the major component of the program to control hypoglycemia.

Is Hypoglycemia Causing Children's Problems?

Some of the clues suggesting that children are suffering from hypoglycemia were mentioned in Chapter 8. These included the occurrence of hypoglycemia among other family members, a craving for sweet or starchy foods, a diet containing large amounts of sweet or starchy foods, an increase in symptoms two to four hours after eating, and a decrease in symptoms right after eating.

In addition there are several symptoms which on their own could suggest any number of conditions, but together with other indications can be considered further evidence of hypoglycemia. Doris Rapp in *Allergies and the Hyperactive Child* summarizes these symptoms: nervous fatigue, exhaustion, depression, confusion, anxiety, dizziness, headaches, muscle aches, trouble sleeping, excessive sweating, tingling skin, cold hands and feet, and midmorning or late afternoon light-headedness.

It should be noted that it is possible for hyperactive children as well as low-energy children to have hypoglycemia.

The Glucose Tolerance Test

Another indicator of hypoglycemia is a positive glucose tolerance test (GTT). Generally, the procedure for the test is as follows:

Children eat as they normally do until after supper the night before the test, at which point only water is allowed. Certain medications which interfere with test results may be stopped for a few days beforehand. In the morning, a sample of blood is taken to find the fasting blood sugar level. After this, a glucose solution (usually from corn) is drunk. Blood and urine samples are then taken at regular intervals, and a record of symptoms occurring during the test should be kept. The test lasts at least five hours, as a three- or four-hour test does not follow the blood curve long enough to be accurate.

Next, the blood and urine samples are analyzed in the laboratory for glucose levels and the results charted on a graph.

The blood sugar curve is then interpreted to decide whether it is consistent or inconsistent with a diagnosis of hypoglycemia. Different doctors may interpret the same test results in different ways, depending on which criteria they use. Many nutritionally oriented doctors feel, due to each individual's uniqueness, that symptoms rather than blood sugar number values should be given the most weight when interpreting a GTT. This does not mean that the numbers should be ignored. Dr. H.L. Newbold in his book *Meganutrients and Your Nerves* (quoted in Doris Rapp's *Allergies and the Hyperactive Child*) gives some useful guidelines:

> Interpreting glucose-tolerance curves is not always uniform by all physicians, but the following may be helpful:
> After drinking the sugar solution, your blood level should double. For example, if the initial level was 80 mg% [that is, 80 milligrams of glucose for each 100 milliliters or cubic centimeters of blood] it should rise to about 160 mg%.

The blood-sugar level should not fall at any point during the test below 60 mg% or more than 20 mg% below the fasting level.

During the test, there should not be a greater than 50 mg% drop during any single hour period. For example, a fall from 140 mg% to 75 mg% in one hour is too much.

If you perspire, become dizzy, weak, confused, depressed, nauseated, or develop a headache or feel your heart beating fast, ask for an *immediate* blood-sugar determination. If this happens, it means that your blood sugar may be too low at that particular time. Fifteen minutes later, your blood level may no longer be low and the correct diagnosis may be missed.

In connection with glucose tolerance tests, there are a few points to be aware of:

• This test might be unnecessary if enough other indications of hypoglycemia exist to make a diagnosis possible, and should be avoided if at all possible. Because they require frequent blood taking and may cause severe symptoms, some doctors do not recommend GTTs until children are at least in their middle teens.

• Some children will feel very unwell at various points throughout the GTT, making it important for someone to be with them at all times. This person should make sure that a symptom diary is kept for the duration of the test.

• A positive test result may in fact indicate an allergy or food sensitivity rather than hypoglycemia. The blood sugar curve of a person allergic or sensitive to the substance the glucose is derived from may be similar to that of a hypoglycemic.

• As with any lab test, mistakes and errors may occur during processing and so results cannot be completely relied upon. In any case, a GTT should not be the only evidence on which a positive or negative diagnosis of hypoglycemia is made.

THE HYPOGLYCEMIA DIET

On the basis of the above clues and indicators, some of us will have decided that our children are quite likely suffering from hypoglycemia. To test this hypothesis we can introduce our children to the hypoglycemia diet; if their symptoms clear up, this is confirmation that our hypothesis is right.

The hypoglycemia diet follows the general basics of good nutrition. (For more information on children's nutritional needs, see Chapter 10.) More specifically, it allows moderate amounts of protein, fat and complex carbohydrates (such as whole grains and vegetables) while restricting all forms of sugar and refined carbohydrates and any foods containing these. The initial hypoglycemia diet, which is to be used either until children's hypoglycemic symptoms are under control or until we have decided our children don't have hypoglycemia, is as follows.

Foods to Avoid

• *Sugar in any form and all foods containing sugar in any form.* This category includes white and brown table sugar, honey, molasses, maple syrup and corn syrup. It is important to note that sugar may not be listed as "sugar" on packages, bottles or cans but as dextrose, fructose, glucose, hexitol, lactose, maltose, mannitol, sorbitol, sucrose, syrup or natural sweetener. We should also note that in addition to the foods one would expect to contain sugar such as baked goods, candies, chocolate bars and soft drinks, many other foods items found in stores also contain sugar. For this reason it is necessary to carefully read the labels of all bottled, canned and packaged foods, including soups, fruits, wieners, bread, crackers, ketchup, peanut butter, fruit juices, salt, cereals, salad dressings, mustard, beans, stews, meat pies and so on. In addition, many children's medicines and vitamins contain sugar.

• *All refined carbohydrates such as white bread, pasta, most commercial cereals and white rice*

• *Food and drinks containing caffeine such as coffee, tea, colas and chocolate*

• *Artificial sweeteners*

• *Alcohol and tobacco*

• *Any foods that produce allergic or other reactions in our children*

What's Left

•• *Vegetables*
•• *Fruit*
•• *Whole grains*
• *Poultry, red meat, fish and seafood*
•• *Milk and dairy products*
•• *Legumes*
•• *Nuts and seeds*
• *Herb teas*
• *Water*

The quantities of the foods marked above with a double bullet (••)

may have to be limited in some children's diets because of their carbohydrate content. (See the next section but one, "Individualizing the Diet," for more information.)

Frequency of Eating

Hypoglycemic children should eat frequently and especially must not miss breakfast. They should also not eat large amounts at any one time. On this diet they will probably be eating six small meals a day (breakfast, snack, lunch, snack, supper, snack), although frequency is a matter of individual needs and some may need to eat even more frequently. This is regardless of how thin or overweight they might be.

Individualizing the Diet

Because every person is biochemically unique, there is no single diet suitable for all hypoglycemic children. For this reason it is important to experiment to find the best possible diet for each child. For example, some children will do better on diets that include large quantities of the allowed carbohydrates while others will do better on diets that include smaller amounts of these foods. Grains, vegetables, fruit, some dairy products, legumes, and nuts and seeds contain significant amounts of carbohydrates and will have to be considered for their effect on hypoglycemic children.

Fruit is the food group most likely to need restricting, especially apples, bananas, grapes, mangoes, dried fruit and fruit juices, which all have a highly concentrated sugar content. In general, fruit eaten at the same time as a high-protein food will be better tolerated.

We should also pay particular attention to milk as many children drink large quantities of it.

Among the vegetables with the highest carbohydrate content are potatoes, sweet potatoes and yams.

To check if children will benefit from a limited carbohydrate intake, we can use the following guidelines suggested by Powers and Presley in their book *Food Power*:

Age	Amount of carbohydrates
two to six	75 grams
six to ten	115 grams
ten to fifteen	135 grams
rapidly growing teens	150–250 grams

As a rough guide, limiting carbohydrate intake to 75 grams a day would allow a child to eat two pieces of fruit, two glasses of milk, two pieces of whole-grain bread and two servings of vegetables. This of course is only approximate and assumes that those foods with a comparatively high carbohydrate content, such as bananas and potatoes, are excluded. For a better idea of what can be included in a carbohydrate restricted diet, refer to books which contain listings of the carbohydrate content of some common foods such as *Nutrition Almanac* and *Laurel's Kitchen*. Also, health departments often have this information available for the general public.

If children don't do well on the amount of carbohydrates we have chosen to start them out with, we can try either increasing or decreasing quantities.

The Maintenance Diet

Many children, after following the diet strictly for a period of time, will be able to tolerate larger quantities of fruit, whole-grain bread and other allowed carbohydrates and to reduce the frequency of their meals, while others will have to be extremely careful to maintain a more limited diet for the rest of their lives. We will only be able to tell which category a child falls into by carefully experimenting.

Our experiments can begin once children have been completely well for a good length of time and have fully adjusted to their new way of eating. Then, we can either slowly increase the amount of allowed carbohydrates in the diet, or add on specific foods one at a time with three days in between each new food addition. (For example, if bananas, potatoes and dried apricots were previously restricted, test bananas on day one, potatoes on day five and dried apricots on day nine.) While doing this we should watch children carefully for the return of hypoglycemic symptoms or general indications of being unwell. We should be aware that the effects of adding on previously avoided foods or increasing total quantities of carbohydrates may not show up until up to three days later. Testing should not be done when children are under stress, either physical (such as infections or lack of sleep) or emotional (such as upcoming exams or quarrels with friends).

It is also important to realize that the diet may need to be readjusted occasionally, as children's dietary needs will vary according to growth requirements, stress levels, amount of exercise, contact with allergens and other factors.

Testing the Hypothesis

To test our hypothesis, children should strictly follow the hypoglycemia diet for three weeks. To begin with, we might want to limit their carbohydrate intake using the guidelines outlined in the section "Individualizing the Diet" (page 197).

How quickly they respond, if they are hypoglycemic, will depend on the severity and duration of the hypoglycemia, as well as how carefully the diet has been observed. Even those children who are suffering from hypoglycemia will most likely not show immediate improvement. On the contrary, initially a worsening of symptoms can be expected. In addition, the greater the addiction to sugar and refined carbohydrates, the more difficulty children will have with this withdrawal phase. To alleviate symptoms which are especially severe, we can try adding on small amounts of allowed carbohydrates, such as an extra serving of fruit a day, another slice of bread or an extra helping of a whole grain.

After this, the situation should improve, although improvement may be somewhat like a seesaw—a little bit better, then worse again, then better. Eventually, though, the hypoglycemic symptoms should clear up and stay cleared up.

If children improve considerably on this diet, then we can safely assume that they are hypoglycemic. If children show only partial improvement, there are two possibilities. One is that their bodies need more time on the diet to readjust. The other possibility is that diet is not the only factor contributing to their hypoglycemia. Food and environmental sensitivities (Chapters 14 and 15), heavy metal toxicity (Chapter 16), unfulfilled nutrient requirements (Chapter 11) and other factors may need to be dealt with before more progress occurs.

In addition to the above, exercise, control of stress and increased self-awareness (discussed in Chapter 18) will also help regulate blood sugar levels and should be included in any hypoglycemia control program.

If children don't improve at all, we should assume that they are not hypoglycemic. It is important, however, to continue restricting the amount of sugar and refined carbohydrates consumed, as sugar and refined carbohydrates in excess are negative influences on health, regardless of whether children are hypoglycemic or not.

Books referred to in this chapter and other suggested reading:

Allergies and the Hyperactive Child, Doris J. Rapp. Cornerstone Books, New York, 1980. For a description, see Chapter 14.

Food Power: Nutrition and Your Child's Behavior, Hugh Powers and James Presley. St. Martin's Press, New York, 1978. A straightforward guide with lots of information on various aspects of nutrition and behavior (concentrating on carbohydrate control).

Hypoglycemia: The Disease your Doctor Won't Treat, Jeraldine Saunders and Harvey M. Ross, M.D. Pinnacle Books, Inc., New York, 1982. Although it focuses on adults, this book is still useful, especially the section on "What Can Be Expected."

Laurel's Kitchen, Laurel Robertson, Carol Flinders, Bronwen Godfrey, Bantam Books, New York, 1978. For a description, see Chapter 10.

Nutrition Almanac, Nutrition Search, Inc. McGraw-Hill Book Company, New York, 1984. For a description, see Chapter 10.

13
YEAST OVERGROWTH

There are many different kinds of yeast. In addition to the yeast which can be used for baking, there is a yeast which is a normal inhabitant of the human body. Kept in check by the body's own defenses and a variety of friendly bacteria, yeast in the body usually presents no problem to health. Many times, even when a yeast infection does occur, it is easily dealt with and beyond a bit of discomfort does not do any serious harm. However, in some cases yeast may proliferate, producing toxins, damaging the immune system and interfering with hormone production. As a result there may be increased susceptibility to illness, increased sensitivity to food substances and chemicals, effects on the central nervous system including learning and behavior problems, and the presence of generalized symptoms such as aches and pains, swelling and fatigue. Autism and schizophrenia have in some cases been linked to yeast overgrowth.

The yeast most commonly responsible for the problems discussed in this chapter is called *Candida albicans*, and the condition where it grows out of control and affects the body negatively is sometimes referred to as candidiasis.

The recognition that yeast overgrowth may be playing a previously unsuspected role in the chronic ill health of some is fairly recent, leaving many questions still to be answered and many conjectures still to be verified through continuing research. However, there seems to be little doubt that many people who have suffered for years, despite undergoing a variety of therapies both traditional and alternative, have been relieved of many of their symptoms only when they started a yeast control program.

The reasons for a yeast overgrowth may include the following:

• The body's immune system is weakened due to illness, nutritional deficiencies or dependencies, or medical treatment with drugs such as cortisone.

• There has been a depletion of friendly bacteria, most often as a result of antibiotics, which tend to kill off not only the bad bacteria but the good as well.

• A too-favorable internal environment is provided for the yeast by a diet high in refined carbohydrates and sweeteners. Such a diet encourages the growth of yeast by providing it with lots of "food." (Yeasts grow extremely well on sugar.)

• There is a high level in the blood of progesterone, generally due to use of the birth control pill, pregnancy and ovulation. Dr. Orian Truss, whose work is responsible for sparking the current interest in yeast overgrowth, writes in his book *The Missing Diagnosis* that the onset of menstruation in girls may exacerbate the yeast problem because of the new fluctuating levels of progesterone.

• Diabetes is present, an ideal situation for yeast because of high blood sugar levels and an impaired immune system.

Is Yeast Overgrowth Causing Children's Problems?

As mentioned in Chapter 8, some of the clues indicating that children might be suffering from a yeast overgrowth include onset of problems preceded by a course of antibiotic treatment; frequent treatment of infections or acne with antibiotics; the consumption of large amounts of sweet foods, highly refined foods, and/or yeast- or mold-containing foods; persistent problems with vaginal yeast infections, oral thrush (yeast infection in the mouth), fungal infections of skin, nails or elsewhere (yeast is a fungus); or chronic problems that have not responded to other treatment programs. Digestive problems, respiratory problems and severe chemical sensitivity may also be symptoms of yeast overgrowth.

Generally, a diagnosis is made on the basis of past history (such as the occurrence of frequent antibiotic treatment), symptoms (such as digestive problems or persistent fungal infection), and therapeutic trial (that is, a yeast control program is implemented and the response noted).

Laboratory tests such as antibody studies are being developed and will be refined as time goes by, but as yet there does not appear to be any consensus on the accuracy of these tests.

Testing the Hypothesis

The hypothesis that children are suffering from a yeast overgrowth can be tested by following a yeast control program (described below) and noting the results. Dr. Truss recommends in his book a trial of six to twelve months minimum; it may be however that a shorter time period such as three months would be adequate, especially where very young children are concerned.

If during this time there is significant improvement, we can assume a strong probability that yeast overgrowth is a factor in our children's problems. If there is only moderate improvement, we should investigate the possibility that other factors, such as those discussed in Chapters 10 through 18, are involved, or that more time is needed to give the yeast control program a chance to work. If there has been no improvement at all, the likelihood is strong that yeast overgrowth is not a factor in our children's problems.

Controlling Yeast Overgrowth

There are a number of methods used to control yeast proliferation, none of which are mutually exclusive. Following is a brief summary of some of these methods:

• NYSTATIN. Nystatin is an anti-fungal medicine considered to be relatively safe because it stays in the gut and does not get absorbed into the bloodstream. It appears to be generally effective against *Candida albicans*, although some people may need to be on it for extended periods of time, and not all are helped by it. It is often recommended that the powdered form be used to avoid additives such as coloring, and that it be refrigerated. (It is also available in tablet, liquid, ointment and cream form.) Dr. William Crook in his book *The Yeast Connection* recommends the following dosages of nystatin for children: "Nystatin, 100,000 to 300,000 units (1 to 4 ml) four times a day for two to three months or longer (nystatin oral suspension—Squibb or Lederle), or nystatin powder, 1/32 to 1/8 teaspoon four times a day." Dr. Crook suggests increasing or lowering the dosage of the nystatin to reduce side effects. He writes that although some people may react to the nystatin itself, side effects are often due to the toxins released when the yeast are dying off in large numbers. This reaction may also occur with other yeast-control methods.

There are other anti-fungal drugs but these may have more severe side effects than nystatin. Some non-drug methods of yeast control that can be used either as alternatives to nystatin (in some situations with very good results) or in conjunction with it are listed below.

• DIET. Whatever other methods are used, a diet eliminating refined carbohydrates and sweeteners such as sugar, honey and corn syrup is essential, as this will help starve the yeast. In some cases it is also necessary to eliminate fruit and milk products, as these also have a high sugar content, until the yeast is under control. (The exception to avoiding milk products may be yogurt, if it does not contain sugar or fruit, and if it does contain live *Lactobacillus acidophilus* bacteria.)

Another aspect of diet that should be considered is the possibility of a sensitivity to yeast or mold in food. (The following information applies to mold sensitivities as well as to yeast sensitivities even when molds are not specifically mentioned; molds and yeasts are closely related members of the fungus family.)

Yeast sensitivity appears to affect a large proportion—though not all—of those suffering from a yeast overgrowth. Although many suffer from both, yeast overgrowth and yeast sensitivity are not identical; a yeast sensitivity is present only when a yeast-containing food causes a reaction after being eaten, whereas yeast overgrowth occurs when yeast is growing out of control in the body.

To test if children are sensitive to yeast in food, keep them off all yeast-containing foods for five to seven days, and on the next day challenge them with brewer's yeast, noting the reaction. Dr. Crook suggests eating a small piece of a brewer's yeast tablet and, if there are no reactions within ten minutes, continuing to eat pieces of the tablet over the space of an hour, then eating another tablet several hours later (stopping immediately if symptoms should occur). For those still symptom-free the next day, he suggests reintroducing yeasty foods to see if there is a reaction.

A reaction following such a challenge would indicate a yeast sensitivity and that yeast-containing foods should be avoided. (However, this would be more certain if the symptoms occurred after eating the brewer's yeast; a reaction to bread, for example, may indicate a sensitivity to wheat rather than to yeast.)

If there seems to be no sensitivity to yeast-containing foods, there is no reason to exclude them from the diet. If in doubt, a repeat trial of elimination and challenge would be in order. (See Chapter 14 for more information on testing for food sensitivities.)

Yeast and/or mold-containing foods include: anything fermented such as wine, beer, sauerkraut, pickles, vinegar (and anything *containing* vinegar, for example condiments such as ketchup and relish); fruit juices unless fresh and made from peeled fruit; malt; the skins of some fruits and vegetables (if necessary, these can either be peeled or washed carefully in a mixture of water and baking soda—or water and bleach—rinsing thoroughly); dried fruit; all yeasted breads, crackers and pastries; cheese; mushrooms; and many vitamin preparations.

Once yeast is under control in the body, in some cases it will be possible to be less rigid with the diet. This is an individual matter, and calls for experimentation to see how much sweet or yeast- and mold-containing food children can tolerate and under what circumstances.

Of course food sensitivities other than to yeast may be involved. Sometimes these will disappear when the yeast is controlled, but other times the sensitivities must be controlled before complete recovery will occur. (See Chapter 14.)

• AVOIDANCE OF ENVIRONMENTAL MOLD. Some yeast sufferers will be bothered by mold spores in the air, and these should be avoided as much as possible. (See page 243 in Chapter 15 for suggestions.) Other environmental sensitivities are also sometimes involved, and as with food, in some cases they may have been caused by the yeast problem and will disappear when it is controlled; in other cases, however, measures of controlling the environmental sensitivities such as avoidance will also have to be used. (Dr. Truss mentions that any neutralizing doses of chemicals whether sublingual or by injection should be stopped in those chemically sensitive if nystatin or yeast vaccine is to be used.)

• LACTOBACILLUS ACIDOPHILUS SUPPLEMENTS. *Lactobacillus acidophilus* is one of the friendly bacteria that may have been destroyed by the use of antibiotics. Resupplying it will help restore the internal balance in a child's body, inhibiting the growth of the yeast.

• GARLIC. Whether raw or in supplement form, garlic appears to be an effective anti-yeast agent. It should be noted that its anti-yeast properties are apparently due mostly to the ingredient allicin, which may have been removed in some deodorized forms of garlic supplements.

• CAPRYLIC ACID. According to Dr. Crook this is a short-chain fatty acid being marketed under a variety of brand names. It appears to be effective in some cases, although, according to Dr. Crook, it may occasionally cause digestive complaints.

• NUTRITIONAL SUPPLEMENTS. Dr. Crook recommends the following nutrients be supplemented in the diets of those with suspected yeast overgrowth: zinc, calcium, magnesium, vitamins A, B-complex, C and E, selenium and essential fatty acids. Yeast overgrowth may both cause nutritional deficiencies and be a result of nutritional deficiencies.

Dr. Jeffrey Bland, in his article *"Candida Albicans:* An Unsuspected Problem," writes that a program including 300 micrograms of biotin three times daily (an adult dose) plus supplementation of other nutrients, two teaspoons three times daily of olive oil (to supply oleic acid), a high fiber diet and one teaspoon three times daily of *Lactobacillus acidophilus* culture has helped decrease symptoms in some people.

• YEAST EXTRACT VACCINES. These may be helpful, but it is important that the doctor be extremely skilled and experienced in their use.

In addition to the methods of yeast control listed above, exercise and stress control (see in Chapter 18) may also be helpful. Wearing loose clothing of natural fibers (such as cotton) to reduce the hot, sweaty conditions that yeasts love (even going bare bottomed for extended periods if diaper rash is a problem) is often beneficial in preventing vaginal or topical yeast infections in children.

Books referred to in this chapter and other suggested reading:

Candida: A Twentieth Century Disease, Shirley S. Lorenzani, Ph.D. Keats Publishing, New Canaan, Connecticut, 1986. Discussion of the condition by someone who has experienced it.

The Candida Albicans Yeast-Free Cookbook, Pat Connolly and Associates of the Price-Pottenger Nutrition Foundation. Keats Publishing, New Canaan, Connecticut, 1985. Recipes and "Rainbow Meal Plan" for dietary control of Candida.

Coping with Candida Cookbook, Sally Rockwell, Nutrition Survival Press, P.O. Box 31065, 4703 Stone Way N., Seattle, 1984. Information about the yeast problem as well as recipes designed to help bring the Candida under control.

The Missing Diagnosis, C. Orion Truss, M.D., P.O. Box 26508, Birmingham, Alabama 35226, 1983. A discussion of Truss's work with *Candida albicans*, including many case histories.

The Yeast Connection, A Medical Breakthrough, William G. Crook, Professional Books, P.O. Box 3494, Jackson, Tennessee 38301, 1986. An extremely helpful and informative book, including chapters on "Health Problems in Children" and "Physical and Mental Problems of Teenagers."

14

FOOD SENSITIVITIES

We are taught from the time we are little that milk is the perfect food, an apple a day will keep the doctor away, bread is a necessary staple to our diet, spinach will make us strong, a sugary treat is a blissful delight, and, if we think about them at all, that additives are "necessary." It may come as a shock to find that the "good food" we have been serving our children—those innocent eggs, that innocuous broccoli, the nutritious pork roasts, the convenient frozen chicken pies, the yummy cupcakes with the pink icing—may in part be responsible for at least some of their behavior problems. Researchers are finding that food sensitivities are a factor in the autism, hyperactivity, retardation and schizophrenia of some children.

Food sensitivities are common; many children exhibit a variety of symptoms both physical and mental when they eat, drink or smell particular foods or food additives. Any part of the body, including the brain and rest of the central nervous system, can be affected by an adverse reaction to a food. The behavior of many children has been dramatically improved by clearing up food sensitivities.

The term "food sensitivities" as used in this book is equivalent to the term "food allergies" in its broadest interpretation (including food "intolerances"). Traditionalists in the medical profession classify as allergies only those reactions caused by an immunological response of the body. However, a growing number of doctors is widening the definition of allergies to include reactions which do not necessarily have an immunological explanation.

There is no doubt that in many cases food-related symptoms are the result of the immune system responding to a food or food by-product as if the body were under attack. However, some children react adversely to certain foods because of problems with digestion and absorption due to the absence of certain enzymes, vitamin deficiencies or insufficient hydrochloric acid. Other children may have toxic reactions to food additives such as coloring and to chemical contaminants such as pesticides, resulting in damage to body tissues or disruption of certain functions. Still other groups of children may be affected by other processes, many of them unknown at this point in time.

Sometimes the food sensitivity can be narrowed down to one constituent of a food. For example, some children are missing the enzyme lactase and so cannot digest the lactose in milk, suffering what is called "lactose intolerance." Other children are affected by the gluten in wheat, rye, oats and barley. Very often it is not the foods themselves that affect children negatively but the additives or contaminants. Dr. Ben Feingold discovered that salicylates, contained in a variety of foods, together with some additives, were causing hyperactivity in many children.

Are Food Sensitivities Causing Our Children's Problems?

Some of the clues suggesting that children are suffering from food sensitivities were mentioned in Chapter 8. These included the occurrence of food sensitivities (including a sensitivity to aspirin) among other family members, aversions to certain foods, cravings for certain foods, frequent consumption of certain foods, the consistent appearance of symptoms after consumption of particular foods, better behavior after a period of not eating, digestive problems such as stomachaches, gassiness, constipation and diarrhea, insatiable hunger, a diagnosis of hyperactivity, the existence of environmental sensitivities, and a strong possibility of a lactose intolerance in children not of Northern European descent.

In addition, as Dr. William Crook writes in *Tracking Down Hidden Food Allergy*, "You can suspect a hidden food allergy when your child . . . has dark circles under his eyes, sniffs, snorts and pushes her nose up, is irritable and overactive or tired, droopy and drowsy, complains of headache, stomachache or leg ache, is bothered by coughing or wheezing, was bothered by colic, rashes and sleep problems."

As can be seen, the symptoms that food sensitivities can cause are varied. It is only fairly recently that people have begun to realize that food sensitivities are not only much more common than previously thought, but that they are also responsible for a much wider variety of symptoms than has previously been accepted. In addition to physical symptoms such as hives, stomachaches, sniffles, eczema and headaches (which because they are painful or at least distracting can lead to behavioral problems), it is now apparent that food sensitivities can be the direct cause of mental and behavioral symptoms as well, such as depression, hyperactivity, confusion, irritability, uncontrollable rages, anxiety and even hallucinations. These symptoms can range from mild to incapacitating, occurring either intermittently or continually. (It should be noted that in some cases severe reactions, such as difficulty breathing, may result from a food sensitivity, leading in some instances to death. For this reason great care should be taken when testing for food sensitivities.)

Why It Is Hard to Pinpoint Sensitivities

In some cases it is easy to pick out which children are suffering from food sensitivities. If a child consistently has a temper tantrum two minutes after devouring an orange (or egg or piece of cheese or chocolate bar), it is obvious that there is a relationship between the food and the behavior.

But in many cases the relationship between cause and effect is not so obvious. Some of the reasons that a search for food sensitivities might be a difficult one are:

• THE RESPONSE TIME IS NOT IMMEDIATE. Children do not always react immediately, or even within hours, to a food. Sometimes reactions do not occur until days later. When two to four days have elapsed before there is a reaction, the link between food and symptom is much less noticeable.

• SYMPTOMS APPEAR INCONSISTENTLY. Sometimes foods provoke reactions only under certain circumstances. For example, in some cases small amounts of a food will not provoke a reaction, while larger amounts will. In other cases, symptoms will appear only if a food is eaten more than once a week. Or, some children will react to a food when it is prepared one way and not another (for example, tolerating cabbage cooked but not raw). It can also happen that exposure to a particular food will cause problems only when a child is at the same time subjected to other stresses (such as certain chemicals, infections or psychological pressures).

• SYMPTOMS ARE CHANGEABLE. Symptoms of food sensitivities do not always stay the same, sometimes changing over time. As Stevens and Stoner write in *How to Improve Your Child's Behavior Through Diet*, "milk may have given your child colic as a baby, caused him to wet the bed at age four, but may make his nose run when he's ten."

• MULTIPLE FOOD SENSITIVITIES ARE INVOLVED. If a child has multiple food sensitivities, symptoms may not clear up unless all of the offending foods are removed from the diet. Removing only one or two may not make any noticeable difference.

• THE SYMPTOM-CAUSING FOODS ARE EATEN FREQUENTLY AND THE SENSITIVITIES ARE OF LONG DURATION. In this case symptoms sometimes become chronic—for example, a continually stuffed nose, constant lethargy, or a seemingly perpetual state of hyperactivity—thereby obscuring the food-symptom relationship.

When addictions are involved, children often crave the foods which are causing their problems. Because their bodies have partially adapted to the harmful foods, they may actually feel better for a short time after eating these foods and experience withdrawal symptoms when they don't eat them. However, if the situation is not corrected, at some point the offending foods may no longer give a "lift," and children may suffer more serious symptoms.

It should be noted that it is easy to mistake addictions for hypoglycemia, as in both cases children may feel terrible (and act terrible) until they are fed.

• COMPLICATING FACTORS ARE PRESENT. When complicating factors are present such as hypoglycemia, yeast overgrowth, metal toxicity or environmental sensitivities, these may have to be dealt with before the food sensitivities will improve.

• THE FOOD-SENSITIVE CHILD IS BREAST-FED. Babies who are breast-fed may react to any of the foods their mothers have eaten. In this case the mothers will have to experiment with their own diets.

Testing for Sensitivities

How do we work our way out of this confusion to find out if foods are in fact affecting our children, and if so, which? Following is a discussion of some of the different methods used to check out food sensitivities. Positive response to the following tests will be further evidence to support the hypothesis that food sensitivities are causing our children's problems.

• SCRATCH-TEST. Test solutions of foods are applied to scratches or pricks that have been made on the skin. If there is more than a mild reaction (usually a raised bump), a sensitivity to that food can be suspected. However, scratch-tests are thought by many nutrition-oriented doctors to be highly inaccurate for foods.

• CYTOTOXIC BLOOD TEST. The suspected food is mixed with some of the child's white blood cells. If antibodies are produced by the white blood cells, a sensitivity to that food is indicated. This method is only useful when the sensitivities are caused by an immune response.

• RAST (RADIOALLERGOSORBENT TEST). Robert Eagle in *Eating and Allergy* writes, "Without going into technicalities, RAST determines whether body fluids or tissues contain antibodies which react specifically to a suspected allergen. The main drawback of RAST is that even if it shows that antibodies are present, there is no certainty that the patient is allergic to that substance. We develop antibodies to many foreign proteins to which we are often exposed, but we do not always become sensitized to them."

• PROVOCATIVE FOOD TESTING. Provocative food testing includes the *subcutaneous* and *sublingual* methods. According to Dr. William Philpott in *A Physician's Handbook on Orthomolecular Medicine* (edited by Williams and Kalita), the subcutaneous method involves injecting food extracts "sufficiently deep into the skin so as to be circulated by blood to all tissues of the body." In the sublingual method, food extracts are placed under the tongue and also end up being carried by the bloodstream to the body's tissues. If symptoms occur, a sensitivity to that food can be suspected. The subcutaneous method might be traumatic for some children, as a number of injections are required.

Concerning accuracy, Philpott writes, "These food extracts have the disadvantage of being aqueous in source, and therefore not carrying all of the qualities of reaction of a complete test food. There is an estimated 80 percent value of a comparison between deliberate food tests and provocative food tests." (Deliberate food tests are when the whole food is tested, such as after a fast or elimination diet.)

• PULSE TEST. Ludeman and Henderson in their *Do-It-Yourself Allergy Analysis Handbook* give directions for doing the pulse test:

"Take your pulse five minutes before eating. Eat all of the food. Then, take your pulse five, ten, twenty and forty minutes after you finish eating. Your pulse may not change for each of these readings. If your pulse varies twelve to twenty points above or below normal, it indicates a reaction to the food you are testing. For example, if your baseline pulse reading is 75, a pulse of 90 twenty minutes after eating would be significant. If your pulse continued to rise, you would know that you were reactive to the food."

• KINESIOLOGY. Again, a quote from Ludeman and Henderson:

"In this diagnostic method, muscle strength is first established. For example, the thumb and index finger are pressed together then the amount of resistance it takes to prevent them from being pulled apart is measured. A food such as chocolate or coffee is then taken into the mouth, and the muscle is immediately re-tested. If there is much less resistance, an allergy to that food may be suspected."

There is controversy about this method of testing, but it does appear to be accurate for some people.

• FASTING. A fast can have serious consequences, making it extremely important that it be done in consultation with a doctor. Many doctors recommend that only older children attempt a fast. We should be particularly wary about subjecting children who are asthmatic, epileptic, diabetic, significantly underweight, physically rundown or very young to a fast.

The first step in a fast suggested by Ludeman and Henderson is this: "Start by ridding your body of as much of the old offending substances and their by-products as possible. Do this by cleaning out your gastrointestinal tract. Use a laxative, like milk of magnesia or Epsom salts, or an enema." Vitamin C in large doses also has a laxative effect on some people.

During a fast, no food or liquid other than purified or uncontaminated water is ingested. When children are symptom-free, generally after four days or more, foods are added one at a time and the effect is noted. There should be a time lapse of at least four hours between each new food. If the food is taken sublingually, the timing between additions may be less as absorption is quicker. Symptoms usually appear fairly quickly after the offending food has been eaten, and generally are more intense than usual.

Blood sugar levels are sometimes tested an hour after the test food has been ingested, as a change in glucose levels is a possible indicator of a food sensitivity. (In some cases food sensitivities may cause blood sugar levels to drop, leading to confusion with hypoglycemia. In other cases, food sensitivities may cause high blood sugar levels, thus being implicated in diabetes.)

We should not expect a fast to be a pleasant experience, although the results may be worth the agony. Ludeman and Henderson write, "As you withdraw from foods to which you are addicted you may experience any number of symptoms. Psychological symptoms such as mood swings and depression may accompany physiological symptoms such as stomachache, gas, headache and sore throat. Withdrawal symptoms usually begin at the end of the first or during the second day, become more troublesome on the second and third day, peak on the fourth day and then taper off. Backache and other muscle and joint aches and pains may occur on the third or fourth day and persist for a day or two. Your sense of smell and taste will probably become more acute. Your pulse rate may go either up or down, and then stabilize. This sequence of symptoms may vary greatly from person to person." Also, energy levels may be below normal.

A fast is probably the most accurate method of testing for food sensitivities, particularly if at the same time exposure to chemicals in the environment—such as gas fumes, synthetics, cleaning agents and perfumes—is minimized as much as possible. This reduces the chance of reactions due to environmental sensitivities. (See Chapter 15 for more information.)

In some cases, a modified fast might be considered. For example, vegetable juices could be given in addition to water, as long as the possibility of a sensitivity to the juices used is kept in mind.

Some of the information contained in the following section on elimination diets also applies to fasts and should be read as well.

• ELIMINATION DIET. An elimination diet is often the best method to use when testing children for food sensitivities. In an elimination diet, one or more food items are not eaten for a period of time (generally until symptoms disappear) and are then reintroduced one by one into the diet. If a reaction occurs, a sensitivity can be suspected. In the case of breast-fed children, the mother can go on the elimination diet.

(If a fairly stringent diet is followed, for example the "rare foods" diet suggested by Dr. Crook, where any food eaten more than once a week is eliminated for one to three weeks, the accuracy of the results should be not too much less than with a fast.)

WHICH FOODS DO WE ELIMINATE?

The first step in an elimination diet is to decide which foods to test. Many children have multiple food sensitivities and it is much better to test all the foods we are suspicious of at once rather than singly. A child who is allergic to three foods—wheat, peanuts and grapes for example—may not show much improvement if only one of these foods is eliminated and the others remain in the diet.

Keep in mind that children may be sensitive to anything they eat or drink, including water. Not all water is the same; water differs according to the minerals, metals, salts and chemical contaminants it contains. Its composition depends on its source (which particular lake, well or spring it was drawn from), what treatment it has received (such as fluoridation, chlorination, carbon filtration, distillation), what kind of pipes it has passed through (picking up lead or copper, for example) and how it has been stored (water can be contaminated by plastic containers).

Noting daily in a symptom diary the foods children eat and drink, and what symptoms they have, may give some indications of which foods (if any) are causing problems. At the very least this will show us which foods children eat most and how often. It is sometimes surprising to find, once eating habits are down on paper, how wrong estimates of the amounts and frequency of food consumption can be.

Another useful feature of a symptom diary is that it provides a written record of a child's behavior, making it easy to compare this behavior before, during and after the elimination diet. Given the faulty nature of memory, it is important to have a written record such as this which describes exactly how rambunctious or slow or confused a child really was, especially when improvement is very gradual. See page 124 in Chapter 8 for an example of a symptom diary chart. (This chart has a column for environmental exposures as well which is useful; many children who have food sensitivities also have environmental sensitivities.)

After a few days of keeping the symptom diary, it is time to compile a list of foods to be eliminated from the following categories of "suspect" foods, remembering that to eliminate *all* categories applicable will increase the likelihood of success:

• Foods that either parent is sensitive to.

• Foods that sometimes appear to cause symptoms, even if irregularly.

• Foods that have previously caused reactions, even if they currently seem to be tolerated.

• Foods that children strongly dislike.

• Foods that are favorites.

• Foods that our children eat frequently. We should be particularly suspicious of foods eaten daily.

• Foods that are most commonly found to produce learning and behavior problems among children: wheat, milk, eggs, corn, sugar, caffeine, foods containing salicylates and foods containing artificial additives.

• Foods that have tested positive on other food sensitivity tests.

• Foods that we are suspicious of for any other reason.

• *We must also add to our elimination list every food that is already known to cause symptoms, and any food that is contaminated with a substance (such as plastic or pesticides) that is known to cause symptoms in our children.*

• *Any foods containing the suspect foods, even in minuscule amounts, must also be avoided.* If children are to stay on medication, we must be sure it does not contain any of the foods or additives we are trying to eliminate.

FOODS CONTAINING CAFFEINE
coffee, tea, cola drinks and chocolate.

FOODS CONTAINING NATURAL SALICYLATES

(as listed in *Children's Nutrition* by Lewis A. Coffin) apples, apricots, berries, cherries, currants, grapes, raisins, nectarines, oranges, peaches, plums, prunes, tangerines, tomatoes, almonds, cloves, coffee, cucumbers and pickles, green peppers, teas, oil of wintergreen, wine vinegar, cider vinegar, chili peppers and malt flavoring.

PLANNING THE ELIMINATION DIET

Once we have decided what to eliminate, the next decision is what to include. Although it may seem that not much is left, many of us will discover there are foods we have never tried before, which will allow us to continue enjoying variety in our diets.

It is a good idea to plan menus a week ahead, making sure to have on hand a good stock of all the food we will need, including snacks.

This would be a good time to start rotating foods, to help prevent the start of new food sensitivities. See pages 220–221 for information on rotation diets.

STARTING THE ELIMINATION DIET

At the beginning of the elimination diet, completely remove the suspect foods from the diet for five or more days, and continue to keep the symptom diary. Be prepared for a less than easy time on the elimination diet for the first few days. Dr. Crook gives a summary of what to expect:

"During the first 2 to 4 days of the diet, he's apt to feel irritable. He may become more hyperactive or more tired and droopy. He may develop a headache or leg cramps. And he may be 'mad' at you (and the world) because he isn't getting foods he craves, especially sweets. (He may act like a two-pack-a-day smoker who's just given up the weed. Children and adults who suffer from a hidden food allergy are often addicted to foods they're allergic to.)

"Usually, if your child is allergic to an eliminated food, he'll feel better by the 4th, 5th or 6th day. And almost always he'll improve by the 10th day. Occasionally, though, it'll take two to three weeks before his symptoms subside completely."

IF THE ELIMINATION DIET DOESN'T HELP

What do we do if symptoms don't disappear? Dr. Crook writes, "If your child fails to improve after following the diet for 14 days, 'turn him loose.' Let him eat what he wants. If his symptoms worsen (such as headache, hyperactivity or stuffiness), chances are one or more foods bother him. And you'll have to do further dietary detective work to find the troublemakers."

If symptoms don't worsen after children have been "turned loose," it is likely that either food sensitivities are not causing any problems, or there are complicating factors. For example, children may be reacting to some of the foods that were not eliminated; environmental sensitivities, hypoglycemia or yeast overgrowth might be involved; or, there were diet infringements (even small amounts of certain foods can cause symptoms, lasting up to four days or possibly even longer, in some children; surprisingly, even odors can sometimes trigger reactions).

If there is no improvement or only partial improvement and we still suspect the possibility of food sensitivities, we can start again, making the conditions even more stringent. For example, we can supervise what children are eating more closely. (Perhaps their friends can come and play at our house instead of our children visiting away from home; even staying home from school for a few days may be necessary.) Next, if it wasn't done the first time around, we can eliminate all the foods included in the suspect categories listed on pages 214–215. Then we can add the following categories to our suspect list:

• Foods that are closely related to known symptom-producing foods (see pages 222–223 for lists of food families).

• Foods that children eat more than once a week.

• Foods that are chemically contaminated. Foods are subjected to many chemicals on the long trip from the farm to our kitchens. For example, plants are often sprayed with pesticides and made to look shiny with wax and mineral oil, and animals are fed hormones and antibiotics. Foods of both plant and animal origin may pick up chemicals from the materials they are packaged in. Water may be contaminated at the source by industrial wastes, by chemicals such as chlorine added to treat it, or by contact with the water pipes. Children may react to any of these chemicals.

In addition to being more stringent with the diet, we can try to control some of the complicating factors that might be interfering with a child's improvement. We can eliminate as many symptom-producing environmental substances as possible (Chapter 14), as food and environmental sensitivities frequently go hand in hand. We can give children small meals every two hours to prevent their blood-sugar levels from falling. (See Chapter 12 on hypoglycemia). We can try to decrease stress levels (pages 269–272 in Chapter 18).

INTRODUCING SUSPECT FOODS

If children do improve, once they have been symptom-free for a couple of days, we can begin the next step, which is to introduce the suspect foods and note the reactions in our symptom diary. The procedure for introducing the foods suggested by Dr. Crook is this:

Give your child all he wants of the eliminated food for breakfast. If he shows no reaction, give him more of the food for lunch and supper (and in-between meals, too).

If he shows no symptoms after adding a food the first day, add another food the second day in exactly the same way, giving him all he wants, *unless he shows a reaction.*

If you think he develops symptoms when you add a food, but aren't certain, give him more of the food until the symptoms are obvious.

If your child shows an obvious reaction after eating a food (such as stuffiness, cough, irritability, hyperactivity, drowsiness, headache, stomachache or flushing), don't give more of that food. *Wait until the reactions subside (usually 24 to 48 hours) before you add another food.*

If the reaction really bothers him, you can usually shorten it by giving him 1 teaspoonful of "soda mixture" (2 parts baking soda and 1 part potassium bicarbonate), or by giving him Alka-Seltzer Gold [Alka-Seltzer in gold foil *without aspirin*] in a half-glass water (2 tablets for teenagers and adults; 1 tablet for children 6 to 12; ½ tablet for children 1 to 5). A laxative such as milk of magnesia will also help terminate the reaction by more rapidly removing the offending food from the intestinal tract.

Please note that the baking soda/potassium bicarbonate mixture should not be used if children have kidney or heart problems. In addition, any child who experiences a serious reaction, such as difficulty breathing, should receive immediate medical attention.

Following are a few more points to keep in mind when testing foods:

• If a child has asthma, suspect foods should be introduced only with the cooperation of a doctor, as a provoked attack may be more severe than usual.

• Test only one new food a day, making sure the food contains no other ingredients. For example, use rice that has been cooked in purified or uncontaminated water with no salt for testing purposes, rather than rice-containing foods such as rice cakes, which sometimes contain millet, sesame seeds and other ingredients.

• Test with food that is not canned or pre-packaged. Otherwise, it will be difficult to tell if a child is reacting to additives that may or may not be specified on the labels, chemicals that the food might be contaminated with (for example if it has been stored in a plastic or aluminum container, can, tinfoil, cling wrap of some sort, or box), or the food itself.

Concerning the nature of the foods being tested, we have two alternatives:

Alternative #1: Testing with foods that are organic and untreated, free from additives and chemical contamination. If this alternative is chosen do not buy food from ordinary grocery stores, as they rarely stock organic food, and it is not known which chemicals the fruit, vegetables, meats and so on they do sell have been exposed to. We will have to do our shopping elsewhere, some possibilities being food co-ops, health food stores or directly from farmers. (See page 51 in Chapter 3 for addresses.) For the duration of the test it is also best to avoid tap water, which usually contains many unfriendly chemicals. Well and spring water are not necessarily more pure.

If children do not react to foods that are organic and additive free, it does not mean that it is safe for them to eat the additive-laden, chemically contaminated equivalent; these will have to be tested separately.

Alternative #2: Testing with food that is not organic. Although we will not be able to differentiate in this case if children are reacting to the food or the contaminants, it makes sense to choose this alternative if it is unlikely, due to cost, availability, energy required or other reason, that we would ever be feeding them organic food as part of their regular diet. However, just for the sake of knowing, if children do react to a food of unknown background, it might be worth retesting with the organic equivalent.

If children do react to a large number of chemically treated foods, we may save ourselves a lot of grief by searching out organic alternatives rather than severely restricting the diet.

• The amount of time it takes for symptoms to appear varies, from minutes up to four days. However, most reactions will occur within a couple of hours if the food has been avoided for five to ten days.

• Incorporate test foods into the diet only after all the testing is done. In other words, children should eat the suspected foods only on the days these foods are tested. Even if the suspect foods appear to cause no symptoms, they are to be avoided until all foods have been tested.

• Test only on days when children are free from physical stresses such as colds and psychological stresses such as exams.

• If children do not react to a particular food, it does not always mean this is a safe food for them. Clear-cut reactions are most likely to occur when a food has been avoided for five to ten days. If more time than this has elapsed, children may not react, or react only slightly, when the food is reintroduced. Unfortunately, symptoms may gradually reoccur when a food is returned to the diet and once more eaten on a regular basis. This is especially important to remember when symptoms take longer than ten days to clear and we are reintroducing foods a couple of weeks after they have been eliminated; in this case we should be even more suspicious than usual.

Testing the Hypothesis

If children test positive for food sensitivities on any of the tests listed above, this is partial confirmation of our hypothesis that food sensitivities are causing at least some of their problems. Keeping in mind that tests can have false positives as well as false negatives, our next step is to test the hypothesis, by following the procedure for the elimination diet as described above. This means eliminating all the foods that tested positive for five to fourteen days and then reintroducing them one by one into the diet, noting the results.

If we have already done the elimination diet, we should confirm our results by retesting, as well as with continued observation. This is particularly easy if we start to follow a rotation diet (described in the following section) and continue on for awhile with our symptom diary.

Some may choose to do the testing and retesting of food in a single- or double-"blind" method, where the food is disguised in some manner—some doctors use capsules—so that the child and/or the person administering the food do not know which food is being tested. This ensures that the child's reaction is a true sensitivity reaction and not due to some other reason, such as disliking the food, and that the person noting the results is not affected by preconceived expectations of what the result will be. If for any reason after testing and retesting with undisguised food we are still unsure of the effect of any particular food, this might be a good method to try.

If children improve considerably when suspect foods are removed from the diet and symptoms return when the foods are reintroduced, our hypothesis has been proved correct. Now that we know that our children have food sensitivities, we can implement the food sensitivity control program described in the next section.

If children improve partially or only minimally, it may be that other factors are involved in causing their problems, such as discussed in Chapters 10 through 18.

If there is no improvement after following these suggestions, we should assume, at least until we have more information, that our children do not have food sensitivities.

Controlling Food Sensitivities

A program to control food sensitivities may include several components, including dealing with any existing complicating factors. In other words, the program may need to include the control of environmental sensitivities, hypoglycemia and yeast overgrowth, elimination and avoidance of heavy metals, and the addition of nutritional supplements. Also, exercise, stress control and self-awareness (all three discussed in Chapter 18) may be found to be extremely helpful in controlling food sensitivities.

Following is a discussion of the two major methods used to control food sensitivities: diet and food therapy.

Diet

GOOD NUTRITION

Children are more likely to be affected by food sensitivities, or suffer more severely, if they are not fed nutritiously. It makes sense that children should be on a diet that follows the general basics of good nutrition. (For more information on children's nutritional needs, see Chapter 10.)

FREQUENCY AND THE ROTATION DIET

It also makes sense to restrict the quantity and frequency of symptom-producing foods in children's diets. How severe the restrictions must be will vary from child to child and from situation to situation.

Some children may be able to tolerate a glass of milk once a week with no ill effects, while others may have a violent reaction simply from eating a half a piece of bread that has whey (a milk product) as one of its ingredients. The same children who can, during a relaxed holiday period, eat corn occasionally, may find that when they are going to school and under more stress, they must completely avoid corn products. For this reason, we may find that a flexible approach to the control of food sensitivities works best.

Once we are confident that the foods children are sensitive to have been identified, they should be eliminated from the diet for about three months. At this point they can be retested. If there are no reactions, they can be reintroduced into the diet as long as we ensure they are not eaten too frequently. Otherwise, symptoms may reappear. We will have to experiment to find out how often our children can safely eat each food and in what quantities. Two apples once every four days may be fine for some children, while others may only be able to tolerate a half an apple once a month. Some foods children will always react to and should be completely avoided.

One way of regulating the frequency of the foods children eat is to follow a rotation diet. In a rotation diet, foods are eaten on a rotating basis, no more often than once every four days. Less often is fine, and in some cases may be preferable. For example, Day 1 of a rotation diet might be a beef, orange, buckwheat and cabbage day, Day 2 might be a fish, melon, millet and green pepper day, and so on. While individual foods must not be repeated more than once every four days, foods from the same family (see food family chart on page 222) need only have one day in between. That is, if apples are eaten on Day 2, pears, which are in the same family, may be eaten on Day 4. A rotation diet is probably one of the best solutions for children with multiple food sensitivities, as it helps to prevent new sensitivities from starting and old sensitivities from re-starting. It can also help pick out sensitivities because it narrows down the possibilities: if Day 5 is always a chicken, rice, banana and carrot day, and on that day children always seem to be flying higher than a kite, chances are the cause is one of the foods eaten that day.

In some cases, it is a good idea to rotate water sources as well.

There is a rotation diet kit available from Sally Rockwell's Nutrition Survival Services which may make it easier. (See page 53 in Chapter 3 for the address.) Some of the books listed at the end of this chapter have sample rotation diets, or we can use the following food family chart to make our own.

The following list of food families is from *The Complete Book of Allergy Control* by Laura J. Stevens:

ANIMAL FAMILIES

Bird: Chicken, pheasant, quail, and their eggs; duck, goose, turkey

Bovid: Beef, goat, lamb, milk products

Crustaceans: Crab, crayfish, lobster, shrimp

Freshwater fish: Bass, herring, perch, salmon, sturgeon, trout, whitefish

Mollusks: Abalone, clam, oyster, scallops, snail

Saltwater fish: Anchovy, cod, flounder, mackerel, sea bass, sea herring, sole, tuna

Swine: Pork and pork products

PLANT FAMILIES

Apple: Apple, pear, quince

Banana: Arrowroot, banana, plantain

Beet: Beet, lamb's-quarters, spinach

Buckwheat: Buckwheat, rhubarb

Cashew: Cashew, mango, pistachio

Citrus: Citron, grapefruit, kumquat, lemon, lime, orange, tangerine

Cola: Chocolate, cocoa, cola

Composite: Artichoke, chicory, dandelion, endive, lettuce, sunflower

Date: Coconut, date

Fungus: Mushroom, yeast

Ginger: Ginger, turmeric

Gourd: Cantaloupe, cucumber, pumpkin, squash, watermelon, zucchini

Grass: Barley, cane, corn, molasses, oats, rice, rye, sorghum, wheat, wild rice

Heather: Blueberry, cranberry, huckleberry, wintergreen

Laurel: Avocado, bay leaf, cinnamon, sassafras

Legume: Alfalfa, bean (garbanzo [chick pea], kidney, lima, navy, pinto, string), carob, clover honey, lentil, licorice, pea (black-eyed, green), peanut, soybean, sprouts

Lily: Asparagus, chive, garlic, leek, onion

Mallow: Cottonseed, okra

Mint: Basil, marjoram, mint, oregano, peppermint, sage, spearmint, thyme

Mustard: Brussels sprouts, cabbage, cauliflower, collards, horseradish, kale, mustard, radish, rutabaga, turnip, watercress

Myrtle: Allspice, clove

Nutmeg: Nutmeg, mace

Parsley: Anise, caraway, carrot, celery, celery seed, coriander, cumin, dill, fennel, parsley, parsnip

Plum: Almond, apricot, cherry, nectarine, peach, plum, wild cherry

Potato: Cayenne, chili pepper, eggplant, paprika, pepper (red, green), potato, tomato

Rose: Blackberry, boysenberry, raspberry, strawberry
Walnut: Black walnut, butternut, English walnut, hickory nut, pecan

The following are food families with only one member each: Brazil nut, grape (raisin), macadamia nut, maple, olive, pineapple, sesame, sweet potato, tapioca, tea, vanilla.

THE FEINGOLD DIET

In this diet, also known as the Kaiser-Permanente or K-P Diet, initially all foods with artificial colors and flavorings are eliminated as well as foods with natural salicylates (the active ingredient in aspirin) and sometimes the preservatives BHA and BHT. Later on, foods with natural salicylates (listed on page 215) may be reintroduced if they are well tolerated. However, Feingold writes, *"From present indications, an individual sensitive to artificial colors and flavors must avoid them throughout his life."*

This diet has good success with hyperactive children. Feingold writes in his book *Why Your Child Is Hyperactive*, "The best estimate, based on careful records, is that 50 percent have a likelihood of full response, while 75 percent can be removed from drug management, even if full response to other symptoms is not achieved."

Generally it takes ten days to two weeks for long-term improvement to occur once a child is put on this diet, although the response time may be shorter or longer. Drugs, Feingold writes, can usually be stopped in two to three weeks, but any changes in medication should be done with the advice of a doctor.

He also writes, and in some cases this will apply to other food sensitivities as well, "The diet must be adhered to 100 percent. Compliance of 80 percent or 90 percent can lead to failure. It is important to remember that often a single bite or a single drink can cause an undesired response which may persist for seventy-two hours or more. An infraction on Sunday and then again on Wednesday can keep the child in a persistent state of disturbed behavior throughout the week."

AVOIDING SYMPTOM-PRODUCING FOODS

Some food substances and additives are extremely common in canned and packaged goods, making it difficult to avoid them. Labels don't always contain complete lists of ingredients, and foods sometimes turn up as ingredients in the most surprising items. Here are some of the things to watch out for:

• Medications for children are often sweetened and often contain artificial flavoring and coloring. Most tablets contain corn. Always check with a doctor or pharmacist for the contents of medications, and if these include symptom-producing foods or additives, ask for an alternative. If there is no alternative, try washing off the color of a capsule or breaking it open. The Feingold Association (see page 53 in Chapter 3) has lists of medications and additives.

• Vitamins and minerals, in all forms (liquid, powdered, capsule, tablet) may contain symptom-producing foods and additives, including artificial flavoring and coloring, sweeteners, preservatives, milk-powder, cornstarch, etc. If in doubt, check directly with the company that produces them. There are some companies now that are conscious of food sensitivities and contain as few extra ingredients as possible. See pages 51–52 in Chapter 3 for addresses.

• Being "label-wise" is crucial. Labels do not always have complete listings of ingredients and are not always clear. See pages 163–164 in Chapter 10 for a discussion of labels. If in doubt about the contents of a food, write the manufacturer.

According to Feingold, it is "a good idea to check the ingredients periodically even on the items you buy routinely. Manufacturers often change the ingredients in the 'additive game.' "

Ludeman and Henderson list on pages 125 to 128 in *Do-It-Yourself Allergy Analysis Handbook* products that may contain common problem-causing foods.

FINDING ALTERNATIVE FOODS

When children are sensitive to many foods, thinking of alternatives is often difficult at first. However, once we start looking, we will probably find a whole world of foods we didn't even know existed. Look through cookbooks of other cultures, browse through ethnic markets and grocery shops (even regular grocery stores are beginning to have more variety), get information from some of the mail-order food suppliers listed on page 51 in Chapter 3, or look through books such as *The Cook's Book* by Howard Hillman.

In addition, cookbooks designed specifically for sufferers of food sensitivities are available in many bookstores and libraries. These contain recipes which avoid common symptom-producing foods. It is also possible to adapt ordinary recipes by replacing ingredients that affect children with those that are safe for them. For example, in many cases lemon juice can be used instead of vinegar, rice flour instead of wheat flour, and soy milk instead of cow's milk.

DEFICIENCIES CAUSED BY FOOD AVOIDANCE

By cutting out a food substance, we may also be cutting out nutrients that are crucial to children's health and growth. For example, we will have to ensure that children who must avoid milk and milk products receive their calcium from other sources. Possible substitutes are soybeans, sesame seeds, almonds, dark green, leafy vegetables or calcium supplements (which should generally contain magnesium as well). Again, it is important to check that these do not contain any foods or additives our children are sensitive to. See the chart on pages 153–156 in Chapter 10 for information on children's nutrient requirements.

Food Therapy

The same methods that are used to test for sensitivities, sublingual and subcutaneous (see "Provocative Food Testing," page 211), can also be used to treat the sensitivities. Doris Rapp in her book *Allergies and the Hyperactive Child* explains:

"Some dilutions of foods appear to cause symptoms, for example, hyperactivity, bellyaches, or a stuffy nose, while other dilutions appear to relieve these same symptoms . . . If a patient has numerous food sensitivities, correct treatment dilutions of several foods can be combined."

Dr. Rapp's experience has been that sublingual food therapy needs to be given three times a day at the outset, but can after a while be cut back to twice a week; subcutaneous therapy is started at once a day but after only a few weeks may be reduced to once or twice a week. While sublingual therapy is clearly preferable when indicated, it is not, Dr. Rapp has found, as helpful for some patients as the subcutaneous therapy.

But initial success isn't the whole story. "Once a patient is well treated, it is not unusual for a parent to forget to give food therapy" with consequent recurrence of the problem.

Dr. Rapp notes that "with food therapy, most offending foods can be ingested in moderation without causing symptoms." But the sailing may still not be smooth, particularly when a child develops a *new* food sensitivity, say to peanut butter. A food therapy devised before the appearance of this sensitivity won't contain peanut and so won't help with this problem. Dr. Rapp suggests that obtaining relief with a bicarbonate preparation may indicate an overlooked food problem.

It can also happen that a child's dosage requirements change, so that symptoms recur when the food in question is consumed, even though the treatment is kept up. Symptoms may also recur when a child's food therapy dosage is reduced too quickly.

If children are sensitive to only one or two easily avoided foods, we might not want to be bothered with the fuss of trips to the doctor. However, if children are sensitive to a large number of foods, some of which involve major food groups, we may want to give food therapy a try. We should be aware that it may be difficult to find a nearby doctor who practices food therapy, as it is not yet completely accepted as a treatment method. In addition, how successful the treatment is depends on the skill of the doctor.

Books referred to in this chapter and other suggested reading:

Allergies and the Hyperactive Child, Doris J. Rapp. Cornerstone Books, New York, 1980. For a description, see Chapter 8.

The Allergy Self-Help Cookbook, Marjorie Hurt Jones, Rodale Press, Emmaus, Pennsylvania, 1984. An excellent sourcebook and cookbook for sufferers from food sensitivities. It includes recipes that avoid the most common food offenders, and has sections on exploring new ingredients, how to plan a rotation diet, allergy-free kitchens, eating out, nutrition basics, and addresses for alternate sources of foods, vitamins and kitchen aids.

Beyond the Staff of Life, Kief Adler. Naturegraph Publishers, Happy Camp, California, 1976. A vegetarian cookbook that is gluten-free and dairy-free. The recipes are simple, always delicious, and written with a touch of humor.

Children's Nutrition, A Consumer's Guide, Lewis A. Coffin, Capra Press, Santa Barbara, California, 1984. For a description see Chapter 10.

The Complete Book of Allergy Control, Laura J. Stevens, Macmillan Publishing Company, New York, 1983. Well-written, very informative and comprehensive.

The Cook's Book, Howard Hillman, Avon Books, New York, 1981. For a description, see Chapter 10.

Coping With Your Allergies, Natalie Golos and Frances Golos Golbitz with Frances Spatz Leighton. Simon and Schuster, New York, 1979. A wealth of information written in a practical style, a book that would make any sensitivity-sufferer's life easier.

Do-It-Yourself Allergy Analysis Handbook, Kate Ludeman and Louise Henderson with Henry S. Basayne. Keats Publishing, New Canaan, Connecticut, 1979. Short and handy, with lots of helpful lists and charts, including recipes and a list of household chemical substitutes.

Dr. Mandell's 5-Day Allergy Relief System,, Marshall Mandell and Lynne Waller Scanlon. Thomas Y. Crowell, New York, 1979. Useful information presented in an interesting manner.

Eating and Allergy, Robert Eagle. Futura Publications, London, 1979. Interesting and informative.

How to Improve Your Child's Behavior Through Diet, Laura J. Stevens and Rosemary B. Stoner. Doubleday, New York, 1979. Includes a very good section on food allergies; has lots of recipes geared to allergy sufferers. A nice informal style, easy to read.

The People's Handbook of Allergies and Allergens, Ruth Winter. Contemporary Books, Chicago, 1984. Contains an "alphabetical listing of allergies, allergens, and other terms related to allergy."

A Physician's Handbook on Orthomolecular Medicine, Roger J. Williams and Dwight K. Kalita, editors. Keats Publishing, New Canaan, Connecticut, 1977. For a description, see Chapter 4.

Sally Rockwell's Allergy Recipes, Sally Rockwell. Nutrition Survival Press, P.O. Box 31065, 4703 Stone Way N., Seattle, Washington, 1984. Contains "no-think pre-rotated allergy relief recipes"—makes cooking and diet planning a lot easier. The recipes are free of the most common sensitivity-causing foods.

Tracking Down Hidden Food Allergy, William G. Crook. Professional Books, P.O. Box 3494, Jackson, Tennessee, 1984. A simple (in the best sense of the word) book that is nicely illustrated and very helpful, managing to include a good deal of information in a few pages. Best of all, it is written for children as well as adults.

Understanding Allergies, John W. Gerrard. Charles C Thomas, Co., Springfield, Illinois, 1977. Nicely written and straightforward.

Why Your Child is Hyperactive, Ben F. Feingold. Random House, New York, 1978. For a full discussion of the Feingold diet, this is the book to read.

15

ENVIRONMENTAL SENSITIVITIES

The term "environmental sensitivities" as used in this book is equivalent to the term "allergies" in its broadest interpretation, and is not restricted to those reactions caused by the immune system. In addition to immunological responses, children's sensitivities may be the result of toxic reactions, yeast overgrowth, nutritional deficiencies or other processes, many of them unknown at this point in time.

Anything that children are exposed to, whether through inhaling, ingestion, skin contact or absorption, can provoke sensitivities. While it is common knowledge that many children are sensitive to dust, pollens, feathers, molds and animal dander, it is not so well known that children may also react to many other substances in the environment such as fumes and odors of gas, oil, cleaning products, toiletries, pesticides, plastics, synthetic fabrics, ozone-producing appliances and foods. Some of these items give off gases that we neither see nor smell, yet their effect on children can be very concrete and sometimes devastating.

Environmental sensitivities can cause a multitude of physical problems from watering eyes to asthma. Because all parts of the body, including the brain and the rest of the central nervous system, can be affected by these sensitivities, a wide variety of mental and behavioral symptoms may occur as well.

Although children can be sensitive to *anything* they are exposed to in their environment, natural products such as 100-percent untreated cotton are often tolerated better than either synthetics or natural substances that have been processed (refined, treated with other chemicals, heated, etc.) Unfortunately, as more and more processed or synthetic substances are produced and introduced into the environment, completely natural unprocessed substances are getting harder and harder to find.

It is not surprising that the increasing pollution of our environment is responsible for an increasing number of serious problems. Out in the open air, children are exposed to, among other things, exhaust fumes from cars and buses, tar and asphalt from road repairs, a large variety of pesticides and heavy-duty emissions from industry. And inside the supposed safety of our own homes children are exposed to a whole other set of dangers. Dr. Theron Randolph writes in A *Physician's Handbook on Orthomolecular Medicine*:

"The gas kitchen stove is the most hazardous device in the American home in contributing to domiciliary air pollution. Following closely are gas-fired fuel oil space heaters, gas dryers, gas-fired warm air furnaces and other fossil fuel burning utilities located within the home. Other major contributing exposures are pesticides; solvents and solvent-containing paints, adhesives and hair sprays: tar containing adhesives; rubber-based paints and sponge rubber bedding, upholstery and padding; plastic constructional materials, toys and furnishing; synthetic carpeting, upholstery, curtains and clothing; certain other cosmetics, pine, creosote, phenol and many others including tobacco smoke."

Cars and other vehicles, in which some children spend a lot of time (going to and from school, on vacations, and so on) should not be overlooked. According to Joseph T. Morgan in *Clinical Ecology*, "The hazards and potential exposures from the automobile include fumes of raw fuel, exhaust emissions, lubricating compounds, synthetic upholstery fabrics, plastics, plasticizers, and foam rubber padding. The person suffering from chemical susceptibility may react adversely on either an acute or chronic basis to one or more of these exposures."

Following is a brief rundown of possible sensitivity-producing environmental substances:

INHALANTS. This category includes dust, molds, pollen, animal dander, fur and feathers.

PETROLEUM HYDROCARBONS AND PETROCHEMICALS. The two major petroleum hydrocarbons are natural gas and oil. An extraordinary number of products, called petrochemicals, are derived from them, and they and many of their derivatives are included in the ingredients for innumerable other products. A partial list of items that *may* be derived from or contain petroleum hydrocarbons and their derivatives includes gasoline, diesel fuel, kerosene, propane gas, asphalt, tar, paint, ink (in newspapers, books, magazines), felt pens, detergents, varsol, paraffin, floor waxes, plastics of all sorts (the more flexible and odorous ones being more likely to cause problems), synthetic fabrics such as polyester and nylon, clothing dyes, Teflon, petroleum jelly, mineral oil, chap stick, hair conditioners, cosmetics, lubricating oils, rubber, pesticides, drugs, edible oil products (for example, nondairy creamers), and artificial food colorings and flavorings. In addition, foods may be inadvertently contaminated by petrochemicals, for example, if they are stored in plastic wrapping or containers.

This category is probably the one most implicated in chemical sensitivities, as well as being the hardest one to avoid.

PINE PRODUCTS. According to Theron Randolph in his book *An Alternative Approach to Allergies*, "Many chemically susceptible persons react to pine and pine products . . . the reason for this may be that hydrocarbon fuels are ultimately derived from great pine forests which were buried aeons ago and compressed into the liquid form we know today." Turpentine is derived from pine, and many cleaning agents are given a pine scent.

SOLVENTS. Eloise Kailin, quoted in *Coping with Your Allergies* by Golos and Golbitz, sums up this category: "These include alcohols, such as rubbing alcohol or ordinary pure ethyl alcohol; fat solvents; xeroxed, dittoed, or other forms of copied material which may contain benzene, ether, acetone, xylene, or toluol . . . Many kitchen cleaners include solvents to remove stubborn fats and oil films."

OZONE. Ozone is a form of oxygen that performs an essential function in the preservation of human life by forming a protective barrier around the earth to block out some of the sun's harmful rays. However, when close enough to earth for us to breathe, it is toxic. It does occur naturally, but can also be made artificially. Many electrical appliances emit ozone, and it also occurs in smog.

FORMALDEHYDE. In *The Complete Book of Allergy Control*, Laura J. Stevens notes the prevalence of formaldehyde in building supplies (particle board, paneling, concrete, plaster, wallboard, resins), furniture (carpets, upholstery, drapes), paper products, medications, insecticides, smoke (coal, wood and tobacco) and smog, wrinkle-resistant fabrics, toiletries—even, she observes, maple syrup, in which formaldehyde is used to promote sap flow.

PESTICIDES. Laura Stevens also comments on the routine use of pesticides since World War II in just about every place we live, shop, work or learn. And, she points out, once they've been used, the residue is almost certainly going to be long-lasting, perhaps permanent. It's difficult to avoid pesticide residues even if you're on the alert for them—furniture retrieved from commercial storage may have been sprayed with insecticide, or newly hung prepasted wallpaper may have been prepoisoned as well, with fungicide, and, of course, pesticides have contaminated much of the food we eat.

PHENOL is present in many pesticides and disinfectants—we may be more familiar with it as carbolic acid. It is also used in cosmetics and even, Laura Stevens notes, in some allergy treatment extracts.

Most tin cans are lined with phenol resins, making phenol another member of the large family of food contaminants.

SMOKE. Tobacco smoke has a list of contaminants as long as a small person's arm, including cadmium and some severe carcinogens. The Surgeon General is only the latest of many to point out the dangers of "passive" smoking—being around the actual puffers—which can be almost as great as active smoking. Smoke from wood and food can also cause symptoms.

There are of course many other categories of substances which may cause problems for children.

Are Environmental Sensitivities Causing Our Children's Problems?

Some of the clues suggesting that children are suffering from environmental sensitivities were mentioned in Chapter 8. These included the presence of environmental sensitivities among other family members; the presence of respiratory problems, skin problems and food sensitivities (food and environmental sensitivities often occur together); the presence of a major source of pollution in the home; symptoms that occur consistently after exposure to specific physical locations, after contact with specific substances or after specific activities; symptoms that occur cyclically; a keen sense of smell or a poor sense of smell; certain odors found either offensive or unusually attractive; the initial onset of symptoms having coincided with exposure to a new location, substance or activity; frequent exposure to specific substances; and improvement in behavior after absences from particular locations or substances.

As with food sensitivities, environmental sensitivities can produce symptoms that include anything from a stuffed nose, rash, asthma, fatigue, headache or moodiness, to extreme restlessness, forgetfulness, irrational fears, unprovoked violence and hallucinations. Symptoms can be mild or severe, constant or intermittent, depending not only on the makeup of the individual child but on changing circumstances in the environment. In some cases symptoms are provoked only after exposure to large quantities of a substance or exposure for a long length of time; in other cases minute quantities of a substance are enough to trigger severe symptoms. Some children are sensitive to only a few substances, others are sensitive to many.

Also similarly to food sensitivities, it is not always easy to narrow down which environmental substances are the ones causing the problems. Briefly, some of the reasons the search might be difficult are:

• Some children do not react immediately to the substances they are sensitive to, with a delayed reaction of up to four or more days.

• Sometimes symptoms occur inconsistently, their appearance depending on variables such as frequency of contact, amount and duration of contact, how old or well washed a substance is, and the presence of additional stresses such as other sensitivity-producing substances and environmental factors, illness or psychological pressures.

• Sometimes symptoms change, the same substances producing different reactions at different times in children's lives.

• Symptoms may not clear up until all existing sensitivities and/or other complicating factors are dealt with.

• If children are in frequent contact with their symptom-causing substances, or if the sensitivities are of long duration, the symptoms may have become chronic and constant, making the cause and effect relationship much less clear-cut.

Testing for Environmental Sensitivities

Despite the difficulties involved, there are a number of methods that can be used to help us pinpoint children's environmental sensitivities. For example, many of the methods used to test for food sensitivities as described in Chapter 14 can also be used for environmental sensitivities. These include the cytotoxic blood test, RAST, provocative testing (both subcutaneous and sublingual), the pulse test (although this may be less reliable for environmental sensitivities than for foods) and kinesiology. The scratch test, which is not recommended for testing food sensitivities, is, according to Theron Randolph, more reliable when testing for sensitivities to pollens, molds, dusts, animal dander and insect residue. The following methods can also be used to pinpoint environmental sensitivities:

OBSERVATION

Keeping a symptom diary such as the one described on page 124 in Chapter 8 is an extremely important part of any attempt to figure out children's environmental sensitivities. (The symptom diary includes food exposures in addition to environmental exposures as food and environmental sensitivities often go hand in hand.) A symptom diary helps us keep track of the substances children have been exposed to and the symptoms they have suffered. Having a written record to refer back to instead of relying solely on memory can be a helpful aid in discovering the origins of children's problems.

To pinpoint which particular substances might be affecting children, try to correlate their symptoms with the following categories:

LOCATION. As children live their days and nights, they pass through many different locations. They may spend most of their nights in their bedrooms; eat breakfast in the kitchen; have a bath in the bathroom; play in the living room, basement, backyard or neighborhood park; go to day care, a baby-sitter's or a friend's house; attend school where in the course of the day they might find themselves in the classroom, gymnasium, lunchroom, art room, home economics room or carpentry or mechanic's shop; visit a library, museum, department store, doctor's office, barbershop or hairdresser's; take a ride in a car, bus or train; walk downtown; attend Brownies or Scouts in a church basement; or end up in any number of other places.

In each location children will be exposed to a variety of substances, some of them common to most of the locations and some of them specific to only one or a few. If symptoms consistently seem to start or get worse either while in or after having been in a particular location, then the following checklist can be used to itemize the substances present in each symptom-causing location. Listing these substances will bring us closer to identifying at least part of what is causing our children's problems:

Insulation: _____
(Urea formaldehyde insulation has been a major source of trouble for many people.)

Method of heating: _____
(Gas is considered the worst because of gas fumes, although oil and coal can also cause major problems; forced hot air systems are also considered poor risks for people with environmental sensitivities because they blow dust and other particles through the house as well as burning particles which come in contact with the high heat and then give off noxious gases.)

Wiring: _____
(Plastic-coated wires when heated can trigger symptoms.)

Floor: _____
(Asbestos tile, vinyl, plastic linoleum, rugs that are made out of synthetic material or have been mothproofed, rubber underpaddings and adhesives can all cause problems; most rugs are serious dust accumulators unless small enough to be washed frequently.)

Walls and ceiling: _____
(Watch out for formaldehyde in paneling and other materials, odorous paint, vinyl wallpaper and wallpaper paste with fungicides.)

Furniture: _____

(Symptoms may be caused by the formaldehyde in particle board, by synthetics such as nylon fabric coverings, polyester filled pillows, foam rubber stuffing, synthetic dyes, as well as by natural substances such as feathers, wool, dust-collecting cotton and kapok stuffings and pine.)

Window coverings: _____

(Again, beware of synthetics.)

Light fixtures: _____

(Plastic shades when heated can provoke symptoms, and fluorescent lights give off ozone.)

Appliances: _____

(Check if they are fueled by gas, give off ozone, or contain mold, plastic parts, oil in motors, or freon gas in fridges and freezers which might leak; as an added note, it should be mentioned that although electric stoves are considered less likely to cause problems than gas, some children may react to them as well.)

Ornaments and decorations: _____

(Keep an eye out for synthetics, dust collectors, and plants whose soil might contain mold.)

Substances used to maintain or protect walls, floors, furniture, ornaments, etc.: _____

(In other words, watch out for stains, varnishes, waxes, polishes, soaps, detergents, bleaches and other cleaning agents and anything that has been Scotchgarded, perma-pressed, mothproofed, drycleaned, treated with fire retardant or sprayed with pesticides.)

Stored materials: _____

(Anything that gives off odors or fumes is suspect, including paint, cleaning materials, pesticides, toiletries and many miscellaneous items.)

Miscellaneous odors: _____

(For example, from air fresheners, tobacco smoke or as a result of activities that occasionally take place in the room, such as gluing, batiking; fires in the fireplace; odors drifting in from other rooms or from outside, such as cooking odors, automobile exhaust, photography fumes and so on.)

Inhalants: _____

(Is the place dusty or moldy, are there pets hanging around or pollens blowing in from outside, or have there been recent renovations with resulting sawdust, plaster dust and so on floating around?)

Other indoor substances: _____

Outdoors: _____

(For any particular outside location be aware of the kind of plants that are growing, the amount of traffic, application of pesticides, road repairs that are taking place, smog and pollen count, industrial emissions and anything else that might be in the outdoor environment. It is important to note that molds are prevalent in soil and dead leaves.)

ACTIVITIES. Certain substances are associated with specific activities. For example, if symptoms worsen during or after time spent developing photos (which chemicals were used?), arts and crafts (were they using glue, paper, paints, felt pens?), having a bath (could it be fumes from the toiletries or cleaning agents, or the chlorine in the water?), vacuuming (reaction possibly either to dust or to the motor oil in the vacuum cleaner), playing with stuffed animals (dust, mold, acrylic fur?), watching television (when plastic coated wires heat up they can give off fumes) and so on. Look to see which substances children were in contact with while doing that activity.

PASSIVE EXPOSURE. Passive exposure includes exposure to clothing (raincoats made of vinyl, shirts of polyester, cotton skirts with synthetic blue dye, perma-pressed pants, rubber shoes, acrylic sweaters, items made of wool which though natural can also be irritating to children).

Passive exposure also includes exposure to substances the clothing has been treated with (detergent, bleach, dry cleaning agent, shoe polish) and substances the clothing has been in contact with (smoke, odors, animal dander, etc.). Toiletries that children use (soap, shampoo, deodorant, nail polish, perfume, bubble bath), and toiletries used by people they come in contact with can also affect children adversely. Weather can also be a factor, for example, breezy days when the wind decides to blow a chemical stew our way, or hot and humid days when exhaust fumes and other lovelies are determined to hang there at nose level. As Doris Rapp writes in *Allergies and the Hyperactive Child*, "Contaminated air can cause particular difficulty on windy or foggy days. Insect, garden, and lawn sprays or fertilizers may be particularly offensive."

TIME. Noting when exposures and reactions occur is valuable in matching up symptoms to the substances that cause them. If every morning children wake up with stuffy noses which clear up during the course of the day, we can suspect something in their bedrooms. If symptoms are worse twice a week after swimming, we can suspect something connected with swimming, whether this might be the bus ride there and back, the water or chemicals in the pool, something in the building, or their regular post-swim snack from the vending machine. If symptoms occur seasonally, the problems may be due to such seasonal factors as pollens or when the furnace goes on. Noting frequency of contact can also provide useful clues—if children are often exposed to specific substances, such as airplane glue or chlorine, this is also something to make us suspicious.

AVOIDANCE AND REEXPOSURE

The best method of testing for environmental sensitivities, if at all possible, is to completely avoid the most likely sensitivity-producing substances until symptoms disappear or for two weeks, whichever comes first, and then reexpose children to the substances. This increases the chances that any resulting reactions will be clear-cut.

This may be particularly important in the case of petroleum hydrocarbons and petrochemicals, since, according to William H. Philpott in *A Physician's Handbook on Orthomolecular Medicine*, "the reaction to petrochemical hydrocarbons may carry the same quality of addiction as that of food."

This concept of addiction that Philpott mentions explains why children often seem to crave certain substances. The craving is a result of their bodies having partially adapted to the offending substances; despite the fact that the substances may be causing them serious harm (to the extent of serious brain damage in the case of glue sniffing and gasoline sniffing), they often get a temporary high from contact with the substances. (This illustrates the difficulty in diagnosing sensitivities when exposure to a substance does not immediately result in negative symptoms.)

If addictions to any environmental substances are present, expect symptoms to worsen during the first part of the avoidance period due to withdrawal symptoms.

Avoiding substances can be done either in a specially set up unit in a hospital (generally called an ecology unit), or in any place that has been made environmentally "clean." To clean the environment requires removing all items which give off odors and fumes, including most cleaning agents, paints, solvents and toiletries; all synthetic products such as plastics, foam rubber or polyester; removing gas stoves and turning off the furnace; sending the dog, cat, budgie, gerbil and plants away; doing a thorough cleaning and airing out (being careful of course to use the most tolerated cleaning agents); not allowing smoking or the use of scented toiletries and cosmetics and so on.

At the same time, it is necessary to avoid all foods that may have any chemical contamination, whether through contact with pesticides, antibiotics, coloring, plastic coverings, etc., as many of the chemicals that pollute the environment also pollute food sources. To do this children can either fast, or eat a strictly organic diet for the duration of the test period. When children start the period of avoidance, we should remember to keep up with the symptom diary.

If we don't have access to an ecology unit due to cost or lengthy waiting lists, don't know anyone who has made their home sensitivity-free, and find it impossible to redo our own homes (it is probably a bit extreme to rip up all the carpets, change the heating system and give away all the furniture without being fairly certain that our children do in fact react to them), then we have several alternatives. One alternative is to pick one room and clear that one up, arranging it so that children sleep in that room at night and spend as much time in it during the day as possible. Odors travel so we should plug any gaps in the door. We should also seal off the heat registers. At the same time, it is important to ensure adequate ventilation (indoor pollution can often be greater than outdoor pollution).

Another possibility is suggested by Theron Randolph in the *Physician's Handbook on Orthomolecular Medicine*: "The effects of sponge rubber, odorous plastics and synthetic textiles in the home are best appraised by placing these materials, one group at a time, in a tightly closed room for about a week. Although the patient may notice changes in symptoms following their removal, the key to the specific diagnosis depends upon what happens upon reentering this room."

Another approach is to compile a suspect list and avoid only the substances included. We should include in our suspect list the following:

• Substances that sometimes appear to cause symptoms, even if irregularly.

• Substances that have previously caused reactions, even if they currently seem to be tolerated.

• Substances with smells that children seem to particularly like.

• Substances with smells that children dislike.

• Strong-smelling substances that children are frequently exposed to.

• Appliances using gas (a common symptom-causing substance).

• Substances that have tested positive on other sensitivity tests.

• Substances that children have been exposed to in massive amounts (for example, if they were present during a crop spraying, home fumigation or major oil spill).

• Substances that we are suspicious of for any other reason.

At the same time, of course, children should avoid any substance that is already known to cause a reaction. Whether avoidance has been total or partial, if children's symptoms clear up or at least lessen considerably, this is a strong indication that environmental sensitivities are indeed a major part of the problem.

If symptoms don't clear up significantly during the period of avoidance, it doesn't necessarily mean they don't have environmental sensitivities. It could be that a longer period of avoidance is necessary (sometimes up to six months), that complicating factors are involved (such as other environmental or food sensitivities, hypoglycemia, yeast overgrowth and so on), or that there was inadvertent exposure to substances on the avoidance list (some of them seem to be everywhere). Despite a lack of improvement during the avoidance period, children may still react to suspect substances upon reexposure to them, indicating that environmental sensitivities are involved in their problems.

If none of the above methods of avoidance are feasible, we can try testing for sensitivities at "a time when symptoms are minimal," as Doris Rapp suggests in *Allergies and the Hyperactive Child.*

We can choose to test either a broad range of substances, or, at least initially, only those substances that we have good reason to suspect. Whichever method of avoidance or non-avoidance is chosen we can follow Doris Rapp's directions for the actual testing, as follows, remembering to write everything down in our symptom diary, and to do the testing in cooperation with a doctor. Doris Rapp writes:

"Do test in a room which can be avoided for several hours if a reaction occurs. Discuss the test with your physician first. Test only if he approves.

"Schedule the test so that it is midway between meals, at 10:10 a.m. or 3:00 p.m. Do no more than one test per day. Observe the patient for any change in activity, behavior, or the onset of symptoms—that is, flushing, pallor, stuffiness, headache, muscle ache, dizziness, and so on. Check pulse before test. If any test produces symptoms, immediately stop exposure. Breathe fresh air or oxygen. Take 1 to 2 tablespoons of baking soda in 2 glasses of water. If no reaction is noticed after the specified time of exposure, stop the test. Continue to watch the patient for an additional half hour for delayed reactions. Take pulse for one full minute every 1 to 10 minutes during entire test. Pulse increase of 12 to 20 may indicate a sensitivity to the item tested."

For liquids and sprays such as turpentine, gasoline, toiletries, floor wax, pesticides, paints and glues (formaldehyde can also be included), Doris Rapp suggests spraying or placing a few drops of the substance on a blotter, and exposing the child for twenty minutes at a distance of two feet. Each item should be tested individually.

For powders such as Clorox and ammonia, she recommends placing one tablespoon in one cup water and exposing the child at twenty feet for four minutes, again testing one at a time.

She gives instructions for other categories as follows:

Foam rubber, polyurethane, soft plastic or plastic polyethylene food or garment bags, freshly cleaned or new polyester clothing
Test each item individually. Expose patient for approximately twenty minutes at two feet.

Gas fumes
Sit two to three feet from a stove which has lighted gas burners and lighted oven for twenty to thirty minutes. Have doors to room closed.

Tobacco
Sit in tobacco smoke-filled room without eating or drinking for twenty minutes.

Newsprint or chemically treated paper (mimeograph, copy machine)
Keep freshly printed paper six inches from face for approximately twenty minutes.

Soap, detergent or fabric softener
Soak washcloth in usual concentration for each item. Squeeze out excess fluid. Keep item six inches from face for twenty minutes. Test each item separately.

Exhaust fumes
Stand near busy bus stop for fifteen to twenty minutes.

Electric blanket or heating pad fumes
Place either on chest for twenty minutes. As plastic-coated wires heat, odors are emitted.

Motor oils
Stand near small motor for ten minutes.

Mothballs or crystals
Expose patient at six feet for twenty minutes.

Carpet, linoleum, tile, upholstered furniture, mattresses or bed sheets
Sit directly upon item for twenty to thirty minutes. Does portion of body in contact with item tingle or feel different?

In addition to the substances and methods mentioned above, William H. Philpott writes, "Pets such as cats, dogs, and so forth can be held close to the nose for sniff testing for three to five minutes. Dust can be determined by vacuuming the house and seeing if there is a reaction during the process . . . Another way to test for petrochemical hydrocarbons is to stand behind a running automobile for three to five minutes to see if symptoms develop. Candles can be sniffed, waxes sniffed, decorative kerosene lamps can be sniffed, magic markers can be sniffed . . . Cosmetics and hair conditioners should be sniff tested. Clothes could be sniff tested after being bleached or the subject exposed to the laundry room during the bleaching process to determine a possible reaction to chlorine . . ."

Particularly if there has been a period of avoidance, symptoms should appear very shortly after reexposure, although as mentioned previously some reactions may not occur until days later.

If children don't improve after a period of avoidance or react when tested with any substances, and if there seems to be no correlation between their symptoms and exposure to particular locations, activities or specific substances, then we can assume either that they don't have environmental sensitivities or that environmental sensitivities are playing a minor role in their problems.

If, however, children either do improve after a period of avoidance or react when tested with specific substances, then we should assume there is a strong possibility that they do have environmental sensitivities, and set about to confirm this assumption.

Testing the Hypothesis

If children develop symptoms when tested with specific substances, we should try to reduce their exposure to these substances for a period of time, either until their symptoms clear up or for ten days and then retest. If symptoms do diminish significantly, this is positive confirmation that they have environmental sensitivities, and if they again react to the same substances when reexposed to them, this is further confirmation.

If children don't significantly improve when they are not in contact with the substances they initially reacted to, we should check out the possibility that other previously unsuspected environmental sensitivities are present, or check whether additional factors are involved such as those discussed in Chapters 10 through 18. If improvement is only minimal but children do react when exposed to the suspect substances, it may be that a longer period of avoidance is needed for full recovery. It sometimes takes up to six months for symptoms to disappear completely.

If they don't react the second time when reexposed to the suspect substances, this could indicate either that the first reaction was coincidence, or that due to the period of avoidance they are not as sensitive as they were and would need to have a longer length of exposure for symptoms to occur.

Controlling Environmental Sensitivities

If environmental sensitivities are confirmed, there are several ways of dealing with them. One is desensitization or neutralization either through injections or sublingually (see Chapter 14); another is avoidance of the offending substances.

How strict the avoidance must be depends on the severity of children's reactions and the degree of sensitivity. Some children are affected by minute traces of a substance, whereas others do not react unless exposed either for a long period of time or to large amounts of the substance. Some children react only with mild fatigue and a snuffly nose, whereas others may have full-blown schizophrenia-like symptoms. In some cases, to regain our children's health, we may have to seriously consider moving to a different house or apartment or location, or doing major renovation work on our present home. In other cases, less extreme measures may be all that are necessary to minimize children's symptoms.

One obvious method of controlling sensitivities is to eliminate as many items causing problems as we can and replace them with better-tolerated alternatives. However, it is not always so easy finding suitable alternatives that are natural and untreated. Labels often do not give complete information on what the item is made of and what chemical treatments it may have received. Even items labeled "hypoallergenic" can provoke symptoms. We should not hesitate to ask salesclerks or managers for more information about any particular item. To be absolutely sure, write directly to the manufacturer. As an extra precaution, especially with major purchases, we can do a tolerance test right in the store by having children sit on or close to the sofa, rug or other item for twenty minutes or until there is a reaction, whichever comes first. (Of course, we will have to take into consideration the possibility that any reaction that occurs may be caused by something in the store other than the item being tested, or that a reaction will occur at home after a longer exposure; but at least this test will give us a rough idea of what to expect.) We should also not be shy about returning items. (Check before purchasing for the store's policy about returns.)

We should note that often the older an item is, or the more it is washed (in tolerated cleaning agents) or aired out, the less it causes symptoms; sometimes old, well-worn synthetic clothing will not cause symptoms although the new equivalent will. (This can occur when a product's surface molecules detach easily into the atmosphere, leaving behind the ones beneath the surface which may be more firmly attached.) In any case, it is a good idea to wash well or air out thoroughly any new items.

If we cannot find new, ready-made items that children can tolerate in local stores, we may have better luck buying things through mail order (see the list of resources starting on page 55 in Chapter 3); making them ourselves or having them made, buying them second hand or searching out more accessible substitutes. (For example, if no commercial toothpastes are tolerated, we can try a baking soda and salt mixture.) Occasionally we will find that the best solution is simply to dispense with an item: it will not be a great hardship for our children if we throw out the spray can of air freshener or pour the perfume down the drain.

Other difficulties in addition to availability include emotional issues, such as deciding whether or not to give away the family dog, and social issues such as requesting guests not to smoke in our homes. Often a major stumbling block is the unhappy question of money and affordability, for example when we have to decide whether to completely replace our current heating system or to attempt toughing it out.

In all of these cases an extremely crucial factor in deciding how much we can compromise is, as mentioned before, the severity of our children's symptoms. In *An Alternative Approach to Allergies* Theron Randolph discusses fumes from gas stoves causing problems: "In cases in which actual removal of the gas range has been impossible, certain halfway measures have proven useful. They have included increased ventilation of the kitchen; installation of a kitchen door, which is kept closed during the time the stove is on, keeping fumes from reaching the rest of the house; or disconnection of the stove, without actual removal. For many people, such measures are beneficial; for the seriously ill, however, there is no substitute for complete removal of the offending appliance."

(If we simply do not have the money for major purchases or renovations, see pages 46–47 in Chapter 3 for suggestions.)

Following are some general suggestions for the control of environmental sensitivities:

VENTILATION. In the kitchen, a stove hood that is vented to the outside will remove any fumes and odors that are created when cooking. Having fans located throughout the house also helps. In addition, unless it is the height of pollen season, the middle of winter or our house faces a major highway or pollution spewing factory, open windows are good ventilators.

AIR PURIFIERS. Good ones can eliminate a large percentage of dust, molds, pollens and some odors such as smoke. Check consumer reports to find which work best, as some are much more effective than others. Also make sure they don't create ozone or give off symptom-producing odors themselves. Some units fit on hot air furnaces and work for the whole house, while others are portable, for individual rooms. Air purifiers can also be used in cars.

CLEANING. Particularly for children suffering from dust and mold problems, frequent cleaning (in other words the usual vacuuming, dusting, washing, scrubbing and laundering), can help alleviate symptoms. Cleaning furnace filters and vents is also helpful. A special effort should be made to clean favorite mold growing spots (the damper and darker the spot the happier is the mold—check bathrooms, basements, closets, drawers, fridges, under the kitchen sink, air conditioning units, humidifiers, dehumidifiers and plants. Reduce the amount of dust in the air by installing a central vacuum system, and block off bedroom heat registers if heating is by forced air. Reducing the number of dust collectors (rugs, knickknacks, books and so on) around the house also makes managing the dust problem easier. Using only cleaning products that children do not react to is a necessity. (Baking soda is a readily available, versatile product that can be used for many cleaning purposes and is generally well tolerated.)

CHECKING REGULARLY FOR GAS LEAKS IN THE HOUSE AND GASOLINE LEAKS IN THE CAR. If children are sensitive to gas or gasoline, this will at least minimize their exposure. If a gas-fired furnace causes them problems, blocking off the heat registers to their rooms might help. (In general, electrical heating systems seem to be better tolerated.)

NEUTRALIZING CHEMICALS. One example of this is given by Golos and Golbitz in Coping With Your Allergies: "A few crystals of sodium thiosulfate changes chlorine in water to chloride; it may be helpful to chlorine-sensitive persons for bathing only—not to be used internally." (In the specific case of chlorine, water filters and distillers and boiling water may remove the chlorine for drinking purposes.)

NATURALIZING. Replacing common sensitivity-causing substances (mainly synthetics and any treated substances) with natural untreated substitutes as quickly as money and energy allow is a good idea. The less stress put on children by chemicals the human body has not yet adapted to the better. The first priority in this changeover should be the bedroom, as this is usually the room where children spend the most time. If necessary, synthetic fabric, plastic and padding can be replaced with natural materials, even in cars.

REDUCING EXPOSURE TIME. If it is impossible to avoid some of the substances our children react to, making sure they spend as little time as possible in contact with these substances will sometimes make a difference in the intensity of symptoms. For example, if riding in a car is unavoidable and causes significant problems, on long trips we can plan to have frequent stops where children can get out of the car for at least a brief respite. Another example would be to allow children to swim in the local pool for only half an hour instead of an hour.

AIMING FOR OPTIMUM HEALTH. Two extremely important components that should be included in a program to control environmental sensitivities are a nutritious diet (Chapter 10) and regular exercise (pages 263–265 in Chapter 18). It is also necessary to control any problems children have with hypoglycemia (Chapter 12), yeast overgrowth (Chapter 13), food sensitivities (Chapter 14), heavy metal toxicity (Chapter 16) or other environmental factors (Chapter 17). Healthy methods of dealing with stress (pages 268–274 in Chapter 18) and an awareness of how each substance in their environment affects them (pages 274–275 in the same chapter) should be encouraged. In addition, we should note that some children find their symptoms decrease when nutritional supplements are added to their diets (Chapter 11).

An integral part of any program attempting to deal with environmental sensitivities that should not be overlooked is prevention. Many times just as we manage to get one sensitivity under control, up pops a new one. Or we may wake up one morning and realize that a sensitivity that not so long ago was only a minor problem has now developed into something quite serious. Many of the above suggestions are good preventive measures, and we should try to follow as many of them as possible.

In line with a preventive approach, even though being sensitive to one item of a particular group does not necessarily mean a sensitivity to all, it is wisest to be particularly watchful of items related to a known sensitivity-causing substance. For example, if children are sensitive to natural gas, we might want to limit their exposure to felt-tipped pens; if they are sensitive to environmental molds, keep an eye out for possible reactions to foods that contain mold, such as cheese, or that are of the mold family, such as mushrooms.

Although after a period of avoidance of a few months or more some tolerance to a substance may be gained, the wisest course seems to be to keep exposure to a minimum as symptoms might flare up again at any time.

It is extremely important to note that many of the substances discussed in this chapter are to some degree toxic to everyone. Whether or not children show overt symptoms after exposure to any of these substances, we should still limit contact as much as possible. This is particularly the case with petroleum products (such as gasoline), tobacco smoke, pesticides and any volatile substances that give off strong odors or fumes (such as solvents).

A final word: the previous chapter on food sensitivities should be read in conjunction with this chapter, as much of the information given on food sensitivities also applies to environmental sensitivities, and frequently children who are sensitive to some environmental substances are also sensitive to some foods.

Books referred to in this chapter and other suggested reading:

Allergies and the Hyperactive Child, Doris J. Rapp. Cornerstone Books, New York, 1980. For a description, see Chapter 8.

An Alternative Approach to Allergies, Theron G. Randolph and Ralph W. Moss. Lippincott & Crowell, Publishers, New York, 1980. Easy reading with lots of case histories. Theron Randolph is responsible for laying a great deal of the groundwork in the field of clinical ecology; a medical approach to health which looks at people in the context of their environments rather than as separate entities.

Clinical Ecology, Lawrence D. Dickey, editor. Charles C Thomas, Publisher, Springfield, Illinois, 1976. For a description, see Chapter 4.

The Complete Book of Allergy Control, Laura J. Stevens. Macmillan Publishing Company, New York, 1983. For a description, see Chapter 14.

Coping With Your Allergies, Natalie Golos and Frances Golos Golbitz with Frances Spatz Leighton. Simon and Schuster, New York, 1979. For a description, see Chapter 14.

A Physician's Handbook on Orthomolecular Medicine, Roger J. Williams and Dwight K. Kalita, editors. Keats Publishing, New Canaan, Connecticut, 1977. For a further description, see Chapter 4.

Why Your House May Endanger Your Health, Alfred V. Zamm with Robert Gannon. Simon and Schuster, New York, 1980. A very helpful book which includes information on both maintaining and building a healthy house. Covers a variety of house-related topics from house dust to electromagnetic waves.

16
HEAVY METAL TOXICITY

There are many metals which not only have no nutrient value for the human body but which can also cause children serious harm, interfering with a number of essential bodily processes and causing irreparable damage, sometimes resulting in death. Side effects caused by metal toxicity may include learning and behavioral symptoms ranging from hyperactivity to mental retardation. Wunderlich and Kalita in *Nourishing Your Child* write, "Foggy thinking, erratic emotions, motor uncoordination and attentional inconstancy may dramatically improve or even disappear entirely when elevated levels of lead, cadmium, mercury or nickel are lowered."

To what extent children are affected by toxic metals depends on a number of factors:

• The degree and length of exposure.

• Method of exposure (eaten or drunk, inhaled or absorbed through the skin).

• The presence of other chemicals or toxins which may significantly increase the ill effects.

• Each child's specific genetic makeup, nutritional status and state of health. For example, children deficient in certain nutrients may be at greater risk to develop metal toxicity.

When metals are mined, smelted, manufactured and put to industrial and domestic use, they end up polluting our air, soil and water, increasing to sometimes dangerous amounts children's exposure to these metals.

One example of a common toxic metal which puts many children at risk is lead. It is well known that lead poisoning can lead to mental retardation, and it is now becoming accepted that lead is in some cases responsible for other learning and behavior problems such as hyperactivity. There have been many studies linking impaired learning ability to increased lead levels.

Wunderlich and Kalita write in *Nourishing Your Child* that lead "blocks proper enzyme activities and can cause the following symptoms in children and adults: weakness, listlessness, fatigue, pallor, constipation, confusion, irritability and abdominal discomfort, anemia, convulsions, headaches, coma and death."

Children are at much greater risk for suffering lead toxicity than adults. As Dr. Allan Cott explains in *Dr. Cott's Help for Your Learning Disabled Child*, "Children are more vulnerable to lead pollution because their body weight is less and they therefore take in relatively greater quantities of lead from the environment. They inhale more air per unit of body weight because of their higher metabolic rates and greater physical activities." In addition, their exposure to lead is increased because they are shorter and lead concentrates closer to the ground.

According to Wallace and Cooper in *The Citizen's Guide to Lead*, "The group of people most sensitive to lead health effects is children under about six years of age, with unborn children and two to three year olds the most sensitive subgroups because of their stage of development and their potential for large exposures."

Common sources of lead are exhaust from automobiles and other vehicles due to lead in gasoline (polluting not only the air and food crops, but also soil and dust which children play in and track into our homes), food contaminated by lead solder in canned goods, industries such as lead smelters, and flaking lead-based paint. There is also lead in cigarette smoke.

Another example of a toxic metal is mercury, which can have devastating effects on the central nervous system. Methyl mercury is the most dangerous form of mercury. However, inorganic mercury can also be a danger as it can be turned into methyl mercury by a certain type of bacteria.

Two common sources of mercury poisoning are mercury-contaminated fish (sometimes a result of disposal of industrial wastes) and food and water contaminated by mercury-containing pesticides. In some instances mercury in dental fillings is also a source of mercury toxicity.

In addition there are many other metals implicated in children's learning and behavior problems, such as aluminum and cadmium. In excess quantities even the essential nutrient copper, also a metal, can affect behavior negatively.

Is Heavy Metal Toxicity Causing our Children's Problems?

As mentioned in Chapter 8, some of the clues suggesting that children are suffering from heavy metal toxicity include the presence of heavy metal toxicity among other family members; living near a major source of pollution such as a busy traffic route, mine, refinery, factory or power plant; living in a house with flaking paint; exposure to large amounts of cigarette smoke; consumption of large amounts of food containing toxic metals such as mercury-contaminated fish, food from lead-soldered cans, water passing through lead or copper pipes, food prepared in aluminum or copper cookware; and symptoms starting during or after the placement of mercury-containing dental fillings.

In addition, the results of neurological tests may suggest whether children are being affected by lead or any other toxic metal.

The main methods of testing for heavy metals are through urine, blood and hair. However, the results of these tests should be taken as indicators rather than as accurate reflections of the status of any particular toxic metal in a child's body, as the amounts that show up in blood, urine or hair may not correspond to the amounts in various body tissues. (Tissue biopsy would be the most accurate method of discovering exact levels of toxic metals, but it is an extreme and unpleasant method requiring surgery, and is not generally recommended for children.) Often a combination of urine, blood and hair analysis will be done to confirm or deny the existence of metal toxicity. It is absolutely essential that any results of testing blood, urine or hair be interpreted by someone knowledgeable and experienced.

The result of any diagnostic test should not be treated as an absolute. For example, the results of hair analysis may vary from lab to lab. This is because different labs use different methods of preparation and analysis of hair samples, as well as different sets of comparative values in interpretation. In addition, some labs may have better quality control than others.

To avoid some of these problems, Elmer M. Cranton and Richard A. Passwater in *Trace Elements, Hair Analysis and Nutrition* suggest "that in choosing a laboratory for performing hair analysis you should inquire if they conform to the standards established by the Hair Analysis Standardization Board, ASETL (American Society of Elemental Testing Laboratories) or other independent standardization boards. But in every case, you should require from the laboratory the exact procedures the laboratory follows for quality control, data interpretation and reporting procedures."

In general it appears that hair analysis is a useful screening method for heavy-metal toxicity. The procedure for collecting the hair sample is to use high quality stainless steel scissors to snip from the nape of the neck about a gram of untreated hair one to two inches in length (measuring from the scalp, not the hair ends).

If it has been confirmed that the amounts of heavy metals contained in the blood, urine or hair have reached levels currently considered to be unacceptable, the likelihood is strong that heavy-metal toxicity is a factor in a child's behavior problems. However, amounts below these levels do not rule out the possibility that children are being negatively affected by the metals. There is a growing recognition that all of us have different levels at which we may be affected by toxins and irritants. In other words, to the individual an arbitrary cutoff point is meaningless. The question also arises whether any amounts of toxic substances in the body can be considered safe, especially where growing children are concerned.

If blood, urine and hair analyses show negative for metal toxicity, children are not exposed to significant amounts of toxic metals through food or in the environment, they are eating a high-quality diet and not suffering from any uncorrected nutritional deficiencies or dependencies which might predispose them to metal toxicity, and none of the clues which might suggest metal toxicity as mentioned on the preceding two pages are present, it is more likely that factors other than metal toxicity are the cause of any problems and these should be investigated.

The Treatment Program

Ridding the Body of Toxic Metals

If the evidence indicates that a child is suffering from metal toxicity, the immediate task is to lower the levels of the toxic metals. The main method used for this is *chelation*.

Dr. Cott writes, "Chelation (the word is derived from the Greek *chela*, meaning 'claw') is the process by which the medication combines with the lead—or with any other heavy metal present in the tissues—to form a new compound that is soluble and can be discharged by the body. I usually administer a high-sulfur amino acid supplement such as methionine or cysteine and suggest that slow-baked beans and/or slow-baked apples be eaten several times a week." He also recommends vitamins C and E as general detoxifiers, and various other nutrients to lower toxic metal levels.

Concerning nutritional supplements and metal toxicity, Wunderlich and Kalita write, "Vitamin C, for example, has an excellent ability to chelate heavy metals from our bodies. Zinc, calcium, selenium and other minerals can also displace the toxic metals cadmium, lead and mercury."

Passwater and Cranton mention that "pectin and algin are effective forms of fiber that decrease lead absorption and show evidence of possibly increasing lead excretion."

In addition to the use of nutritional supplements, implementing a high quality diet is very important, as the healthier a body is, the better able it is to deal with any toxic assaults.

Penicillamine (except for those sensitive to penicillin) and EDTA (ethylenediaminotetracetic acid) are chelators sometimes used to treat metal poisoning on a short-term basis. Because of their potential toxicity they are unlikely to be used with children except in very severe cases of poisoning. Dr. Abram Hoffer writes in a personal communication, "Both penicillamine and EDTA would have to be used very, very carefully in children, and only under very strict supervision from a physician who knows exactly what these compounds can do."

In the case of mercury, *removal of mercury-containing fillings* may be indicated especially if these give off a negative charge. Dr. Hal A. Huggins and Sharon A. Huggins in their book *It's All In Your Head* stress that removal of mercury-containing fillings should be done sequentially; that is, the fillings in the quadrants of the mouth with the highest negative charges should be removed before those with positive charges. They also recommend that a nutritional program be initiated before removal. As alternatives to these so-called silver fillings, they recommend either light-cure or chemical-cure composites, which are basically plastic.

Wunderlich and Kalita write that *exercise* "promotes perfusion of body tissues with oxygen, better distributes nutrients and utilizes the musculo-skeletal system that otherwise would remain dormant. Lactic acid, formed as a by-product of muscular exercise, is a chelating agent that cleans the body of toxins." (See pages 263–265 in Chapter 18 for more information on exercise.)

Preventing the Recurrence of Metal Toxicity

Once metals have been removed from a child's body, the next step is to ensure that levels of toxic metals do not have a chance to build up again. This can be done by correcting any nutritional deficiencies that may be making children more susceptible to metal toxicity, and by removing the sources of any metal toxicity.

There are indications that certain metals are more likely to cause problems if children are suffering from nutritional imbalances. For example, children deficient in calcium may retain more lead in their systems than other children, those with low zinc levels may be more susceptible to copper excess, and children eating diets containing large amounts of highly refined foods may have higher cadmium levels. As Wunderlich and Kalita point out, optimum nutrition is extremely important in preventing metal toxicity. Even when deficiencies do not exist, taking nutritional supplements is often a wise preventive measure, especially if we live in a high pollution area. (For further information on nutrition and nutritional deficiencies, see Chapters 10 and 11.)

Another integral part of a treatment program for heavy metal toxicity in addition to nutrition is the identification and, whenever possible, elimination of the sources of children's toxicity. Following is a brief discussion of common sources of heavy metal toxicity:

TOXIC WASTES. Waste by-products of mines, smelters, refineries, factories and power plants contain toxic metals which contaminate the surrounding atmosphere, waters and soil. The specific metals involved and the nature of the environmental pollution (that is, whether wastes are dumped into nearby rivers or lakes, buried in dumps to leach into the nearby water table or soil used for plants, emitted into the atmosphere in gas form, and so on) depends on the type of factory, etc.

If pollution from a local industry is causing major health problems, moving to a less polluted area should be seriously considered. If this is not possible, the long-term solution is to work with others for a reduction in the amount of toxic wastes being produced and/or safer disposal of these wastes, plus an environmental clean-up.

More immediately, we should take sensible precautions such as finding out the degree of contamination of air, water, soil and food (whether this be vegetables from the garden, wild berries in the bush or fish in a nearby lake). If necessary, we will have to find alternative sources to contaminated water and food and avoid planting gardens in contaminated soil. We can obtain information about toxic metal levels either from the appropriate government department, or by independently getting water, soil or food samples tested at a laboratory.

It is often useful to refer to the appropriate government standards outlining safe or acceptable levels of toxic metals when deciding what action to take. If the contamination exceeds the acceptable level set by the standards, obviously immediate steps must be taken to safeguard children's health. However, it should not be assumed that any contamination falling below acceptable levels set by the standards can be safely ignored. These standards are helpful in providing guidelines with which to judge the seriousness of the contamination, but should not be seen as absolutes. Each person is different and what is safe for one may not be safe for another.

In addition, amounts of exposure will vary from person to person according to individual circumstances. For example, some children may eat much more of one type of food than other children. Also, the point has been made many times that a toxin, metallic or otherwise, may be considerably strengthened in its ill effects by the presence of other factors (such as other toxins); this means that an accurate assessment of the toxin's danger is not possible if only the measured level is considered. Another consideration is the growing evidence indicating that low levels of exposure to toxins over a long period of time, even those considered to be well within accepted safe limits, may have serious effects. In other words, it is not necessarily only high levels of exposure that are dangerous.

LEAD EMISSIONS FROM VEHICLES AND INDUSTRIES. A major source of lead for many is living in close proximity to a heavily used traffic route. The lead from the resulting exhaust contaminates the air children breathe, dust tracked into houses (which particularly endangers curious toddlers who love to chew their fingers and everything else that looks of interest), and soil (thereby contaminating food crops as well as increasing the levels of exposure of any children playing in the dirt). Lead from lead smelters and other industries may pollute homes, gardens and children's play areas in the same way.

One parent who is a nutritionist suggests, "If you live in a heavy traffic area get your soil tested. [See chart on page 255]. Lead content may be too high to grow garden vegetables—plant a hedge or put a fence around garden to keep out auto exhaust . . ." She passes on the advice of another parent she knows who has discovered that "the best way to stop lead tracking through the house, besides removing shoes at the door, is to damp mop—better at removing lead than vacuuming . . ." In addition, Barbara Wallace and Kathy Cooper give the following directions for reducing house lead levels in *The Citizen's Guide to Lead*:

"If you have reason to think the level of lead in your house dust may be high, you might wish to do a thorough 'decontamination' cleaning and then follow it regularly with the dustbusting routine [see box on facing page]. 'Decontamination' cleaning involves wet cleaning with a phosphate detergent or cleaner (phosphate seems to help loosen lead particles from surfaces) in every nook and cranny of your house. Make sure that no children are exposed to the dust that gets disturbed or to the dirty water. Change the cleaning water frequently and/or go over the surfaces a second time with clean water. Carpets should be cleaned twice using a commercial carpet cleaning machine: follow the directions using a hot water-phosphate-detergent mixture, wait 24 hours, and then repeat the entire cleaning process using the regular commercial cleaning solution. If the carpet is removable, do both sides and the floor underneath."

(The following chart is reprinted from *The Citizen's Guide to Lead* by Barbara Wallace and Kathy Cooper.)

DUSTBUSTERS

• Use a damp mop and damp cloths for cleaning and dusting.

• Sweep only when absolutely necessary and in a careful manner.

• Clean near windows and doors frequently since dust in these areas tends to have a high lead level.

• Use window shades that can be wiped clean and washable curtains.

• Vacuum or wash window screens periodically.

• Vacuum rugs often. Cover them with a sheet when babies play on them. If your vacuum expels dust, don't vacuum when children are around. Flat-weave carpets and bare floors collect less dust than shag, pile or looped rugs.

• Have a professional clean your forced-air heating ducts periodically.

• During the heating season, clean or replace furnace filters every month.

• Try to keep the humidity level between about 35–50%. Drier air encourages dust to fly around and wetter air encourages mould growth.

• Brush house pets often. Their coats collect dust and dirt. Groom them outside and keep them out of young children's rooms.

• Clean children's bedrooms or other play areas often. Remove dust-catching items or store them in closets or drawers. A covered toy box keeps toys cleaner and makes cleaning easier.

• Cover furniture with washable covers.

• Clean shoes or remove them when you come inside.

MAKE DUST CONTROL YOUR GOAL

Source: Adapted from *Dustbusters: Tips for controlling lead exposure through housedust*. Used with the permission of the Toronto Department of Public Health. Readers may reproduce this table provided the Toronto Department of Public Health is acknowledged.

Some of the suggestions that Wallace and Cooper make for reducing contact with lead include keeping children's hands and fingernails clean, as well as play areas and plush or fabric toys, and covering all bare-soil play areas with, for example, grass, sand or wood chips.

Children should be exposed as little as possible to high traffic areas. This can be accomplished in part by walking or bicycling along back streets and lanes rather than heavily traveled roadways, making sure children restrict the amount of time they spend in any playground, empty lot, front yard, sidewalk or other place which is near a busy street or major intersection, and so on.

WATER. In addition to industrial wastes, another source of water pollution is the pipes that the water passes through. Some pipes are made of lead, especially old ones, and some pipes contain cadmium. Copper pipes are now common and may cause problems for some children. If we live in a soft-water area, a higher proportion of metal from the pipes will be leached into the water than in hard-water areas. (If a water softener is used, it should be attached to the hot water only.)

If water is contaminated, our options as mentioned in Chapter 10 are to find an alternative source that is less contaminated, rent, borrow, or buy a home water distiller or purifier (remembering that with the distillation or purification good minerals will disappear along with the bad and may need to be supplemented, and that these processes do not necessarily eliminate all the toxins), or run drinking water a few minutes every morning before using to decrease levels of toxic metals.

FOOD. As mentioned in Chapter 10, how contaminated our food is depends on the toxic metal content of the soil, water and air that nourish it, the acidity of the soil and the type of crop or animal being grown or raised. Fertilizers and pesticides may also contribute toxic metals to the food supply, as may sewage sludge when used to grow food in. Aluminum in its various manifestations is a food additive popular with the food industry, and some food may be inadvertently contaminated with other metals as a result of food processing. The containers food is cooked, stored or served in sometimes contribute to excessive levels of toxic metals in children as well. Copper or aluminum pots and pans and lead in improperly glazed pottery (plates, pitchers, etc.) can contaminate food.

Certain foods are more likely to be contaminated with high levels of metals than others. Foods from lead-soldered tin cans are a major source of lead; grains and cereals, tomatoes, potatoes, liver, kidney, oysters, clams and large ocean fish such as swordfish and tuna may be high in cadmium; fresh-water fish from mercury-contaminated lakes and large ocean fish are likely to contain significant amounts of mercury.

To reduce children's exposure to heavy metals in their food, we should reduce consumption of canned goods, remove food from opened cans and store in glass or stainless steel containers (for example, if canned apple or tomato juice is used, after opening the can it is safest to pour the remainder into a glass bottle before storing in the fridge), restrict consumption of food likely to contain large amounts of toxic metals such as fish from mercury-polluted lakes or food grown in highly contaminated soil, and read labels for the presence of aluminum-derived additives.

Concerning cookware, copper pots and pans should never be used (except when the copper is only on the bottom where it is not in contact with the food). It is also a good idea to phase out aluminum pots; although this can be done gradually, cooking high-acid foods such as tomatoes and fruits in aluminum cookware should be avoided. Stainless steel (with or without copper bottoms) or iron pots and pans are good alternatives to pots and pans made out of copper or aluminum. In addition, only pottery that is properly glazed should be used.

The relationship between soil lead levels and the advisability of planting specific vegetables, reprinted from *The Citizen's Guide to Lead* by Barbara Wallace and Kathy Cooper:

GARDENING GUIDE

Roots: Beets   Carrots   Bulb Onions   Potatoes   Parsnips
Leafy: Lettuce   Celery   Broccoli   Cabbage   Chard
Fruiting: Tomatoes   Cucumbers   Squash   Peas   Beans

Soil Lead Level in PPM	Kinds of Vegetables		
	roots	*leafy*	*fruiting*
0–500	OK	OK	OK
500–1000	NO	OK-NO*	OK
over 1000	NO	NO	OK

*OK if garden is not near a main traffic route or smelter, and NO if it is.

Foods that are safe to grow (and eat) in soils containing different amounts of lead. OK means safe; NO means not safe.

Source: Adapted from City of Toronto Department of Public Health, *Get the Lead Out*.

• NUTRITIONAL SUPPLEMENTS. Some supplements may be contaminated with heavy metals, just as food often is. For example, lead is sometimes found in dolomite and bone meal, although generally the amounts are no greater than would be found in food. (This does not of course mean that these amounts are any more acceptable in supplements than they are in food.) The level of contamination may vary from brand to brand. If there is any concern about contamination, check with the appropriate government agency to find the legally allowed limits of toxic metals in supplements and how closely these limits are monitored, with the manufacturer for the exact levels of toxic metals contained in their particular product, and/or with an independent lab for an analysis of the toxic metal content of the supplement in question. When deciding what is an acceptable level, individual circumstances must be taken into account, such as how often and in what dosage the supplement is taken, the availability of other less contaminated sources of the particular nutrient, amounts of toxic metals ingested from other sources, and so on.

• CIGARETTE SMOKE. Even second-hand smoke can contribute to children's lead and cadmium levels, and smoking when children are present should be avoided.

• PAINT. When there is old, flaking, lead-based paint on interior or exterior walls, young children sometimes put paint flakes in their mouths, or pick up dust containing lead from the paint as they are playing or crawling around indoors on the floors or outside in the dirt. Keeping walls in good repair and repainting with nonlead-based paint is helpful, as are damp-mopping to get rid of the dust and washing children's hands frequently.

A favorite painted toy that children love to chew or suck may also contribute significant levels of lead and should not be allowed.

Painted wood should not be burned in fireplaces or stoves.

NEWSPAPERS AND MAGAZINES. These contain toxic metals (particularly pages with color), and children should not be allowed to chew on them. Neither should they be burned in fireplaces or stoves.

HOBBIES AND RENOVATIONS. Wallace and Cooper make the following comment in *The Citizen's Guide to Lead*:

"Hobbies and renovation activities may be the most frequent source of additional lead exposures to both children and adults. If renovations, soldering, stripping or painted furniture, stained glass work, or some hobby activities involving lead are occurring in your home, make sure that these activities do not cause an increase in lead exposure to children. Old painted surfaces may have very high levels of lead. Even recently painted surfaces can have a lead level that is risky for young children. A single small chip of leaded paint may have ten times more lead than a child's usual total daily diet. Keep children away from renovation, soldering, or similar lead-related activities and be very careful to clean up any scraps or debris from this kind of work."

DENTAL FILLINGS. Mercury-containing fillings may be a source of mercury toxicity. Dr. Hal Huggins and Sharon Huggins warn that this is particularly the case with high copper amalgams which apparently emit mercury even more quickly than the regular kind.

Obviously prevention is the best policy. Making sure all nutrient needs are met, avoiding sweets and sticky foods such as raisins; and brushing and flossing regularly will help prevent cavities. When fillings are needed, ones that don't contain mercury should be considered.

TOXIC DUST FROM THE WORKPLACE. Dust of toxic metals may be transferred from workplace to home in clothing. If possible clothing should be removed and washed before being brought home.

Getting Better

It may take weeks or months to rid the body of toxic metals, and in general it should be expected that improvement will also take time, with symptoms decreasing in severity gradually. If despite evidence of metal toxicity children show only partial improvement after following the treatment program, it may be that other factors such as those described in Chapters 10 to 18 are involved and should be investigated.

Books referred to in this chapter and other suggested reading:

The Citizen's Guide to Lead, Barbara Wallace and Kathy Cooper. NC Press, Toronto, 1986. A useful primer on the lead situation in North American communities covering historical, legal, economic and health aspects. Lists sources of contamination and ways to decrease lead exposure, as well as explaining some of the issues involved in the politics of decreasing lead exposure on a societal level.

Dr. Cott's Help for Your Learning Disabled Child, The Orthomolecular Treatment, Allan Cott, J. Agel, E. Boe. Times Books, New York, 1985. For a description, see Chapter 8.

It's All In Your Head, Hal A. Huggins and Sharon A. Huggins, P.O. Box 2589, Colorado Springs, Colorado 80901, 1985. Discusses the relationship between dental fillings and mercury toxicity, including diagnosis and treatment.

Nourishing Your Child, Ray C. Wunderlich, Jr. and Dwight K. Kalita, Keats Publishing, New Canaan, Connecticut, 1984. For a description, see Chapter 8.

Trace Elements, Hair Analysis and Nutrition, Richard A. Passwater and Elmer M. Cranton, Keats Publishing, New Canaan, Connecticut, 1983. A valuable book containing a fairly comprehensive discussion of minerals and toxic metals, including their sources, role in health and illness, relationships to other elements, ways of reducing toxicity and how to interpret hair analysis values.

17 OTHER ENVIRONMENTAL FACTORS

There are factors in the environment other than those discussed in previous chapters that may affect children's behavior. These include fluorescent lighting, negative ion depletion and radiation. Following are brief descriptions of each of these:

Fluorescent Lighting

Fluorescent lighting is widely used in schools, other public places and sometimes at home, because it is less expensive than incandescent lighting. It has, however, been implicated in children's learning and behavior problems. There are three reasons why fluorescent lights may cause problems:

• Fluorescent lighting that is not shielded gives off two kinds of radiation—X-ray and radio frequency—which may have negative effects on some children.

• Cool-white fluorescent lights, the type used most commonly, do not give off some of the wavelengths of light that are given off by natural sunlight. According to John Ott, who has done extensive research on light, radiation and health, some of these omitted wavelengths appear to be necessary for certain biological processes and their absence may be detrimental to some children.

• Most fluorescent lighting, according to John Ott in his book *Health and Light*, has a 60-cycle flicker that "is recognized as contributing to headaches, eye strain, and fatigue, and which may be a factor in seizures in those subject to epilepsy."

In general it seems like a good idea to encourage children to play outside on a regular basis so that they can gain some of the benefits of exposure to natural sunlight. (Unfortunately sunlight can also be harmful, especially now with the destruction of the world's ozone layer resulting in increased rates of skin cancer. This makes it extremely important to use moderation and common sense to avoid sunburn and other ill effects of overexposure.) Either full-spectrum incandescent or full-spectrum fluorescent lights can be used when artificial lighting is necessary. In addition to being full-spectrum, fluorescent lights should have their ends shielded with lead to prevent any escape of X-ray radiation from the cathodes, and John Ott also suggests a "combination 'egg crate' and wire grid screen" for the purpose of grounding the radio frequency radiation. To prevent the fluorescent lights from flickering, John Ott describes a full-spectrum fluorescent stabilizer which changes AC line current to DC.

Depletion of Negative Ions

Ions are molecules with either positive or negative charges. Fred Soyka and Alan Edmonds write in their book *The Ion Effect* that there is an optimum ratio of positive to negative ions in our environment which if disturbed causes some people to suffer ill effects. Unfortunately, in modern society this ratio is often disturbed and there are generally an overabundance of positive ions and a scarcity of negative ions.

This imbalance may occur as a result of certain winds, or it may occur when negative ions are depleted due to:

• exposure to friction, such as when air is forced through heating ducts

• attraction to particles of dust and pollution to which the negative ions attach themselves, thus losing their charge

• static electricity, which is caused by, among other things, the use of synthetic materials and the use of certain technologies such as visual display terminals (VDTs)

According to Bob DeMatteo in his book *Terminal Shock*, "Scientific research on the biological effects of static electric fields indicates that effects are caused by the depletion of negative ions resulting from static buildups. This research, which has been recently summarized by Dr. Charles Wallach of the Faculty of Medicine at the University of California, indicates that negative ion depletion can cause biochemical changes in the body." These changes include disturbance of the sodium/potassium ion exchange, of the binding of calcium ions in brain tissue, of the serum levels of the hormone serotonin, and of the functioning of the thyroid gland. As a result of these changes, muscle function and nerve impulses may be affected.

The number of negative ions in the atmosphere can be increased by running water, such as in a shower, and by negative ion generators. (Unfortunately, though, some negative ion generators may also produce ozone.) Soyka and Edmonds mention that even spraying water out of a container used to mist plants may be helpful. Replacing synthetic carpeting and other synthetics with natural materials may reduce static electricity and the resulting number of positive ions. DeMatteo mentions in his book that mesh filters placed on the screen can reduce the static electricity associated with VDTs.

Radiation

There are many different kinds of radiation, and children's exposure to a variety of radiation sources is increasing. As mentioned previously, fluorescent lighting gives off radiation. So do television sets, microwave ovens, electric power lines and VDTs, just to mention a few other sources.

Most people are aware of the dangers of ionizing radiation such as X-rays, particularly with respect to causing cancer. Less well-known are the dangers of non-ionizing radiation.

Although it is disputed by some, there is evidence that non-ionizing radiation at very low frequencies (VLF), radio frequencies, microwave frequency and possibly extremely low frequencies (ELF) can seriously affect the central nervous system (as well as affecting other body systems such as the reproductive, cardiovascular and immune systems).

We should especially be aware of the possible dangers where children are concerned. As Bob DeMatteo writes, "Children, in large numbers, are now being exposed to radiation with the growing use of VDTs in homes, in schools and in coin-operated video game parlors. A radiation survey of VDTs used in the City of Toronto school system showed that over one half of the VDTs used by the children were emitting VLF radiation levels of over 300 V/m."

DeMatteo notes that home VDT buyers often go for economy and so may get a model that's not shielded; others, who hook their computers to an old color TV, risk higher levels of X-ray and VLF emissions.

At the same time, he points out, electromagnetic radiation is a particular danger to growing children. The rapidly growing cells of the organs and nervous system are highly vulnerable to damage, which may result in cancer or impaired organ function.

Research indicates, DeMatteo writes, that the central nervous systems of children are at special risk from electromagnetic fields and pulsating visible radiation. "For example, there is evidence to suggest that pulsating visible light from TV receivers can trigger changes in brain wave patterns, epileptic seizures and even contribute to hyperactivity in children. These kinds of effects are just now being explored in relation to pulsed VLF and ELF emissions from VDTs and TVs."

DeMatteo gives directions for shielding VDTs to reduce radiation. Another reasonable precaution is to limit the amount of time children are exposed to sources of radiation such as television and VDTs, and to inquire about levels of radiation, which vary from manufacturer to manufacturer, when purchasing such items.

Books referred to in this chapter and other suggested reading:

Health and Light, John N. Ott. Pocket Books, New York, 1976. Describes the important relationship of light to health.

The Ion Effect, Fred Soyka and Alan Edmonds. Bantam Books, New York, 1977. An interesting and informative discussion of how people are affected by an imbalance of negative and positive ions.

Light, Radiation and You, John N. Ott. The Devin-Adair Company, Old Greenwich, Connecticut, 1982. A discussion of the effects of different forms of light and radiation, including connections with hyperactivity.

Radiation Alert, A Consumer's Guide to Radiation, David I. Poch. Doubleday, New York, 1985. A survey of the different types of radiation we and our children are exposed to at home, work, in the environment, and through medical use; their sources, potential dangers and side effects, and how we can minimize their effects.

Terminal Shock, Bob DeMatteo. NC Press, Toronto, 1985. An excellent review of the possible dangers of video display terminals (including effects on the central nervous system) and how to minimize them.

18

RELATED FACTORS

There are many factors such as regular exercise and sufficient sleep which play a crucial role in the health of a child. These factors help maintain the efficient functioning of body systems, ensure the proper utilization of nutrients and other essentials to well-being such as oxygen and minimize the effects of physical and emotional stresses. Because they greatly increase the effectiveness of nutritional and environmental health measures, they should be considered important components of a child's treatment program. Following are brief descriptions of some of these related factors:

Exercise

Regular exercise is vital to physical and mental health and well-being. It keeps the body "tuned up," and operating efficiently. Some of the benefits of regular exercise may include improved muscle tone and strength, a strong heart, increased circulation and oxygen utilization, and effective digestion and metabolism. It helps correct poor posture and sleep problems, and is a major method of minimizing the effects of stress.

It is also a mood elevator. Martha Davis, Elizabeth Robbins Eshelman and Matthew McKay write in *The Relaxation & Stress Reduction Workbook*, "Research is just beginning to explain why exercise is effective in reducing general anxiety and depression. Fifteen to twenty minutes of vigorous exercise stimulates both the secretion of neurochemicals called catecholamines into your brain, and the release of endorphins into your blood. Depressed people are often deficient in catecholamines. Endorphins are natural pain killers and mood elevators."

An important spin-off benefit of regular exercise is that along with improvement in coordination, stamina and general well-being comes an increase in self-confidence.

There are four basic types of exercise: those that increase muscle strength, such as push-ups and sit-ups; those that promote cardiovascular fitness, such as running, bicycling and swimming; those that improve coordination and other physical skills, such as gymnastics; and those aimed at general conditioning, such as stretches, warm-ups and cool-downs.

What type or types of exercise should parents encourage their children to do? According to Martin I. Lorin in *The Parents' Book of Physical Fitness for Children from Infancy Through Adolescence,* such a decision "will depend upon several factors. First, for what goals are we striving? If health, energy and the prevention of disease are our goals, then those exercises that increase endurance and improve cardiovascular fitness would be of the highest priority. Some general conditioning exercises would also be important. For most children this should be the case . . .

"The second step is to analyze what sorts of physical activities the child already engages in and then to design a program to supplement what is missing. A child who already spends a great deal of time running, swimming, or cycling does not need as much emphasis on endurance as the child who almost never exerts himself and rarely works up a sweat."

The child's individual physique and capabilities also have to be taken into account, Lorin says: the big, strong child probably should concentrate on skill and endurance, while the graceful, nimble skinny child, on the other hand, would do well to work on increasing strength.

As much as possible, exercise should be integrated into a child's daily activities, such as by walking places instead of being driven in a car, using stairs instead of escalators, helping with strenuous house and yard work rather than sticking to the light stuff (depending of course on age), spending leisure time skipping, bicycling and playing leapfrog rather than watching television, and so on. For some children this nonregimented manner of exercise will be enough to maintain good health, but for others a regular exercise program will be needed as well.

There are a number of physical activities to choose from which may appeal to children and can either be incorporated into an exercise program or simply encouraged as healthy leisure-time activity. Running, swimming, bicycling, skipping, bouncing on a rebounder (a mini-trampoline), dancing, skating and a variety of group sports, such as soccer, all provide good exercise, and, very importantly, emphasize cardiovascular fitness.

It is important to remember that an exercise program has the best chance of success if it is based on the physical activities children most enjoy, the ones which seem like play rather than work. Adding music will make an activity more enjoyable for every age group, and for younger children it is possible to make some exercises into games, such as hopping around like bunny rabbits, bouncing like kangaroos or playing tag. Also, doing activities with other family members or friends will make any kind of exercise more fun.

Children should work into their exercise programs slowly and gradually increase either the length of time they spend exercising or the intensity of their exertions, or both. Their exercise sessions should take place on a regular basis at least a few times a week. Once children have achieved a degree of comfort doing exercises at one level of difficulty, they should push themselves to work a little harder. To quote Dr. Lorin, "Remember that for a child, the same performance each day actually represents less and less of an achievement as growth occurs!"

Dr. Lorin stresses that it is important for children to do warm-up exercises before workouts, not to become overheated or restrict fluid intake, and not to exercise immediately before eating or to do a major workout until two hours after eating.

He makes a point of noting that girls and boys are much the same with respect to physical activity: "The mistaken notions that girls need less physical activity and that they can accomplish less in the way of sports and athletics than boys have prevailed in our society for a very long time. Only now are such ideas beginning to give way to a more rational and understanding philosophy . . . The fact is that girls have always had the same needs and basic abilities as boys, but they have had less training and fewer opportunities."

Lorin emphasizes strongly that girls' fitness potential is high and can and should be developed through training programs as strenuous as those undergone by boys; they deserve the physical and mental benefits produced by such programs and should not be unjustly and needlessly denied them.

Age should not be a barrier to a regular exercise program either. Lorin writes that, up to the age of a year, all that is necessary is to encourage children's natural inclination to activity. However, "Running and jogging can be started by two years of age. Walking, riding a tricycle, skating, and swimming are all healthful physical activities which can be initiated before the age of three."

In addition, the presence of a physical handicap should not be allowed to prevent most children from exercising. The book *Reach for Fitness* by Richard Simmons describes many exercises for those who are physically challenged.

Digestion

Digestion is a major factor affecting children's nutritional status and overall health. If the digestive system is not functioning properly, nutrients may be incompletely absorbed, toxins produced which interfere with bodily processes, and wastes eliminated inefficiently. Poor digestion may be the underlying cause of many conditions such as vitamin and mineral deficiencies and food and environmental sensitivities.

If illnesses or physical disorders such as diabetes are not present, then the possible origins of digestive problems may include, among other things, inadequate diet (Chapter 10), food sensitivities (Chapter 14), nutrient deficiencies or dependencies (Chapter 11), yeast overgrowth (Chapter 13), lack of exercise (pages 263–265), emotional stress (pages 268–274), and poor eating habits (such as eating in a rush, eating when tense or anxious, or not chewing food thoroughly).

Imbalances in pH levels in the digestive system (pH measures the degree of acidity or alkalinity) are also a possible cause of digestive problems. Correction of pH imbalances should be done only under medical supervision.

A high-quality diet containing adequate amounts of fiber and water as well as regular exercise are both extremely important in avoiding digestive problems.

Breathing

Breathing is a bodily function that is usually taken for granted, yet improper breathing can affect health and well-being. As a result of lack of vigorous exercise, poor posture or clothing that is too tight, some children breathe shallowly and therefore suffer the effects of lack of oxygen. According to Davis, Eshelman and McKay in *The Relaxation & Stress Reduction Workbook*, "When an insufficient amount of fresh air reaches your lungs, your blood is not properly purified or oxygenated. Waste products that should have been removed are kept in circulation, slowly poisoning your system. When your blood lacks enough oxygen it is bluish and dark in color, and can be seen in poor complexion. Digestion is hampered. Your organs and tissues become undernourished and deteriorate. Poorly oxygenated blood contributes to anxiety states, depression and fatigue, and makes each stressful situation many times harder to cope with. Proper breathing habits are essential for good mental and physical health."

Exercise and paying attention to posture (slumping will ensure inefficient breathing) are two ways of improving breathing habits. Breathing exercises, such as described in *The Relaxation & Stress Reduction Workbook* and in many yoga books, will also help children regain the natural breathing patterns they had in babyhood.

Sleep

Sleep needs vary but generally children are more likely to get less sleep than they need rather than more. Not getting enough sleep can cause any child to be cranky, irritable and unreasonable, so it is important to make every effort to ensure that children receive adequate amounts of sleep.

Some children seem to fall asleep easily, any time and any place, regardless of disruptions such as noise, and stay asleep for a sufficient amount of time. Others have difficulty falling asleep, sleep restlessly and may wake up before they have fulfilled their sleep requirements. Unfortunately many children affected by nutritional/environmental factors suffer from sleep disturbances; however, these should improve as treatment progresses. In the meantime, however, following are a few suggestions which may improve a poor sleep situation:

• CREATE CONDITIONS THAT CHILDREN WILL ASSOCIATE WITH SLEEP. Children like everyone else are creatures of habit and, if a regular sleep routine is set up, they will likely have less trouble falling asleep. According to Richard Ferber in *Solve Your Child's Sleep Problems*, some children need to have certain conditions met before sleep will come, such as the presence of familiar surroundings (their own bed, pillow, favorite blanket and teddy bear), the observance of a nightly bedtime ritual (snack, bathroom, bedtime story, good-night hug and kiss), and adherence to a regular bedtime or naptime. If these conditions change from night to night or naptime to naptime, children may feel that something is not quite right and have trouble relaxing into sleep.

Although we should not try to force children to sleep longer hours than are necessary, we should take responsibility for enforcing reasonable bed and naptimes. Children are often so eager to continue their activities that they will strenuously deny they are tired, even when they are drooping with fatigue.

Just as children can get into the habit of falling asleep at certain times, they can also get into the habit of waking up at certain times, such as the middle of the night (for example, to nurse or feed long past the age when there is a need for it). The nice thing about habits, though, is that they can be broken gently—gently being the operative word.

• MAKE SURE SLEEP CONDITIONS ARE COMFORTABLE. It is easier to fall sleep when comfortable. This means controlling temperature (generally nighttime temperatures are more comfortable when lower than daytime temperatures); humidity (using a humidifier or dehumidifier as necessary); amount of light (dark enough to be conducive to sleep, light enough to reassure those who are scared of the dark; the problem of early morning sun in the summertime can be solved by using blinds or garbage bags on the windows to keep the light out); air circulation (a stuffy room increases the possibility of a poor-quality sleep) and amount of noise. Other factors contributing to comfort are the quality of the mattress and the presence or absence of sensitivity-producing substances (such as dust, molds, plants, animals and so on).

• ENCOURAGE RELAXATION AND CONTROL OF STRESS. A tense child will find it much more difficult to fall asleep and to have a restful sleep. Winding-down activities before bedtime such as reading or drawing (not playing frisbee or haunted house) and utilizing relaxation techniques such as massage, tightening and loosening muscles, deep breathing and listening to calming music may be helpful. Control of stress is sometimes extremely important in decreasing sleep problems. (See the following section for more information on control and reduction of stress.)

• INSTITUTE A REGULAR EXERCISE PROGRAM. Exercise enhances the ability to fall asleep and the quality of sleep, as long as it is not done right before bedtime.

• INCLUDE SPECIFIC FOODS AND NUTRITIONAL SUPPLEMENTS IN THE DIET. Certain foods, such as turkey, cheese and bananas, contain the amino acid tryptophan which is a sleep inducer. Giving these foods as a bedtime snack is sometimes helpful. Nutritional supplements, such as those mentioned on page 172 in Chapter 11, are also helpful in some cases.

Control of Stress

Day and night children are subject to a number of physical and emotional stresses. Pollution, extremes of temperature, insect bites, junk food, vitamin deficiencies and infections all cause stress, as do the ordinary events of life (crossing a busy street, arguing with a friend, writing an exam) and the extraordinary events of life (the death of someone close, moving to a different country). Any kind of change, whether perceived as negative or positive, is stressful.

Whether the origin of the stress is physical or emotional, the effect on the body is the same: the adrenal gland kicks into high gear, preparing the body for "fight or flight" with, among other changes, increases in blood pressure, heart rate and energy. If the stress occurs frequently and its physiological responses are not diminished through either physical action or relaxation, a wide variety of physical and emotional problems may eventually result, such as poor digestion, disruption of sleep, nutrient loss, increased susceptibility to injury and infection, depression, anxiety, hostility, fatigue, apathy and muscular tension. (Stress that is not dealt with may in some cases be a factor in illnesses such as heart disease and cancer.) More specific symptoms of excessive or inappropriately handled stress may include diarrhea or constipation; frequent urination; dry mouth; stooped posture; sweaty palms; cool, clammy skin; loss of appetite; restlessness; teeth grinding; nail biting and tics.

Just as the body affects the mind, the mind affects the body, making it essential to include reduction and control of emotional as well as physical stress in the nutritional/environmental treatment program. Reduction and control of physical stresses such as food sensitivities and environmental toxins are discussed in detail in Chapters 10 to 17; the rest of this section concentrates primarily on reduction and control of children's negative emotional stresses.

What Can Parents Do to Reduce Children's Stress Levels and Minimize the Effects of Stress?

How children react to stress will differ according to the state of their physical health, how well prepared they are to deal with stress, the type of stress they are subjected to (some children are affected worse by some types of stress than by other types), and what their optimum stress levels are (children vary in how much stress they can cope with). In other words, it is important for us to make sure our children are as physically healthy as possible, to teach them methods of handling stress, to reduce as much as possible the types of stress they are most adversely affected by, and to keep the amount of stress in their lives at the level that is best for them.

Following are a few specific suggestions of what we as parents can do to reduce the emotional stress in our children's lives and to minimize the effects of this stress:

• ENSURE A HIGH-QUALITY DIET WITH THE POSSIBLE ADDITION OF NUTRITIONAL SUPPLEMENTS. According to *Nutrition Almanac*, "Many of the disorders related to stress are not a direct result of the stress itself but a result of nutrient deficiencies caused by increased metabolic rate during periods of stress." For this reason, although a high quality diet is always a good idea, it is especially crucial during periods of greater than usual stress. In some cases adding nutritional supplements to the diet, if these are not already a part of a child's program, may be necessary. If children are already taking supplements, Dr. Abram Hoffer writes in a personal communication, "I do think it is important to increase some of the water soluble supplements during stress, particularly vitamin C and some of the B vitamins, but one does not have to go up too high with the B vitamins. Also it might be a good idea if a child is taking zinc to increase that a little bit for the duration of the stress." (See Chapter 11 for more information on nutritional supplements.)

• ENSURE ADEQUATE SLEEP. Being short of sleep makes it difficult to cope with stress effectively. Thinking is often less clear, emotions more volatile, reactions hard to control. Unfortunately a vicious cycle sometimes occurs where excess stress makes it harder to get to sleep and to stay asleep, with the resulting insufficient hours of sleep causing increased stress. When this occurs it is important to concentrate on relaxation techniques at bedtime as well as other methods of stress reduction. For more information on sleep, see the preceding section.

• PROBLEM-SOLVING TO ELIMINATE EXCESS OR NEGATIVE STRESS. The best way of dealing with excess stress, especially of a negative kind, is to eliminate its source. We should encourage children to join us in working out appropriate solutions to problems by thinking through all available options and alternatives. Eventually children will learn that a bit of time and creativity can go a long way toward solving at least some of their problems, whether these be how to neutralize a bully, handle teasing about a birthmark, prevent the weekly loss of library books, improve punctuality or earn enough money to buy a skateboard.

It is very important to keep in mind that if children's most serious problems are caused by any of the nutritional/environmental factors mentioned in this book, then following the nutritional/environmental treatment program is a crucial step in removing a great deal of negative stress from their lives. When problems stem directly from disturbances in sight, hearing, thought, mood and so on, as a result of nutritional/environmental factors, *these problems will not be resolved until the basic causes are dealt with.* As children improve on the program they will generally find it easier to make friends, do well in school and cope with life's ups and downs.

• ENCOURAGE A POSITIVE ATTITUDE. There is nothing worse than feeling that a bad situation will never change. The sense of power-lessness this engenders, plus the weight of hopelessness, are very stressful. Unfortunately, change rarely happens quickly. It will be helpful to emphasize that patience and determination are needed for change, point out all positive signs that indicate a situation is im-proving, however slowly, and encourage children to recognize the good aspects of their lives (taking care not to deny the validity of their negative feelings).

In connection with stress caused directly by nutritional/environmental factors, it is a good idea to remind children that, as they continue to follow the treatment program and their worst symptoms disappear, their physical comfort, learning capacity and social relationships will improve. Knowing that there is hope that unpleasant situations will change for the better is crucial in the reduction of stress.

• REDUCE EXCESS STIMULATION. One way to reduce the stress-load of some children with behavior problems is to limit the amount of stimulation they receive; very often the more severe their prob-lems are the more important this is, especially when perceptual problems such as faces changing shape and sounds coming out of nowhere are involved. (In some cases of course children will need more stimulation rather than less.) In practice, reducing stimulation means having a regular structured daily routine, restricting the num-ber of activities children are involved in, limiting the number of new experiences they are exposed to, keeping social situations simple (for example, socializing in a small group setting rather than a large group), decreasing visual stimulation by physically removing or covering with a white sheet all toys or other distracting items cur-rently not being used, and generally creating as calm an atmosphere as possible. Limiting stimulation helps children feel more secure as they know better what to expect from each day and have fewer variables to deal with. Once children start improving on their treat-ment program, limiting stimulation will of course be much less necessary.

• ELIMINATE BOREDOM. Some children do not find enough that is challenging to them in their environments and have not yet learned how to use their creative energies constructively. Sometimes they end up creating stress for themselves in the form of fears, anxieties and obsessions. Children who are involved in activities that are engrossing to them, whether sports, reading, painting, researching dinosaurs or collecting stamps, feel better about themselves and spend less time in destructive worrying and brooding.

In connection with both reducing excess stimulation and eliminating boredom, it is important that we be aware of what our children's optimum stress levels are until they are able to sense for themselves when they are being under- or over-stressed.

• REPLACE CRITICISM WITH POSITIVE FEEDBACK. Children with behavioral problems are often faced with problems such as difficulty in making and keeping friends, poor school performance, and constant pressure to change (often in the form of anger and overt criticism), which naturally give rise to chronic feelings of rejection, self-dislike, failure and frustration. However, children who feel good about themselves are more likely to handle stressful events and problems in a constructive way. This makes it important to emphasize their positive qualities and abilities while keeping criticism to a minimum. Reassuring children often that they are lovable and worthwhile people will help them build positive self-images.

• SPICE THEIR LIVES WITH HUMOR. It is becoming well accepted that laughter is good therapy, releasing tension and diminishing worries and fears. Most children love jokes, riddles, funny stories and films, making it easy to tickle their funny bones.

• INITIATE COUNSELING. A good counselor who is sympathetic to a nutritional/environmental approach will often be able to help children find positive ways of dealing with problems and decreasing stress.

• USE TOUCH. Many techniques of stress control are best suited to older children, but even infants benefit from touch. Touch can include among other things massage (of feet, shoulders, neck, back, forehead or wherever feels best), or the close physical comfort of holding our children on our laps and giving frequent hugs. One parent recommends repetitive moving of body parts with younger children, for example moving their legs in a bicycling motion or crossing their arms over their chests and then straight out to the sides.

What Can Children Do to Minimize Harmful Effects of Stress?

We cannot protect children from all stress because there is not always a completely satisfactory solution to every problem. Also, stress is an unavoidable result of even positive changes which may be necessary for a child's well-being, such as reducing the amounts of sugar in a diet. In other words, it is not possible to have life without stress. However, listed below are some methods of minimizing the *effects* of stress, which we can help children integrate into their daily lives. (Many of these methods and more are described in detail in *The Relaxation & Stress Reduction Workbook*.)

• REGULAR EXERCISE. In addition to all its other benefits, a program of regular exercise is a very effective method of controlling the effects of stress. (For more information see pages 263–265).

• CONSCIOUS MUSCLE RELAXATION. It is difficult to feel tense when muscles are relaxed. Children can learn to be aware of muscular tension and ways of relaxing muscles. Practiced daily, tightening and relaxing each muscle in turn from the toes up to the scalp is one exercise that may be helpful.

• DEEP RHYTHMICAL BREATHING. In times of stress the rate of breathing tends to speed up and become more shallow. Consciously controlling breathing by slowing it down and breathing deeply from the abdomen will help children relax, as will breathing rhythmically. One deep-breathing exercise children might find relaxing is to lie on the floor face up and breathe in through the nose, filling the abdomen with air to the count of five (or whatever number is comfortable), and then breathe out through the mouth to the count of the same number; they should repeat breathing in and out in this manner for a few minutes. (See pages 266–267 for more information on breathing.)

• USING IMAGERY. When children are feeling bad it may help if they use their imaginations to transport themselves to a calming situation. Some might like the idea of floating down a gentle stream on a raft on a sunny day, others might prefer the thought of being snugly wrapped in a warm, feather-soft cocoon.

Imagery can also help improve children's concept of themselves. For example, spending a few minutes each day picturing themselves as they would like to be, such as effortlessly reading a book, answering a question correctly in class, playing happily with children they like, walking away from people they are angry with rather than hitting or kicking them, and so on, may prove to be beneficial.

Another use of imagery is to prepare for stressful situations. For example, before an exam children could picture themselves coolly and collectedly going into the classroom, sitting down at the desk, receiving the test, writing it, etc.

• ASSERTIVENESS. Children who act aggressively may hurt others (either verbally or physically) and children who act passively allow themselves to be hurt, ignored or taken advantage of. In addition, aggressive and passive behavior seldom achieve satisfactory results.

On the other hand, children who act assertively have learned how to state their needs and stand up for their rights without harming others, with more effective results and a resulting decrease in stress; assertive children have more control over their lives and therefore feel better about themselves and about any potentially difficult situations they may find themselves in.

To be assertive requires first of all that children recognize that they are worthwhile and likeable people with valid needs and desires (just as the worth and needs of others must be recognized and respected), and secondly that they recognize that assertiveness is an effective approach to life which will benefit them more than aggression or passivity. Practicing being assertive in pretend situations (role playing) can help children act assertively when faced with real-life situations.

• EXPRESSION OF FEELINGS. Expressing fears, anxieties and other feelings often clarifies problems and puts them in perspective, making them seem more manageable. Sometimes the act of expression frees a solution that otherwise would remain buried. At the very least some pressure is relieved by expressing feelings and emotions.

The best method of expression depends on the individual child and the specific situation. Some children will find it easiest talking to us or to others they feel comfortable with. (To encourage this see page 36). Others will prefer to express their feelings by drawing pictures, keeping a diary or writing stories. Acting out feelings or situations with dolls and through dance and movement are other possibilities.

• RELAXATION. Many methods of inducing relaxation have already been mentioned such as massage, exercise and deep breathing. Children should explore other methods as well, such as listening to music, soaking in a warm bath and different forms of meditation, in order to discover what works best for them.

Self-Awareness

Children who are in tune with themselves physically and mentally understand their real needs, nutritionally, emotionally and otherwise, and can act accordingly. For example, they are more likely to know which foods they can safely eat at any particular time and in what quantities, which muscles are getting tense and need relaxing, which odors bother them and must be avoided, and when a social situation is affecting them negatively and must be dealt with. They are more likely to know when their judgment is reliable and can be trusted, and when their judgment may be faulty because nutritional/environmental or other factors are distorting their perceptions, thinking processes and emotions.

They are more likely to know these things because they pay attention to the signals given to them by their bodies and minds and have learned, for the most part, how to interpret these signals correctly.

Signals can range from the blatant, such as the onset of a headache warning that no more apples should be eaten for a few days, to the subtle, such as a vague feeling of unease at the thought of a long bus ride. Tickles in the nose, stiff necks, stomachaches, feelings of anger, depression or restlessness, sore eyes, lightheadedness, sleepiness, even dreams—all these contain messages of one sort or another.

The first step children must take in order to become more closely in touch with their feelings and bodily sensations is to understand that what they eat, breathe and touch, how they interact with people and how they spend their time, can be either positive or negative influences on their health and well-being; in other words, that they are involved in a relationship with the world around them. The next step is to increase awareness of the feelings and bodily sensations they experience, and the third step is to learn how to interpret these feelings and sensations.

Self-awareness can be developed by conscious observation of physical and emotional reactions and sensations. For example, does this orange taste good or bad? Is working out math problems an experience that is frustrating, pleasurable, boring or a combination of all three? Which physical and emotional feelings are present just before an exam? Are there any manifestations of discomfort associated with being exposed to paints? Observing the difference in feeling between a hand that is first clenched into a fist and then shaken loose will help illustrate the difference between a tense muscle and a relaxed one. Noting differences in how children feel before and after any particular activity or event will help make connections between symptoms such as stomachaches, stuffed noses, fuzzy heads, irritability and lack of concentration, and possible causes such as swimming in a heavily chlorinated pool, being yelled at by the teacher, spending time in a dusty room and eating a hot dog.

In general, keeping a symptom diary such as the one described on page 124 in Chapter 8 can be an invaluable aid in the development of self-awareness.

Following is a description of how one child has developed her awareness to the point where she is able to tell which foods are safe for her to eat and which are not:

Marla has always been aware of the fact that she has allergies and must show some concern about what she eats.

If she comes across a food she is not used to, or is not sure what the food is, she will smell it. She then makes the decision as to whether or not she should eat it based on the smell of the food. Surprisingly enough she is able to pick out things containing foods she is allergic to simply by smelling the food. It is by sense of smell that she has avoided eating foods with eggs in them, for example custards.   —Marla's mother

Books referred to in this chapter and other suggested reading:

Aerobics Basics, Karen Liptak, Prentice-Hall, Englewood Cliffs, New Jersey, 1980. Written for children, this book concentrates on aerobic dancing and includes a variety of different dance routines with suggested music.

Aerobics Fun for Kids, David Steen, Fitzhenry and Whiteside, Markham, Ontario, 1982. Includes exercises (many in the form of games and suitable mostly for school age children) that can be done individually, in pairs or in groups.

The New Holistic Health Handbook, Shepherd Bliss, editor. The Stephen Greene Press, Lexington, Massachusetts, 1985. A good introduction to the variety of alternative approaches to health, with lots of references.

Nutrition Almanac, Nutrition Search, Inc. McGraw-Hill Book Company, New York, 1984. For a description, see Chapter 10.

Parents' Book of Physical Fitness for Children from Infancy through Adolescence, Martin I. Lorin. Atheneum, New York, 1978. An excellent book with general information about exercises, sports and fitness for children plus specific activities for each age group.

Reach for Fitness, Richard Simmons. Warner Books, New York, 1986. A book of exercises for people of all ages who are physically challenged (with specific information for those with cerebral palsy, Down's syndrome, spina bifida, cystic fibrosis, etc.) This book shows that people in wheelchairs or who have missing limbs, poor coordination or balance can still exercise and have fun doing it.

The Relaxation & Stress Reduction Workbook, Martha Davis, Elizabeth Robbins Eshelman and Matthew McKay. New Harbinger Publications, 2200 Adeline, Suite 305, Oakland, California, 94607, 1983. A very helpful book which, though aimed at adults, contains useful information that can be adapted for children.

Solve Your Child's Sleep Problems, Richard Ferber. Simon & Schuster, New York, 1985. An excellent book containing information on how to encourage good sleeping habits and eliminate bad ones.

Suzy Prudden's Exercise Program for Young Children, Suzy Prudden. Workman Publishing, New York, 1983. For children four weeks to four years; has exercises for each age group including baby massage, with photos accompanying the directions; the exercises have appealing names such as "the pretzel" and "monkey walk."

19

PREVENTION

The benefits of prevention are obvious, and the importance of prevention in a nutritional/environmental approach should not be overlooked. It is not enough to help children overcome existing behavioral problems; we also want to prevent new ones from starting. In addition, we want to ensure that other children will never suffer from preventable problems caused by nutritional or environmental factors. It is much easier to stop a problem from starting than to solve it once it has taken root.

Prevention, to be truly effective, must take place on both an individual level and a community or societal level. Following are discussions of these two aspects of prevention.

Prevention on an Individual Level

Although there is much that is beyond our immediate control concerning prevention, there are some preventive measures, described below, which may help minimize behavioral and other problems:

Good Prenatal Care

Ideally, prevention on an individual level starts even before conception occurs. If both future parents follow the precepts of good health, this will help ensure the healthiest possible egg and sperm and prepare the parents for the demands of pregnancy. Although the focus concerning conception, pregnancy and birth is often almost entirely on the woman, the importance of the male's contribution to the well-being of the embryo and future baby, in terms of the quality of his sperm as well as his ability to give practical and emotional support to the mother-to-be, should not be overlooked. All the components of a healthy lifestyle as listed on page 282 in this chapter are important—eating nutritiously, exercising regularly, avoiding drugs and environmental toxins as much as possible, practicing reduction and control of stress, and dealing effectively with health problems.

Another point to consider is the growing feeling that a good all-round program of nutritional supplementation should be started several months before conception in order to provide the optimum amount of nutrients.

In addition to following a healthy lifestyle, it is also important to check for any possible problems such as heavy metal toxicity, nutrient deficiencies, food and environmental sensitivities and lack of immunity to German measles. (If there is lack of immunity and a vaccination is given, conception should not take place until at least three months have passed.)

Groups such as Foresight, a group dedicated to the promotion of pre-conceptual care (see page 54 in Chapter 3), can provide valuable information and assistance.

When conception has taken place, the mother should continue to follow a healthy lifestyle. She must also be careful to fulfill the extra requirements of pregnancy, in order to supply her own needs and those of the growing fetus.

A weight gain of at least 25 to 30 pounds is often recommended during pregnancy to ensure sufficient nutrients for mother and child and an adequate birth weight for the baby (low birth-weight babies are at greater risk). In other words, pregnancy is an inappropriate time to diet.

Pregnant women generally need more protein (roughly 75 grams in total), more fiber (due to a more sluggish digestive system), and more iron, folic acid and calcium. Many other nutrient requirements also increase.

In addition to following a nutritious diet which takes into account the increased requirements of pregnancy, it is frequently recommended that the diet be supplemented with iron (60 milligrams are often suggested) and folic acid (at least 0.8 milligrams), as well as about 1,200 milligrams daily of calcium if the mother is unable to eat or drink milk and milk products.

Many doctors recommend that a general program of nutritional supplementation be maintained throughout pregnancy (starting before conception) to protect against the effect of environmental pollution and the widespread deterioration in the quality of food. Such a program might include, for example, the full complement of B-complex vitamins, vitamins A, C and E, a balanced multi-mineral preparation, and a good source of essential fatty acids (making sure of course that adequate amounts of the previously mentioned folic acid, iron and calcium are included).

Sheila Kitzinger in *The Complete Book of Childbirth and Pregnancy* stresses that in general most nutrient intake should come from food during pregnancy, but adds that, "Certain women are at 'nutritional risk' and need to pay special attention to diet; for them vitamin and mineral supplements may be useful. The ones particularly at risk are those pregnant during adolescence (while they are still growing themselves), women who are underweight when they become pregnant, women who are overweight because of excess consumption of carbohydrates and fats, those living on a very restricted range of foods like a macrobiotic diet, women who have lost a baby from miscarriage or stillbirth before, and women who have had three pregnancies within two years. Also included in this high risk category are women suffering from some chronic diseases involving the regular use of drugs, women who smoke, heavy drinkers and those with multiple pregnancies." Kitzinger goes on to mention research which "demonstrated that taking a multi-vitamin preparation for at least one month *before conception* and up to the second missed period helps to prevent spina bifida and anencephaly (both known as neural tube defects)."

Some of us who need extra nutrient supplementation to maintain health even when in a non-pregnant state should, in consultation with our doctors, continue taking nutritional supplements during pregnancy.

The most crucial development of the fetus and future child takes place during the first three months, requiring that the greatest of care be taken in this time period to avoid contact with anything which might be harmful to the growing fetus. In other words, this is not the time to be exposed to X-rays, chemical fumes, most prescription drugs and many over-the-counter medications as well as many illegal substances; in fact, the list of things that may harm the fetus is growing constantly. Caution is by far the best approach, and this of course applies to the whole length of the pregnancy. Even though the fetus is most sensitive during the first three months, it is still vulnerable for the remaining six and must be protected as much as possible.

It is important to note that everyday substances such as caffeine (found in coffee, tea, cola drinks and chocolate), tobacco and alcohol may also be harmful to the fetus and should either be avoided or used only in small quantities. For example, there are indications that large amounts of caffeine may cause birth defects and behavioral changes. Due to the number of variables which may be involved in such damage, it is impossible to tell what quantity, if any, is safe. Probably the wisest course is to eliminate caffeine totally from the diet, or at least to drastically reduce its intake.

Concerning alcohol and tobacco the *Boston Children's Hospital Parents' Guide to Nutrition* states,

"Alcohol is extremely dangerous to the baby. As little as two drinks a day can cause low-birthweight babies and developmental and learning difficulties. Chronic excessive drinking can lead to Fetal Alcohol Syndrome, which involves extensive mental and physical defects. Most experts, therefore, recommend that alcohol be avoided during pregnancy.

"Cigarette smoking can depress the appetite and is associated with low-birthweight infants. Furthermore, nicotine is harmful to the fetus, and carbon monoxide from cigarette smoke reduces the oxygen supply to the baby's red blood cells by constricting the blood vessels in the placenta. Abstention from smoking during pregnancy, therefore, is also strongly advised."

Prenatal classes are often very helpful, and continuing care by a doctor or midwife with regular checkups is extremely important.

Because labor and delivery are also times when mother and child are at risk, advance thought should be given to the kind of birth we would like to have. This means choosing where we give birth, who will be present at the birth, whether we want enemas, episiotomies, fetal monitors or pain killers, which positions we would like to use during delivery (lying on our backs or squatting) and so on. We might of course want to change some of these decisions after labor and delivery have begun due to changing circumstances, but it is important to be aware of our options.

Careful Selection and Introduction of Food to Babies

It is not necessary for babies to have solids until around the age of six months. Until then breast milk or formula are adequate. From the point of view of health and nutrition, breast milk is by far the best choice, but there are of course other considerations and all of us must decide on the basis of our own individual circumstances. If we would like to breast-feed but encounter difficulties, helpful suggestions and advice are often available from other mothers who have nursed their children, members of La Leche League (a support group for nursing mothers with numerous local branches—see pages 53 and 54 in Chapter 3), doctors or nurses sympathetic to breast-feeding, and books on breast-feeding. Many of us have overcome problems such as cracked nipples, engorged breasts and a baby's awkward nursing habits; some women have even successfully lactated and nursed their adopted infants.

It is important to note that the food and medicine (including in both cases additives and contaminants) a nursing mother consumes can affect her baby. For example, babies who are sensitive to cow's milk may react with stomach cramps or stuffy noses when their mothers drink or eat milk products, or a baby sensitive to artificial additives may show indications of hyperactivity if these are included in the mother's diet. If a sensitivity is suspected, the mother can follow the procedure for an elimination diet as outlined in Chapter 14 to discover which foods are causing the problems, and then either eliminate them from her diet or rotate them. Concerning medication, mothers should check with their doctors or La Leche League for possible effects on breast-fed babies. In a few cases it may be a good idea to test breast milk for levels of concentration of pesticides and other toxins, for example, if the mother has been exposed to particularly high levels of pollutants through working in a factory or eating contaminated food; a 24-hour sample should be used to ensure accuracy. In general, in addition to many other benefits, children who have been breast-fed develop fewer allergies than those who have been bottle-fed.

Babies can also have reactions to their formulas, and some experimentation may be needed in order to find one that is tolerated. In some cases rotation of formulas may be necessary.

Around the age of six months a baby's iron reserves are depleted and more calories are needed. For this reason somewhere between four to seven months is the time to start introducing solid foods, the exact time depending on the individual baby. In most cases it is a good idea to wait until babies are able to sit up on their own and indicate they are full by refusing more food. It is important to note, especially when there is a family history of allergies, that the later a food is introduced the less likely it is to cause sensitivities.

The best procedure for the introduction of solids is given by Laura J. Stevens in *The Complete Book of Allergy Control*: Begin with a teaspoon of the new food the first day, two teaspoons the next day, four teaspoons the day after, until the baby is receiving a full serving. A new food should not be introduced more often than once every three days; some doctors recommend, for allergic babies, serving each food only once every four or five days.

Symptoms of food sensitivity to be on the lookout for, Stevens writes, are fussiness, wheezing, diarrhea, rashes, vomiting, colds and coughing—though, of course, they may be the result of other conditions. She recommends keeping a complete diary of the baby's food consumption and reactions (noting the baby's age throughout). Overfrequent or over-large portions are not advised; neither are food mixtures which make it impossible to isolate the individual food that produces symptoms.

Louise Lambert-Lagace suggests in *Feeding Your Child* that cereal grains be introduced first, vegetables second, fruits third, and protein sources (such as meat, poultry, fish and legumes) fourth, remembering to test only one food within each group at a time.

It is a good idea to test *last* foods that are most likely to cause allergies such as eggs, wheat, citrus fruits, nuts and nut butters.

Following a Healthy Lifestyle

From the day children are born to the day they are grown we should give them as much support and help as they need to enable them to follow a healthy lifestyle. Some of the major components of a healthy lifestyle include the following:

• Eating a nutritious diet, with the addition of nutritional supplements as necessary. (See Chapters 10 and 11 and the section above on introduction of solid foods.)

• Exercising regularly. (See pages 263–265 in Chapter 18.)

• Avoiding contact with nutritional and environmental toxins and pollutants as much as possible. (See Chapters 10, 15 and 16.)

• Avoiding overuse of drugs (including alcohol, caffeine and tobacco as well as antibiotics, tranquilizers, patent medicines and illegal substances).

• Practicing stress reduction and control. (See pages 268–274 in Chapter 18.)

• Dealing immediately and effectively with health problems in the best way possible. Children must learn how their bodies work and to listen to what their bodies are telling them. (See the section on awareness on pages 274–275 in Chapter 18.) As parents, we should also be aware of warning signs and what to do about them. In addition, we must know which resources (doctors, clinics, self-help and support groups, and other sources of information) and choices of treatment are available.

Prevention on a Community or Societal Level

In theory everyone is in favor of prevention, but in practice it is usually given only token support. Any practical preventive measures that are emphasized by the government, media, health organizations, health professionals and others are almost certain to be on an individual rather than societal basis. As important and crucial as individual preventive measures are, it is only when society as a whole is involved that a preventive health program can be fully implemented.

An effective preventive health program on a societal level would include the following components:

• MAKING NUTRITIOUS FOOD WIDELY AVAILABLE. Good nutrition is crucial to physical and mental health, yet it is getting increasingly difficult to eat nutritiously. Grocery stores overflow with food that is refined, sweetened, laced with artificial additives, sprayed with chemicals, full of antibiotics and hormones, and contaminated with pesticides and toxic metals, while food that is fresh, whole and unadulterated is a rarity. If we want to put prevention into practice, then food that is health-promoting must become as easy to find as food that is health-destructive. Good food must become affordable to everyone regardless of income.

• REDUCING POLLUTION OF THE ENVIRONMENT. A clean environment is as essential to health as good nutrition. The quality of the soil that our food grows in, the water that we drink, the air we breathe and other environmental conditions all have a tremendous influence on the quality of our physical and mental health. We are paying the penalty of a polluted environment with illness and disease, and the problems are getting worse. Drastically reducing pollution by initiating effective pollution controls and practicing conservation would be a major preventive health measure.

Changes Necessary Before a Preventive Program Can be Implemented

Unfortunately, it is not enough to know what needs to be done. The simple two-pronged plan of prevention briefly outlined above will never be achieved unless many other things change first. A preventive health program stressing improvement in the quality of food and the environment as well as individual preventive measures will only occur when there is a major shift from a narrow technological approach to a more holistic approach. A dramatic reordering of societal priorities is needed so that prevention and the needs of children are seen to be as important as the needs of industry. More community involvement in decision making is needed as well. Following are discussions of some of the changes that are needed before an effective preventive program will ever be implemented.

A Major Shift in Approach

Few would disagree with the statement that life is a web of complex interrelationships. In practice, however, the approach that is acted on is one that reduces life to a set of isolated elements and explains life in terms of quantities. This narrow and rigid perspective ignores the importance of prevention and is responsible for the misuse of technology, which causes many of the health problems we are facing today.

(For the most part, the term "technology" is used in this chapter in its broad sense as the application of scientific knowledge. For example, the knowledge that is applied may either be concerned with how to use organic farming techniques to avoid polluting the environment and increase a crop's nutritional quality, or how to best use chemicals for a greater crop yield.)

To any one problem, there are usually several solutions. However, some of the solutions may in turn cause other problems; the trick is to find the solution that causes the least amount of harm. In most cases, simple preventive measures such as sanitation and seat belts are more effective than having to rely on fancy techniques and expensive gadgets to put Humpty-Dumpty back together again.

A preventive holistic approach (that is, an approach which takes into account the myriad interconnections among all aspects of life and attempts to work as much as possible with nature rather than against nature) may achieve results more slowly than an approach which depends on short-sighted technological quick-fixes. But in the long run the preventive approach would cause much less damage and more effectively eliminate the sources of illness and disease than the quick-fix approach.

This is not a commonly accepted view, however, as we often see solutions applied without adequate thought or knowledge and little concern for long-term consequences, an obvious example being the use of X-rays, which when first introduced were said to be completely safe. Rather than prevention being a focus, the emphasis in our society is on patching people up with drugs, surgery, transplants, rehabilitation, and where these don't work, long-term care. Food is regarded as a commodity to be sold and profited from like neckties and panty hose, and pollution of the environment is seen as the necessary price to pay for material progress. Only lip service is paid to the concept of food and the environment as integral factors in the quality of health.

Unfortunately, the inappropriate application of technology to agriculture has had devastating effects on the quality of our food and thus our health. In *Dr. Mandell's 5-Day Allergy Relief System*, Marshall Mandell traces the beginning of the problem to the success of the work of the German chemist Justus von Liebig in the middle of the last century. Based on his analysis of the mineral ash of plants, under the mistaken assumption that this contained all a plant's nutrient requirements, artificial fertilizers were developed. As it turned out, these nitrogen-potassium-phosphorus fertilizers produce a large crop yield but do not contain the full spectrum of nutrients necessary for a healthy crop.

The Industrial Revolution in the United States caused other problems. "A machine could clear more land than a farmer, his family, and any helpers could clear in ten times as much time. Huge machines rolled across the land, plowing and fertilizing. The amount of land devoted to crops increased; the forests and hedgerows began to disappear. *The birds left*; they no longer had as many places to nest. *The insects and pests stayed*; they multiplied without the birds to keep them in reduced numbers. And therefore insecticides and pesticides began to be used across the fields. These chemicals left toxic residues in the food that were totally foreign to our body chemistry. Not only did we eat the food, but we fed our animals with it and then ate them. We took the seeds from this contaminated food and planted them for the following year's crop."

In the meantime, Dr. Mandell continues, the microbe population of the soil diminished, along with insects and pests. As the interaction of the rootlets of plants with microbes provides a substantial portion of the nourishment the plants need, their nutritional value dropped. This nutritional loss affected the seeds of the new generation of plants, so that deficient seeds were planted in deficient soil, perpetuating a downward spiral which was intensified when the nutrient-poor plants were used to feed animals which were then used to feed humans.

The common practice of multiple spraying of a crop during its growing season, up to fifteen times. Dr. Mandell notes, results in the insecticide permeating the fruit right through to the pulp—there is no way to get rid of it.

And it is not only the food crops that these agents poison. They are washed by rainfall from the soil where they were deposited into streams, waterways and reservoirs. "Now, not only are we eating food contaminated with insect and weed poison, we are also drinking water that has been chemically polluted with these toxic agents."

The prevailing attitudes toward technology need to be reevaluated and the alternatives considered. For example, there are already many farmers successfully farming organically, and the concept is gaining both popularity and respectability, as indicated by a foundation award of over a quarter of a million dollars in July 1988 to Dr. Garth Youngberg of the Institute of Alternative Agriculture in Greenbelt, Maryland—the Institute is the chief U.S. advocate of organic farming. Certainly the potential for large-scale use of organic farming methods should be explored. A more holistic approach would mean using technology only where appropriate according to local conditions such as weather, geography, plant and animal life, social and cultural attitudes and organization of the human communities involved, and available resources including raw materials, supporting technologies, money, information and expertise. Attention must be paid not only to the existence of these conditions but to how all of these variables interact and affect each other; it is absolutely necessary to give thorough consideration to both short-term and long-term effects on the ecosystem, human health and the social structure, and to seriously examine all alternatives before deciding which solution is best.

To do this requires that we question whether the results of scientific studies can always be trusted, as very often decisions are made on the basis of these results. In general, unfortunately, scientific studies provide the justification for the continued use and expansion of inappropriate technology and in some cases the justification for the suppression of more appropriate technological approaches.

The scientific method can, if used properly, provide extremely helpful information. However, it must be used with caution. The objectivity of science is a myth; results of studies depend on whether all important variables are being considered, whether the method of the study is appropriate to the subject, what questions are asked, the accuracy of the observations, how meticulously or carelessly the study is carried out, the honesty and competence of the researchers, and the interpretation of the results, which can differ widely depending on who is doing the interpretation. In addition, just as with fashion, there are trends in science and an unpopular subject may never get the funding or facilities to be tested, or even the exposure to make knowledgeable discussion possible within the scientific community.

Many major decisions affecting health are made on the basis of laboratory experiments which do not even attempt to replicate all the variable conditions and complicated relationships of real life. Michael F. Jacobson describes in *The Complete Eater's Digest and Nutrition Scoreboard* some of the shortcomings of these experiments:

"Laboratory experiments are almost always conducted with well-fed, pampered animals, the kind that might be most resistant to the effects of marginally toxic chemicals. Humans, on the other hand, suffer infections and diseases and are frequently malnourished. Diabetes, alcoholism, hypertension, food allergies, and dozens of other problems could increase the toxicity of a chemical."

Jacobson notes two other deficiencies in laboratory experiments. One is that substances are tested in isolation, as "one food additive in an otherwise 'pure' diet." The fact that the American diet contains an awe-inspiring mixture of additives and pollutants, with an incalculable potential for chemical interaction, is almost never taken into account. A second limitation of laboratry tests is that many possible effects, particularly those on the brain—slight memory loss, impaired coordination—are not concidered. Tests do exist which can assess the effect of additives on behavior, but such tests are not required by the FDA.

Ross Hume Hall in his book *Food for Nought* discusses the shortcomings of research with specific reference to pesticides:

"How did these 900 pesticides come into existence? Were they carefully researched for their selective action on target organisms and their subsequent fate in the ecosystem? Did the chemical companies understand fully the physiology of the target organisms they were trying to eliminate, as well as the nontarget organisms that would come in contact with their products? Not likely, for industrial research is tied in with the economic goals of the industrial organization, goals designed to produce results in as short a time as possible.

"The approach of industrial research is empirical. Large numbers of chemists with Ph.D. degrees are hired who unquestioningly synthesize thousands of compounds in the laboratories; these compounds are then tested by another set of specialists against insects designated pests, under laboratory and field conditions. Their only criterion of success is body count. Little attempt is made to study the field situation in depth or to learn the habits of the target organisms themselves. Chemical companies in North America and Europe have put large sums of money into this type of research and have been rewarded handsomely by the increasing sales of their new products."

As part of the justification for inappropriate technology, the current short-sighted approach to science has resulted in the concept of the "allowable" or "tolerance" level, considered safe because it is set lower than the level where toxins or other environmental factors supposedly begin to cause negative health effects. Theoretically this provides a margin of safety in cases of special circumstances such as extra sensitivity.

However, there are many problems with an analysis which relies only on numerical values to define what is a safe or hazardous level of any specific chemical or kind of radiation. For example, there may not be a safety margin large enough to account for individual differences, which may occur due to a variety of variables including health, age (children, who are still growing and changing, are particularly vulnerable to negative nutritional and environmental conditions); length of exposure (what is safe at one level for a short period of time may have cumulative effects and be harmful after a longer period of time); diet, and the presence of other factors which may increase the potency of the nutritional or environmental influence in question.

The fact that allowable levels are sometimes meaningless and out of line with reality is illustrated by the following quote from Anne Montgomery in her article "America's Pesticide-Permeated Food" (in the June 1987 issue, Volume 14, Number 5, of *Nutrition Action Health Letter*, published by the Center for Science in the Public Interest):

". . . FDA bases its tolerance levels for many pesticides on wildly inaccurate estimates of how much produce some Americans eat. Take cantaloupe, for example. FDA's 'average' diet assumes that Americans eat no more than 7.5 ounces—about one-half of a single melon—*per year*. Similarly, the agency assumes we eat only one avocado, 1½ cups of cooked summer squash, 2½ tangerines, one mango, 1¾ cups of cooked winter squash, and 1½ cups of cooked Brussels sprouts, among dozens of examples. In other words, eating more than 7.5 ounces of these fruits and vegetables could conceivably expose the consumer to a level of risk above what the government considers 'safe.' "

An essential element missing from much of science and by extension technology is an ethical perspective. Neither science nor technology is neutral, making it necessary for everyone to consider the implications of any scientific research and its applications. Two key questions in connection with a particular line of scientific research or application of technology must always be asked from both a short-term and long-term point of view. Who will benefit: industry, an elite group of "haves," or the population at large? Who, or what, will be changed or harmed?

Obviously these questions are rarely asked, at least out loud, and the ethical component is neglected. Instead, a quantitative approach to the world is followed. How large, how many, how fast and how much are the questions which are perceived as crucial, leading to the viewpoint of acceptable risks. For example, the dangers of nuclear power plants have been illustrated graphically with the serious nuclear power plant accidents at Three Mile Island and Chernobyl, yet countries continue to keep current plants in operation and in some cases build new ones. The risks to human life and the environment, based on probability, are said to be less important than the benefits. Ignored are the facts that the world's energy requirements could be easily reduced, that safer technologies could be developed to fulfill our energy needs, and that the number of people actually benefiting from nuclear power (primarily members of the nuclear industry) are few and the number of people taking the risks are large. The same risk/benefit analysis applies to most other industries as well; a few people benefit (mainly economically), and many are put at risk.

In replacing a narrow technological approach with a more holistic approach, many practical difficulties would almost certainly arise, and reorganization of agriculture and other industries would probably be necessary. But with patience and the channeling of our energy, imagination and resources from the inappropriate use of technology to the appropriate use of technology, there is no doubt that most obstacles would be overcome, in a more satisfactory way than before.

A Reordering of Priorities

In this society, the needs of industry are given precedence over the prevention of health problems, and are often dramatically opposed to effective preventive health measures. In the search for expanding markets and greater profit margins, industry totally ignores the effects of the industrial process on the quality of our food, environment and health. Industry daily disposes of large amounts of toxic wastes, uses large amounts of chemicals in its agricultural practices, and produces large amounts of garbage in the form of disposable or poorly made products and packaging, all of which results in serious pollution of our atmosphere, water and soil. It also produces products such as automobiles which themselves poison the environment, and food which is of low nutritional quality (highly refined, dosed with sweeteners, salt and artificial additives and contaminated with pesticides, other hazardous chemicals and toxic metals).

From industry's point of view it is all very straightforward. Produce a commodity, whether this be food, energy, computers, medicine or table cloths, as cheaply and expediently as possible and sell it as widely and as expensively as possible. It is only logical that anything that cuts into profits and causes even minor disruptions, such as the institution of preventive health measures, would be strongly resisted.

For example, the orientation of the gigantic health industry (responsible for drugs, research, hospital and medical equipment, training of health personnel, treatment and care of patients and construction of health facilities such as hospitals and clinics) is toward cure rather than prevention; much time, energy and money have been invested in the search for "magic bullets" and the development of a system of care to deal with those for whom no magic bullet has been found. Changing the focus from cure to prevention would neither be easy nor particularly profitable for most parts of the health industry.

Prevention is not in the interests of the food industry either, as there are greater financial costs associated with nutritious foods than with less nutritious food in terms of growing, shipping, packaging, manufacturing, storage and quantity of sales (the latter due in large part to manipulative advertising and to the addictive qualities of sugar and salt). And if agricultural practices were to change from their dependence on inappropriate technology, there would be huge losses for companies who manufacture fertilizers, pesticides, and so on. Polluting industries never spend any more money on pollution controls than they have to, and conservation, from the current industry point of view, must be actively discouraged; if goods and resources were made to last longer, used more sparingly and recycled, this would result in loss of revenue.

As with the health industry, though, it is not simply a fear of economic loss that makes these other industries resistant to accepting prevention as a major consideration. Also playing a role in industrial reluctance are the very real (though not insurmountable) difficulties, both psychological and practical, involved in changing from one approach to another.

(It should not be thought that government ownership of any of these industries would necessarily improve the situation, as governmental corporations are often motivated by the same economic factors, empire-building impulses and dislike of change as private corporations. In addition, governments may tend to enforce health standards even less stringently when an industry they own is involved.)

The rationale for putting the needs of industry first is that the greater the economic productivity of industry the more everyone will benefit in terms of employment, individual comfort, convenience and improved treatment and health care. This is partly true, and in general people in industrialized nations do benefit from longer life spans and higher standards of living. On the other hand, despite massive support of and concessions to industry, there are many people in our society who cannot find work, are unable to afford the comforts and conveniences of modern-day industrial society (including what most of us consider necessities such as sewage systems and running water), and do not have access to top quality medical care (in addition to those who do not respond to current treatments or have been made worse by them).

In other words, giving industry top priority has not eradicated poverty (of either the jobless or the working poor), yet poverty is a major contributing factor to the ill health of many children. For example, children from low income families are more likely to have a low birth weight, which is the single most common cause of infant mortality, and to suffer from infectious diseases, dental caries, iron deficiency anemia and low body levels of vitamin C, vitamin A, folic acid and calcium.

To have a truly preventive health program, the needs of all children regardless of income level must be met, and at least as much energy should be devoted to this end as to meeting the needs of industry. From a health point of view, some of the needs of children include:

• NUTRITIOUS FOOD. Even in affluent North America children are going hungry, and the nutritional needs of children in low income families are especially unlikely to be met when special diets are required. Low income families are often limited in the selection of food they are able to afford. (For example, potatoes, carrots and cabbage are a lot cheaper than eggplants, avocados and asparagus, and organically grown food is usually more expensive than chemically grown food.) In addition, in poorer neighborhoods or smaller centers there is generally a smaller selection of food available (in terms of quality as well as type) than in other areas. It is not only lack of money that is a problem, however, as lack of time is also often in short supply in low income families. Searching around for the most nutritious ingredients and cooking from scratch rather than relying on convenience foods is healthier but may be difficult in, say, a household where there is only one adult who must be breadwinner, cook, chauffeur, housecleaner, repairperson, shopper, launderer and chief emotional support to any young children. (For some immediate ways of reducing costs and saving time see page 46 in Chapter 3 and page 22 in Chapter 1.)

• HEALTHY LIVING CONDITIONS. Many children are exposed daily to a variety of health hazards in their homes and neighborhoods because their parents cannot afford to move or otherwise improve their living conditions. A partial list of the health hazards which put children at risk are flaking lead paint, contaminated water supplies, lack of running water, inadequate heat, poor ventilation, damp and mold, overcrowding, high noise levels, and pollution from busy traffic routes, pesticides, factories, mines and smelters.

• GOOD MEDICAL AND DENTAL CARE AS REQUIRED. Good dental health is extremely important to overall physical health, yet, due to the expense, many children rarely see a dentist let alone have regular dental checkups. In the same way, many medical problems get to a critical stage before they are caught because poor children often have limited access to knowledgeable doctors or other health professionals. Although drugs should be used sparingly they are sometimes necessary; in some cases, however, they are beyond a family's income. This applies also to nutritional supplements, which are sometimes expensive especially if large amounts are needed. Health aids to enable sick or injured children more flexibility are another example of medical help that a low-income family may not be able to afford.

• REASONABLE STRESS LEVELS. As mentioned in the section in Chapter 18, stress can play a major role in illness, and there is no doubt that poverty is highly stressful. It is not only physically stressful in terms of poor nutrition, greater exposure to pollution, and lack of adequate medical care, but is also extremely stressful psychologically.

This chapter should not be interpreted as a blanket argument against industry, but as an argument in favor of a prevention-oriented industry which functions in the long-term interests of the world and its inhabitants. Taking a narrow perspective of industry's role in society rather than viewing it in a holistic context is extremely dangerous to all of us.

It is clear that until our order of priorities is reversed, and prevention of health problems is given precedence over the current goals of industry for growing profits and expediency, many of us will continue to suffer from illness and disease.

The disruption that a change of this magnitude would cause could be minimized considerably with planning and forethought. Although not easy, this redirection of society and industry to give first consideration to prevention would be well worth the effort, and fears of economic disaster would turn out to be unfounded. Different industries would spring up resulting in the old jobs being replaced with new ones, such as cleaning up the environment, developing the use of renewable resources (for example solar and wind power), producing goods which are safe and long-lasting, implementing recycling and conservation principles, farming ecologically, distributing nutritious food (of which with a holistic approach to life there would be more than plenty), educating people about health and prevention issues, and so on. At the same time, there would no longer be the incredible financial (and social) costs associated with the massive degree of ill health afflicting our current society.

Industry would probably have to decentralize, but this should not be a problem; most people would agree that the present state of large centralized monopolies is not of benefit to society anyway. On the contrary, it is likely that the decentralization of industry would be a positive step, resulting in a better and stronger economic system, as well as making it more possible for those affected by any particular industry to have more say in its actions.

Any loss of individual convenience and comfort (say, fewer cars) could be compensated for (improved public transportation systems), and would be more than offset by the gains of better health, a cleaner environment and a general improvement in quality of life.

More Community Involvement in Health Decisions

As our society grows larger and more complex, it becomes increasingly difficult for most of us to have any input into decisions that affect our health. More and more our choices are limited to deciding between brands X, Y and Z in the supermarket, and between living in an area polluted by industry or living in an area polluted by agriculture.

Major decisions relating to health issues are, for the most part, made by government (elected representatives and administrative officials) on the advice of experts (professionals such as scientists, doctors, lawyers and other specialists) and industry.

There are at least two main reasons for this state of affairs. One reason is that elected representatives and administrative officials are as susceptible as the rest of us to the mythical infallibility of the expert (impressed upon us by our education system and the mass media), and the second is that they are often genuinely sympathetic to the needs of industry (because many of them are friends or acquaintances of the industrialists involved, come from a business or business-associated background themselves or feel that a healthy economy with all its spin-off benefits is dependent on industry being catered to).

Unfortunately, almost always the experts and industry are united in an anti-prevention bias, and governments usually make their decisions accordingly.

Despite the fact that the prevention of ill health is not a concern of industry, governments generally accept without question the information given to them by industry, often basing crucial decisions on this information. That such faith is not necessarily warranted is illustrated by the following quote from Michael F. Jacobson in *The Complete Eater's Digest and Nutrition Scoreboard*:

"One of the biggest problems is that most testing of food additives is done by the manufacturers themselves. Companies either test chemicals in their own facilities or contract the work out to private testing laboratories whose financial solvency may depend upon delivering favorable results to their clients. One would not be surprised if companies used lax experimental protocols or overlooked an occasional tumor. At the subtle end of the spectrum, industry scientists might unthinkingly interpret ambiguous results in a way that absolves the chemical of any harmful effect. At the other end of the spectrum are the horror stories about lying, cheating, greedy laboratories."

It is not difficult to understand why scientists, researchers and other specialists dependent on industry tend to reflect industry attitudes in their work. The immediate concerns are often how to further a career/not get fired/maintain good relations with employers and fellow employees/get more funding/not rock the boat. In addition, experts have their own biases which may get in the way of their judgment. If they have had a pet theory for 20 years, it is unlikely they will seriously examine contrary evidence.

Commenting on the tendency of specialists to become emotionally attached to their individual specialties, Ross Hume Hall writes in *Food for Nought*, "The emotional involvement is usually masked because it is expressed in scientific terms: The specialist cites experimental proof that this particular technologic pathway is the only one to tread. However, he is equally careful, perhaps unconsciously so, to design experiments and improve his technology in a way that can only support his contention."

The origins of the anti-prevention biases of government experts and administrators are somewhat more obscure, but, as described in the following quote by Michael F. Jacobson, often can be traced to a combination of apathy and strong industry ties:

"One of the big problems with FDA [Food and Drug Administration] —and other federal regulatory agencies—is that the employees have no great incentives to find or act upon problems. In fact, most of the incentives run in the opposite direction. Let's say that a scientist thought he or she found a problem with an existing food additive (or drug or cosmetic preparation). The first thing the scientist would have to do is persuade other agency employees . . . who, perhaps, had been involved in the original decision to declare the chemical safe."

Making such waves, Jacobson points out, involves facing opposition both within the agency and outside—from the industry involved and often with Congress and the media—inconvenience and effort, and quite possibly a black mark on the record as a troublemaker. There is also what Ralph Nader has called the "deferred bribe," the understanding that "good" behavior while in government will be rewarded with a cushy job upon leaving it.

Another factor weakening the regulatory effectiveness of government agencies is the fact that many of their staff are drawn from the industries they regulate, which gives them excellent knowledge of how the industry runs, but also "a philosophy that has excessive respect for industry's interests."

The minor role most of us play in making decisions about health-related issues is to a certain extent a result of our faith in professional expertise, lack of confidence in our own abilities, and a feeling of powerlessness in the face of massive bureaucratic, industrial and technological forces.

However, it is becoming more obvious all the time that reliance on experts is misplaced, and that in matters which affect us deeply such as health, more trust should be put in the judgment of critical and well-informed communities (which means us, our families, our friends, our neighbors).

Clearly, the mechanisms which are now in place for making important decisions do not work to protect our food, environment or health adequately, and alternatives should be found. If the premise is accepted that those who are going to be affected by a decision should have a say in it, it is only logical to increase community involvement in decision making with regard to health issues. Although a large amount of discussion and experimentation would be necessary to put a workable solution into practice, greater community involvement certainly is feasible; community review boards, neighborhood health committees and rotating membership on government policy-making teams are just some of the possibilities.

Making good decisions relating to food, environmental and other health issues is not hard if we have access to relevant and accurate information presented in a comprehensible form (rather than, say, as masses of unorganized data), have developed the ability to think critically and independently, and engage in widespread public discussion. Good decision making also depends on maintaining respect for the intricate and delicately balanced interrelationships which shape our world; giving recognition to the mutual interdependence of all the various segments of humanity and the interdependence of humans and the rest of nature will in the long run serve all our interests best. Very important of course is a positive attitude towards our own abilities, recognizing that if given a chance we are capable of making good judgments, and that if we make errors they will certainly not be worse than those being currently made by others in our names.

What Can We Do To Make Changes?

Although it may feel as if we are totally powerless to make necessary changes, it is not actually so; the more of us there are working together the more power we have to affect nutritional, environmental and other health issues.

A good start to a preventive health program can be made by taking the time to inform ourselves, our children and others about health-related issues; to practice prevention (eating nutritiously, exercising regularly, recycling, avoiding the use of polluting products, and so on) as much as possible in our own lives; to think for ourselves and question even the "experts"; to insist that the media fulfill their function of watchdog and become more critical and informative; to use consumer power by shopping selectively and complaining loudly; to work for creative solutions as much as possible; and, at the very least, to be supportive of other people's attempts to either practice prevention individually or to encourage the practice of prevention on a society-wide level.

There are many groups around working for a preventive approach to health (Chapter 3) which welcome new members, or, with other concerned people we can start our own. Groups have an extremely important role to play in making prevention a major priority in our society: producing educational material including newsletters, pamphlets and films; distributing information through the mail, in schools, on radio talk shows, at shopping centers and via public meetings; initiating programs such as increasing the nutritional quality of school lunches, the environmental safety and quality of classrooms, and recycling projects; lobbying governments for a greater say in deciding important health-related issues and the institution of effective preventive health measures; pressuring industry (from the corner store up to the head offices of multinationals) for more nutritious food, stricter pollution controls, implementation of conservation principles, and a more appropriate and holistic use of technology; providing support for individuals who are attempting to overcome health problems; and so on. The projects we spend our energies on do not have to be major, as even small changes are a step forward.

Effective prevention of health problems is a dream which many of us hold for our children and future generations. It is not an impossible dream, but a dream which by believing it is possible and working together we can make into a reality.

Books referred to in this chapter and other suggested reading:

Boston Children's Hospital Parents' Guide to Nutrition, with Susan Baker and Roberta R. Henry. Addison-Wesley Publishing Company, Reading, Massachusetts, 1986. An informative book if one overlooks its unfounded bias against "megavitamins."

The Complete Book of Allergy Control, Laura J. Stevens. Macmillan Publishing Company, New York, 1983. For a description, see Chapter 14.

The Complete Book of Pregnancy and Childbirth, Sheila Kitzinger. Alfred A. Knopf, New York, 1983. A very lovely book, comprehensive and supportive, dealing with all physical and emotional aspects of pregnancy and childbirth.

The Complete Eater's Digest and Nutrition Scoreboard, Michael F. Jacobson. Anchor Press/Doubleday, New York, 1985. For a description see Chapter 10.

Dr. Mandell's 5-Day Allergy Relief System, Marshall Mandell and Lynne Waller Scanlon. Thomas Y. Crowell, New York, 1979. For a description see Chapter 14.

Feeding Your Child, Louise Lambert-Lagace. General Publishing, Toronto, 1982. For a description, see Chapter 10.

Food for Nought, Ross Hume Hall. Harper & Row, Publishers, New York, 1974. A thought-provoking in-depth discussion of food issues.

Total Nutrition During Pregnancy, Betty Kamen and Si Kamen. Keats Publishing, New Canaan, Connecticut, 1986. Contains good information on nutrition and pregnancy, including menus.

INDEX